D1233703

MEDICINE
FOR THE
OUTDOORS

MEDICINE
FOR THE ✴ ✴ ✴
OUTDOORS

A Guide to Emergency Medical
Procedures and First Aid
Revised and Updated

PAUL S. AUERBACH, M.D.

With illustrations by Christine Gralapp and Alexandrine Bartlett

Little, Brown and Company
Boston   Toronto   London

REVISED EDITION

Library of Congress Cataloging-in-Publication Data

Auerbach, Paul S.
    Medicine for the outdoors: a guide to emergency medical procedures and first aid / Paul S. Auerbach; with illustrations by Christine Gralapp and Alexandrine Bartlett. — Rev. and updated.
        p.   cm.
    Includes index.
    ISBN 0-316-05932-3 (hc)
    ISBN 0-316-05931-5 (pb)
    1. Outdoor life — Accidents and injuries.
    2. Medical emergencies.   3. First aid in illness and injury.   I. Title. [DNLM: 1. Emergencies.
    2. Environmental Exposure.   3. First Aid.
    4. Recreation.   QT 250 A917m]
    RC88.9.095A94   1990   616.02'52 — dc20   90-13339

HC: 10   9   8   7   6   5   4   3   2   1

PB: 10   9   8   7   6   5   4   3   2   1

MV

Published simultaneously in Canada
by Little, Brown & Company (Canada) Limited

PRINTED IN THE UNITED STATES OF AMERICA

Preface

Medicine for the Outdoors should be an encouragement to go outside and experience the good life. Diving adventures in exotic oceans and camping expeditions on forested mountainsides are rewards well deserved by those who struggle each day to stay on-line in our technological society. For me, a tired mind and unexercised body are restored when I hoist a scuba tank and explore underwater or slip on a backpack and take off for the woods. Yet, as much as I like to hide the stethoscope on these occasions, I frequently need to practice medicine. It has become clear to many of us who educate physicians about wilderness medicine that we have an equal responsibility to laypersons, whose companions may become ill or injured in tough environments and who may be hours or days from a doctor's care. It is to everyone's advantage for all outdoor persons to have a heightened sensitivity to safety, proper rescue techniques, and sound first aid principles.

It is a pleasure to complete the revised edition of *Medicine for the Outdoors*. I have learned a great deal in the past few years, and I am particularly grateful for the chance to utilize information gathered for the most recent edition of *Management of Wilderness and Environmental Emergencies* (C. V. Mosby, 1989) and the *Journal of Wilderness Medicine*. In this updated version of *Medicine for the Outdoors*, I have attempted to respond to reviewers' suggestions by expanding the technical how-to information, as well as offering more details about such topics as infectious diseases, medical equipment, and injury prevention. As before, the tough part was not gathering information to put into the book, but deciding what to leave out. To provide as much information as possible in a limited space, I have avoided philosophizing.

Although writing *Medicine for the Outdoors* was a pleasant task, it was a lot of work. My family and friends gave me momentum, for which I am tremendously grateful. The spirit and editorial support of Chris Coffin, Ellen Denison, and Roger Donald at Little, Brown have been delightful. As before, Stan, Chris, and Scott Steindorf provided technical expertise and suggestions that made the text tighter and much more useful. My thanks also go to Ken Kizer, Jeannine Courtney, Doug Gentile, Julia Morris, and Tom Jackson. I would especially like to acknowledge the extraordinary curiosity, wisdom, and kindness of Sherry Auerbach and Charlie Houston. Their enthusiasm for life and their love of the outdoors have been constant inspirations. This edition is dedicated to Sherry, Brian, and Lauren, who accompany me whenever possible on adventures in the outdoors.

Contents

Introduction

GOING outside is spirited recreation for those who seek good health and exhilaration. However, as with everything else, there are associated hazards. Major and minor accidents, poisonings, insect stings, reptile and animal bites, exposure, sunburn, exhaustion, and natural disasters sooner or later affect everyone who explores in the wildlands or vacations in the out-of-doors.

The purpose of this book is to provide the reader with brief explanations of a wide variety of medical problems and to offer understandable solutions. The five parts of the book are arranged to make the information easy to retrieve. The index lists most disorders by common name as well as by medical name. Part One outlines basic principles of health care and recreational planning that should be applied to all travel situations. Parts Two and Three describe first aid procedures, beginning with life-threatening situations and covering in turn the major and minor medical problems one might encounter. Part Four discusses specific disorders related to various wilderness settings. Part Five covers additional practical information, such as evacuation guidelines and techniques, water disinfection, drug injection techniques, and recommendations for immunization. The appendixes provide details about drugs and doses, and further sources of information about wilderness medicine. The glossary explains medical and technical terms used in the book.

To keep this book to a reasonable size, I have assumed that the reader has a basic knowledge of how the body and its organs (brain, heart, lungs, etc.) are supposed to work. By intention, the explanations are brief and to the point. This is neither a survival manual nor a biology text, nor is it a sports medicine encyclopedia. Rather, it is a book meant to be carried on a journey as a ready reference for those who have assumed responsibility for the medical rescue and relief of their companions. I have included the information that is necessary to make simple, accurate diagnoses and to act on them.

The material presented here cannot transform the layperson into a physician. Many doctors argue that a little knowledge can be dangerous. However, it is my feeling that no knowledge is more dangerous. Unfortunately, there are times when medical help is miles or sometimes days away, and total medical ignorance can be catastrophic. No intervention is completely without risk, but some familiarity with diseases and injuries can minimize that risk. Although some of the techniques and drugs discussed in this book could worsen a situation if misapplied or incorrectly administered, the treatments presented are current and well accepted. The reader should use this book for guidance in difficult situations when a formally trained medical professional is not present or cannot be rapidly reached. *The recommendations for therapy and drug administration should never be considered a substitute for prompt evaluation by a physician.* In no case should the reader forget the caution necessary to perform first aid. Legally, a rescuer is always liable for his actions. He should never take any unnecessary risks. At any time when the diagnosis is uncertain, or a victim appears to be more than minimally ill, all efforts should be directed at seeking a professional medical opinion.

The basic therapies recommended are not those that could be rendered by physicians with sophisticated equipment and a large armamentarium of drugs. For this reason, I have not described every infectious or tropical disease that could possibly be contracted. However, the diagnosis and management of illnesses such as schistosomiasis, malaria, Lyme disease, yellow fever, dengue fever, and Rocky Mountain spotted fever are relevant to many persons who travel abroad in wilderness areas, and have therefore been considered. Only drugs that are commonly available are discussed, including a number of prescription items. *To use any medical reference to best advantage, the pertinent sections should be reviewed prior to the expedition.* Manual skills such as the application of splints and slings should be practiced until one is confident.

On occasion I have deviated from a strictly medical format to provide information that is as important as medical knowledge. This includes such topics as how to avoid drowning and injury from lightning, and what to do if caught in a flood zone or near a forest fire.

I hope that the reader finds this material enlightening and useful, and that good luck prevails.

PART ✤ ONE

GENERAL INFORMATION

How to Use This Book

IN order to use this book to best advantage, read the appropriate sections *before* you embark on a trip. At a minimum, you should read all of Part One and Part Two ("Major Medical Problems"), so that you are familiar with potentially life-threatening situations and their therapy. In this way, you will remember where to find information in case of an emergency. Use the index to locate specific topics, such as bee stings, frostbite, or choking. When reading about different problems, you will often be referred to general instructions for medical aid, which are outlined in Parts One and Two. All readers are encouraged to participate in formal first aid courses, such as those offered by the American Red Cross, Outward Bound, and American Heart Association CPR training. There is no substitute for hands-on education in these techniques.

A brief glossary of medical terms follows the appendixes and precedes the index.

Whenever drug doses are not specified in the text, refer to Appendix One for recommendations. Many of the drugs are available only through a prescription provided by a physician, who will explain their uses and side effects. All pregnant women should consult a physician prior to any expedition for current advice on the advisability of immunizations and the use of particular drugs (see "Drugs and Pregnancy" in Appendix One). For estimation of body weight, 1 kilogram (kg) equals 2.2 pounds (lb).

In a number of places, I have advised the reader to administer oxygen. Although most people do not have ready access to oxygen tanks and masks, I have mentioned it anyway as a reminder to those who are so equipped.

If you wish to learn more about wilderness medicine, additional sources of information are cited in Appendix Two.

Before You Go

BE PREPARED

There is no substitute for preparedness. Adherence to this basic rule will prevent or ease the majority of mishaps that occur in the wild. Proper education prior to situations of risk allows the participant to cope in a purposeful fashion, rather than in a state of fear and panic. At least two, and preferably all, members of a wilderness expedition should understand first aid and medical rescue. One responsible adult on a casual family outing should be skilled in first aid. Manual skills, such as mouth-to-mouth breathing, cardiopulmonary resuscitation (CPR), and the application of bandages and splints, should be practiced beforehand. Become familiar with technical rescue techniques pertinent to the environment (e.g., high-angle rock, swift water, avalanche). Be certain to carry appropriate survival equipment, such as maps, a compass, waterproof matches, a knife, nonperishable food, a flashlight, and adequate first aid supplies. Suitable education and planning will minimize the need for improvisation in critical situations.

COMMON SENSE

Many accidents occur because people do not anticipate problems or ignore obvious danger signs. California coastal shark attacks have occurred when surfers violated the traditional feeding habitat of the great white shark; nonswimmers have drowned while participating foolishly in hazardous whitewater rafting expeditions. *Pay heed to rangers, posted warnings, weather reports, and the experience of seasoned guides.* Prepare for situations of risk (technical rock climbs, prolonged scuba diving expeditions, exploration in the forest) by developing your skills in less challenging conditions. Wear recommended personal safety equipment, such as a flotation jacket, safety harness, or climbing helmet. Do not tolerate horseplay in dangerous settings.

CONDITIONING

Cardiovascular (heart and lungs) and muscular fitness are the cornerstones of athletic performance. Many health hazards of wilderness travel can be avoided by a reasonable degree of strength and endurance that can be acquired only through conditioning. Soundness of body and mind are developed through regular, moderate programs of exercise and attitude adjustment.

EQUIPMENT

In all cases, be prepared for foul weather conditions. Carry warm clothing and waterproof rain gear. Break in all footwear and take care to pad rough edges and exposed seams. Always assume that you will be forced to spend an unexpected night out of doors. All expedition leaders should carry safety and first aid supplies for the most likely mishaps. Depending on the situation, this may include items such as shelters, ropes, lanterns, matches, helmets, inflatable rafts, and flare guns. Be certain to carry extra eyeglasses or contact lenses. Bring coins for emergency telephone calls. Medical supplies must be arranged so that they may be rapidly located and deployed. Recommended first aid items are listed in Part Five (see page 328).

COMMUNICATION

Before every expedition, prepare a trip plan (itinerary) and record it in a location (trailhead, ranger station, marina, etc.) where there is someone who will recognize when a person or party is overdue and potentially lost or in trouble. Similarly, determine beforehand a plan for getting help in an emergency, whether it involves radio communication, ground-to-air or ship-to-shore signals, or simply knowing the location of the nearest telephone, ranger station, or first aid facility. If mobile rescue-grade radio equipment is to be utilized, it should be checked and double-checked prior to departure, and regularly scheduled communications prepared. At least two members of any expedition should be able to fashion standard ground-to-air distress markers (see page 351). Make sure that children wear an item of bright clothing and carry a whistle that they know to blow if they are frightened or lost. If you carry a radio, know how to tune in to a weather information channel. The National Weather Service issues a "watch" when a storm is approaching and a "warning" when its arrival is imminent.

TRIP PLANS

In most cases of miraculous ocean or wildland survival, the first chapter of the story includes the account of how the victim lost his way. An ounce of prevention is worth hundreds of hours of search and rescue, risk to life and limb, and thousands of dollars in expense. All wilderness travelers should carry maps, be proficient with compass routing, and know in advance where they intend to explore. Local trailblazing is exciting, but it needs to be as well thought out as an exotic jungle expedition. Similarly, do not plan an overly rigorous expedition; fatigue and exhausted supplies lead directly to physical mishaps.

Persons with specific medical disabilities, such as chronic severe lung disease, may be advised by a physician to avoid certain stressful environments, such as high altitude.

MEDICINES

There is no need to carry a drugstore on a day hike. On the other hand, those drugs necessary to treat established medical problems (such as nitroglycerin tablets for a person with angina) should always be on hand. It is the responsibility of the trip leader to be aware of any potential problems and to insist that persons in obvious poor physical condition not undertake vigorous activity that might endanger themselves or others. All persons with allergies, diabetes, epilepsy, or special medical instructions should wear medical identification bracelets (such as those from Medic Alert Foundation International, Turlock, California 95380-1009, phone 800-344-3226). Anyone who takes medication regularly should carry a list of drugs and doses. It is wise for travelers to foreign countries to carry an adequate supply of routine medications, as well as a note from a physician stating their necessity, should the traveler be questioned or need refills. All persons should receive adequate tetanus and other locally required immunizations prior to the trip (see page 334). Basic medical supplies are listed in Part Five (see page 328), descriptions and dosages in Appendix One.

NUTRITION

Anyone who undertakes vigorous physical activity should consume adequate calories in a well-balanced diet. Debilitating weight-reduction programs should not be continued in the wilderness when a rescue might depend on extraordinary effort, endurance, and a clear mind.

To avoid dehydration and exhaustion, take adequate time to eat, drink, and rest. Most adult males require 3,000–5,000 food calories each day in order to sustain heavy physical exertion. Women require 2,000–3,500 calories. A nutritious diet can easily be maintained with proper planning. Don't plan to "live off the land" unless you are a survival expert. If you don't starve, you will probably poison yourself (see page 304). Anticipate your dietary needs, and carry adequate supplies.

FLUID REQUIREMENTS

Fluid requirements have been well worked out for all levels of exercise. They are discussed in the section on heat illness (see page 232). Encourage frequent rest stops and water breaks. If natural sources of drinkable water (springs, wells, ice-melt run-off) will not be encountered, you should carry at least a 48-hour supply. Carry supplies for water disinfection (see page 323).

General First Aid Principles

I N *all first aid situations, the rescuer must remain calm.* If you panic, you will lose control of the victim as well as of yourself. It is important to establish your authority by acting calmly and purposefully.

Do not endanger additional inexperienced rescuers. If you cannot get to the victim easily, send for help. Approach all victims safely; don't allow the sense of urgency to transform a sensible rescue into a series of risky or foolhardy maneuvers. If it appears that the victim is too ill to be moved, set up camp immediately. In all cases, protect the victim from the elements.

Always assume the worst. Assume that each victim you encounter has a broken neck or a heart attack until proven otherwise. Always be conservative in your treatment and recommendations for further evaluation or rescue.

Never administer medicines or perform procedures if you are not sure what you are doing. The good samaritan has legal protection for his actions so long as he operates within prudent limits and takes reasonable care. This book will not make you a doctor. A good rule to follow is *primum non nocere* ("first of all, do no harm"). If you are not certain what to do and the situation isn't worsening, don't interfere. Explain to the victim that you are not a physician but will do your best to get him through whatever crisis he has encountered, to the best of your knowledge and ability. If you encounter a victim who may be seriously ill, seek an expert opinion as soon as possible. Even if your treatment seems successful, a good general rule to follow is to consult a physician if you would have done so ordinarily. *Never move a seriously injured victim unless he is in danger from the environment or needs to be moved for medical reasons.* Don't encourage a victim to "get up" and "shake it off" until you have examined him for a potentially serious problem.

EVALUATE THE VICTIM

Immediately determine if the patient is breathing, if his heart is beating, and if he has any obvious major injuries. Techniques and procedures for treatment are covered in Part Two.

LISTEN AND FEEL FOR BREATHING. Put your ear close to the victim's mouth and nose, and try to detect if he is moving air into and out of his lungs. Watch for chest wall motion. In cold weather, look for a vapor cloud or feel for warm air moving across your hand. If the victim is not breathing well (or not at all), you must manage the airway (see page 18) and begin to breathe for him (see page 24), *taking care to protect the neck if there is any chance of a cervical spine injury* (see page 31). Record the number of breaths per minute; "normal" is 12–18 per minute in adults and 20–25 per minute in small children.

FEEL FOR A PULSE. Place your fingers gently on the radial artery in the wrist. If you cannot detect a pulse there (particularly if your fingers are cold), move your fingers quickly to the femoral artery in the groin or the carotid artery in the neck (see page 25). If no pulse is detected in any of these locations (and the patient is not breathing), you will need to begin chest compressions (see page 26). Record the pulse rate; normal is 60–90 per minute in adults and 80–110 per minute in small children. The pulse rate is faster with excitement or fear and slower in trained athletes. A rapid, weak pulse is a sign of impending shock, usually due to excessive bleeding.

LOCATE BRISK BLEEDING. Quickly survey the patient (taking the neck precautions mentioned above) to locate any obvious sources of brisk bleeding. Quickly apply firm pressure to these areas (see page 49).

Once you have dealt with these life-threatening problems, begin a careful examination of the victim. Take care to touch, look, and listen.

IF THE INJURY IS MORE THAN ROUTINE, EXAMINE THE WHOLE PATIENT (obviously, someone who has a fishhook in his finger doesn't need a complete physical examination). Particularly dangerous situations include falls, blows to the head, neck, chest, or abdomen, altered mental status, difficulty with breathing or shortness of breath, and injuries to children. In these cases, or whenever the diagnosis is not readily apparent, take the time to evaluate the patient from head to toe. Assume nothing, and you will miss nothing. Weather and appropriate modesty permitting, be sure to undress the victim sufficiently to perform a proper examination.

Examine the neck. Without turning the victim's head, feel each cervical vertebra from behind and note tenderness or muscle spasm. Check for swelling. If there is a chance of neck injury, immobilize the neck (see page 31).

Examine the spinal column. Run your hand down the length of the spine to elicit any tenderness. Check for spinal cord injury by having the victim voluntarily move his arms and legs and report his sense of feeling.

Examine the head. Feel the entire scalp for raised areas or cuts; look into the ears for bloody drainage; feel the nose for obvious instability; look into the eyes to see if the pupils react to light and are equal in size; have the victim open and close his mouth to see if the teeth fit properly; check the teeth for looseness or breaks and the tongue for cuts. Ask the victim if he can swallow.

Check the victim's mental status. If he is awake, determine if he is oriented to time, place, and person. ("What is the date? Where are you? Who are you?") If the answers are in any way abnormal, suspect a head injury or intoxication and maintain constant observation of the victim until all of his responses are appropriate.

Examine the skin. Look for sweating, color (normal, pale, dusky blue, reddened, mottled), bruises, rashes, burns, bites, and cuts; note the skin temperature.

Examine the chest. Observe whether the chest expands fully and equally on both sides with breathing; feel for tenderness or deformation. Place your ear against each side of the chest to listen for breath sounds.

Examine the back and abdomen. Gently press in all areas to elicit tenderness. Examine the buttocks and genitals.

Examine all bones. Gently press on the chest, pelvis, arms, and legs to elicit any tenderness. Observe for any deformation or discoloration.

SEND FOR HELP EARLY. As soon as you have determined that a situation will require extrication, rescue, and/or advanced life support, initiate your prearranged plan for communication and transportation. Don't assume that someone will call for help; you must assign this task to a specific individual.

Take an adequate history. Listen carefully to the patient; in most cases he will lead you to the affected organ system. Inquire about allergies, previous surgeries, previous illnesses, medications, and the current event. Ask if the patient has any recent or chronic medical problems.

Reassure the patient. Most disorders are not life-threatening and will allow you plenty of time to formulate a treatment plan. Avoid making comments such as "Oh my God!", "This is a hopeless situation," or "Whoops!" Let the victim know that you are capable and in charge. Be sure to introduce yourself to the victim, and explain what you are doing in a direct fashion. Accentuate the positive aspects of the situation. Do not argue with other rescuers in the presence of the victim. Be particularly gentle, parental, and reassuring with children. Always warn the victim before you do anything that might cause pain.

Keep a written record of all medications given. If possible, also record symptoms and objective measurements (such as temperature) with times noted. Don't trust your memory.

Remove all constrictive clothing or jewelry from any injured areas. If the victim has a hand wound, all watches and rings should be removed before swelling makes doing so impossible. In particular, rings left in place can become inadvertent tourniquets on swollen fingers.

ALWAYS REMEMBER TO REEXAMINE AND REEVALUATE A VICTIM AT REGULAR INTERVALS. Persons may not get into difficulty until after a time delay, particularly if the problem is related to a head injury or internal bleeding. If you are concerned enough about someone to examine him once, wait awhile, and examine him again. *If someone has an altered mental status (particularly after a head injury), he requires your constant attention.*

Medical Decision Making

THE art of outdoor medicine absolutely depends upon observation, anticipation, and resourcefulness. The cardinal rule is to act conservatively and not take unnecessary risks when making the decision to continue a journey or to postpone travel and seek formal medical attention. Similarly, one must decide whether to carry out a disabled victim or to stay put and signal or send for help.

Although every situation is unique, all decisions begin with an accurate assessment of the victim's condition. The situation should be categorized as trivial (small cuts, sting without allergic reaction, mild diarrhea), minor (sprained ankle, small burn wound, sore throat), moderately disabling (broken wrist, kidney stone, bronchitis), potentially severe (chest pain, severe abdominal pain, high fever), totally disabling (seizure, broken hip, severe high-altitude illness), or life and limb threatening (uncontrolled bleeding, extensive frostbite, poisonous snakebite with symptoms). In all cases that are other than trivial or minor, it is proper to insist upon prompt evacuation or rescue for thorough medical evaluation. Never overestimate your abilities as a healer or count upon good fortune. *The assumption you must operate under is that clinical conditions will deteriorate, particularly in harsh environmental settings.* No adventure is worth a lost life or permanent disablement.

If more than one victim is injured, you must set priorities and attend to the most critically injured. While discussions of disaster management and complex triage are beyond the scope of this book, two points bear mention. First, continue to reevaluate each victim, to detect improvement or deterioration over time. Second, do not focus on situations that you cannot control. For example, if a victim is near death from severe burns, decide if there is really anything you can do to save him, and if not, get busy with the persons you can help. These are emotionally charged and extremely difficult decisions, even for those of us who make them every day.

The rescuer may have to decide whether to evacuate a victim or to wait for a rescue party. In some instances, this is an easy decision, as when a victim must be carried to a lower altitude to treat severe mountain sickness, or when the transport route is short and easily negotiated. In many cases, it is a judgment call based on weather conditions, the nature and severity of the injury or illness, and the distance that needs to be covered. Transportation of the injured is fully discussed in Part Five (see page 342), but again, there is no substitute for careful planning. You can't possibly anticipate every eventuality before your trip, but you should play out a few emergency scenarios in advance. Although the worst case is not likely to happen, it is wise to have a plan.

PART ✤ TWO

MAJOR MEDICAL PROBLEMS

This section describes common disorders that may be life threatening. The problems are often present in combination, and require prompt recognition and management.

An Approach to the Unconscious Victim

A NY disorder that causes decreased supply of oxygen or sugar to the brain, brain swelling, bleeding into the brain, or alteration of critical body chemistries can cause unconsciousness. Thus, virtually every major illness or injury can ultimately cause a person to become unconscious. The rescuer who comes upon someone who cannot be awakened must rapidly assess the victim for any treatable life-threatening conditions and then try to discover the cause of the altered mental state. Loss of consciousness should be considered a manifestation of serious illness, and the victim should not be moved until you carefully perform the following examination in sequence. UNTIL YOU ARE ABSOLUTELY CERTAIN THAT THE VICTIM DOES NOT HAVE A NECK INJURY, DO NOT ATTEMPT TO AROUSE HIM BY VIGOROUS SHAKING METHODS.

1. Evaluate the airway (see page 18).
2. Evaluate breathing (see page 23).
3. Check for pulses (see page 25).
4. Protect the cervical spine (neck) (see page 31).
5. Control obvious bleeding (see page 49).
6. Examine the victim for chest injury (see page 35), broken bones (see page 62), and burns (see page 90).
7. Consider shock (see page 53), head injury (see page 54), seizure (see page 59), low blood sugar (see page 118), stroke (see page 120), fainting spell (see page 134), hypothermia (see page 221), heat illness (see page 232), high-altitude cerebral edema (see page 247), poisoning, and alcohol (drug) intoxication.
8. Remove contact lenses (see page 147).
9. Transport the victim to medical attention (see page 342).

AIRWAY

Airway obstruction is one of the leading causes of death in victims of head injury, and a frequent complication of vomiting in the unconscious patient. Adequacy of the airway and breathing must be attained rapidly in every patient.

The anatomy of the respiratory system is diagramed in Figure 1. Air enters the mouth and nose (where it is warmed and humidified), traverses the pharynx (throat), passes through the trachea (windpipe) and bronchi, and normally proceeds into the lungs with each breath. During swallowing, the epiglottis and tongue cover the entrance (via the vocal cords or voice box) to the trachea, so that foodstuffs enter the esophagus and do not enter the airway.

Obstruction of the path at any level can interfere with the

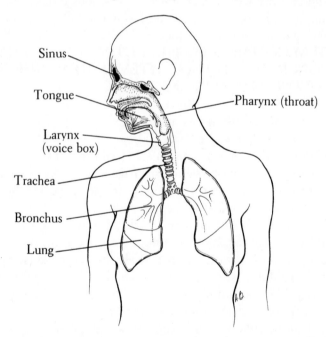

FIGURE 1. *Anatomy of the respiratory system.*

passage of air, delivery of oxygen via the lungs to the blood, and exhalation of carbon dioxide. The mouth and pharynx may fill with blood, vomitus, or secretions. With facial injury, deformation of the jaw or nose may hinder breathing. In the supine unconscious victim, the tongue may fall back into the pharynx and occlude the opening to the trachea. Inhalation of a portion of food or teeth can obstruct the opening between the vocal cords and cause rapid suffocation.

Symptoms of airway obstruction include sudden inability to speak, blue skin discoloration (cyanosis), choking gesture (hand held to the throat), harsh raspy noise that comes from the throat during breathing (stridor), and difficulty with breathing as evidenced by struggling and profound agitation. All persons who collapse suddenly or who have been in an accident should be examined rapidly for airway obstruction. If oxygen is not supplied to the brain until after a period of 4–5 minutes has elapsed, irreversible brain damage may occur.

1. UNDER NO CIRCUMSTANCE SHOULD THE NECK BE MANIPULATED IF THERE IS A POSSIBILITY OF INJURY TO THE SPINE OR SPINAL CORD. If the patient is unconscious and has suffered a fall or multiple injuries, it is safest to assume that the neck is broken. If this is the case, keep the airway open by gently but firmly lifting the jaw, either by grasping the lower teeth and jaw and pulling directly forward, or by maintaining a forward pull on the angles of the jaw (Fig. 2). Do not bend the neck forward or backward.

2. IF THERE IS NO CHANCE OF A BROKEN NECK, maintain the airway with the jaw lifts previously described, or by tilting the head backward while gently lifting under the neck (Fig. 3).

3. Keep the airway clear of blood, vomitus, loose dentures, and debris. This can be accomplished by sweeping the mouth with two fingers, or by continuous suction with a bulb syringe or field suction apparatus. Take care not to force objects deeper into

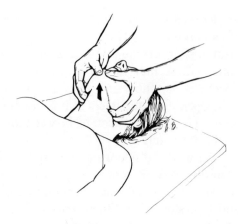

FIGURE 2. *Jaw thrust method to open the airway. Grasping the angles of the lower jaw firmly, the rescuer pulls forward to lift the tongue out of the throat.*

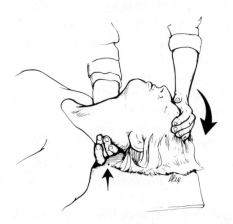

FIGURE 3. *Positioning the head to control the airway. The forehead is gently pushed back while support is maintained under the neck.* NEVER manipulate the head or neck if a broken neck is suspected.

the throat. If the tongue appears to be the problem, wrap the end of the tongue in a cloth or gauze bandage, grasp firmly, and pull it out of the mouth (Fig. 4). If it cannot be held in this manner, a large safety pin or wire may be passed through the tongue and used to improve the grip (Fig. 4 inset), taking care to avoid the large visible blood vessels at the base of the tongue. In most cases, the jaw lift will carry the base of the tongue out of the airway.

4. If the victim is unconscious, and there is no chance of a broken neck or back, do not leave him lying flat on his back. Turn him on his side, so that if vomiting occurs, the fluid can drain from the mouth and the victim won't drown.

5. CHOKING is a life-threatening condition in which the upper airway (above the vocal cords) is obstructed by a foreign object (tongue, broken teeth, food). The choking person is profoundly agitated (before he becomes unconscious from lack of oxygen), frequently grasps at his throat in a "choking" gesture, cannot breathe, and is unable to speak. If someone suddenly chokes on a piece of food or other foreign object, you must respond rapidly:

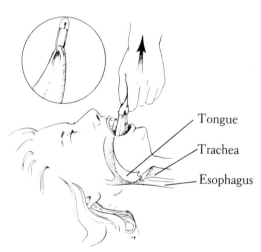

Tongue

Trachea

Esophagus

FIGURE 4. *Manual tongue traction. With a cloth or safety pin (inset) to secure the grip, the tongue is lifted out of the mouth to clear the airway.*

Sweep the mouth with one or two fingers to remove any foreign material. Take care not to force material farther into the throat. Quickly remove loose dentures.

Using an open hand, give the victim two to four rapid sharp blows on the back between the shoulder blades. This may be more effective if the victim is lying on his side or is bent forward at the waist. If a small child is choking, perform this maneuver while holding the child facedown or upside down.

Perform the HEIMLICH MANEUVER (Fig. 5). Position yourself behind the victim and encircle him with your arms, clasping hands in a fist in the upper abdomen just below the ribs. Squeeze the victim suddenly and firmly ("bear hug") two or three times, in an attempt to produce a violent exhalation (cough) and

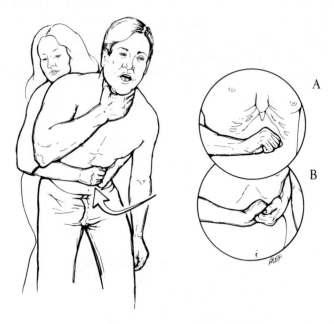

FIGURE 5. *The Heimlich maneuver. (A) A hand is placed in the upper abdomen. (B) The second hand interlocks to create a tight grip. A sudden forceful squeeze ("bear hug") causes the victim to cough.*

ejection of the foreign body. If the first attempt is unsuccessful, alternate back blows with the Heimlich maneuver. If *you* are the victim and no one is present to help you during a choking episode, you can throw yourself against a log or table edge in an attempt to perform a "self" Heimlich maneuver.

6. If necessary, begin artificial respiration (mouth-to-mouth breathing) (see page 24).

BREATHING

People cannot live without oxygen. The continued supply of this gas depends upon the ability to breathe, the delivery of oxygen to the lungs during inhalation, the ability to exchange oxygen for carbon dioxide in the lungs, the ability to remove carbon dioxide during exhalation, and the ability to carry oxygen in the bloodstream. Of these factors, the one most frequently affected by an injury is the ability to breathe.

The rate and depth of breathing are controlled by the oxygen and carbon dioxide content in the blood, by the body's oxygen demand, by the ability of the blood to unload oxygen to the tissues, by brain and brainstem regulatory sensory systems, and by emotional factors. If there is head or spinal cord injury, the central nervous system stimulus for breathing may be lost. In many instances, this is only transient, and thus it is imperative to provide artificial respiration for a period of time before giving up hope.

A direct chest injury (broken ribs, fractured breastbone, bruised or collapsed lung) may render respirations inadequate because of pain or mechanical dysfunction. The accumulation of fluid in the lungs because of inhalation (e.g., drowning or burn injury) or the obliteration of the smaller branches of the airway (e.g., asthma or allergic reaction) may make the work of breathing overwhelming for the victim. In all of these cases, the rescuer must be able to provide support by the best means available. ·

HOW TO ASSIST BREATHING (MOUTH TO MOUTH)

1. Position the victim's head in the "sniffing position" by gently placing one hand under the neck and the other on the forehead, to lift behind the neck and tilt the head backward (Fig. 3). If a broken neck is suspected, do not move the victim's neck, but merely lift the jaw.

2. Quickly sweep two fingers through the victim's mouth to remove any foreign material. Remove loose dentures.

3. Pinch the victim's nose closed and cover his mouth with your own (Fig. 6). For mouth-to-nose breathing, close the victim's mouth and cover his nose with your mouth. For small children and infants, cover both the mouth and nose with your mouth (Fig. 11C).

4. Blow air into the victim until you see the chest rise. With infants and small children, proceed gently.

5. Remove your mouth and allow the victim to exhale passively. Repeat the cycle every 5 seconds for adults and every 3 seconds for children.

6. If it is difficult to blow air into the victim's lungs, check your positioning and reclear the mouth. If it is impossible to blow

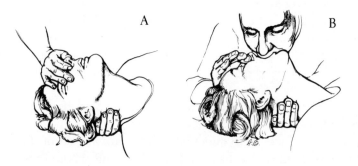

FIGURE 6. *Mouth-to-mouth breathing. (A) While the neck is supported with one hand, the nose is pinched closed. (B) The rescuer covers the victim's mouth with his own and forces air into the victim until the chest rises.*

any air into the lungs, it might be that he has something caught in his airway. Turn the victim on his side, and deliver four sharp blows between the shoulder blades or perform the Heimlich maneuver (see page 22).

7. If the victim's stomach fills with so much air that it becomes tense and you cannot expand the lungs, turn him quickly on his side and press on the abdomen. This may make him vomit, so be ready to clean out the mouth.

CHECK FOR PULSES

ASSESS THE NEED FOR CARDIOPULMONARY RESUS-CITATION (CPR). Check for pulses at the neck (carotid artery: Fig. 7C) or groin (femoral artery: Fig. 7D). Do not rely upon the wrist (radial or ulnar artery) for the determination of heartbeat (Figs. 7A and 7B). The carotid artery may be located at the level of the Adam's apple between this structure and the large muscle (sternocleidomastoid) that runs from the base of the ear to the collarbone (Fig. 7C). Pulsations from the femoral artery may be felt below the abdomen in the groin crease where the front of the leg attaches to the trunk, two fingerbreadths medial to the midpoint in the line from the hipbone (anterior iliac spine) to the bony region directly under the pubic hair (the pubic symphysis) (Fig. 7D). Other locations where the pulse may be felt (often with great difficulty) are on the inner aspect of the elbow (brachial artery: Fig. 7E), behind the knee (popliteal artery: Fig. 7F), directly behind the bony prominence (malleolus) on the inner side of the ankle (posterior tibial artery: Fig. 7G), and centrally on the top of the foot (dorsalis pedis artery: Fig. 7H). A normal pulse rate is 70–90 beats per minute for adults and 90–110 beats per minute for small children. A well-conditioned athlete will often have a pulse rate of 45–50 beats per minute. Do not use your thumb to feel for a pulse, because this finger often has pulsations of its own, which may be confused with the victim's pulse. Failure to feel a pulse means that the heart is not

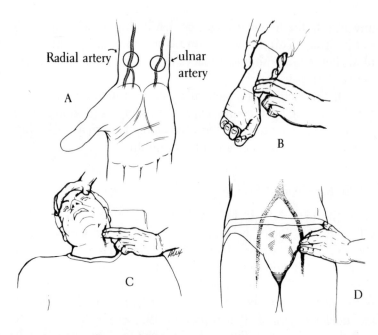

FIGURE 7. *Location of the pulses. (A) Radial and ulnar arteries in the wrist. (B) Taking a radial artery pulse. (C) Carotid artery in the neck. (D) Femoral artery in the groin.*

beating (cardiac arrest), the pump (heart) is not squeezing with sufficient force (profound shock or hypothermia), there is an injury to the artery (from a fracture or severe cut), or you are feeling in the wrong place.

IF NO PULSE IS DETECTED (AND THE VICTIM IS UNCONSCIOUS AND NOT BREATHING), SEND SOMEONE FOR HELP AND BEGIN CARDIOPULMONARY RESUSCITATION (CPR). It is performed as follows:

1. Place the patient on his back on a firm surface, and position the heel of one hand over the center of the breastbone (Fig. 8A). The heel of the second hand is placed over the bottom hand. Interlock the fingers (Fig. 8B).

2. The rescuer's shoulders should line up directly over the

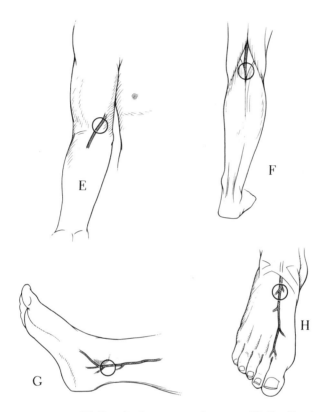

FIGURE 7 (CONT.). (E) *Brachial artery in the arm.* (F) *Popliteal artery behind the knee.* (G) *Posterior tibial artery on the inner aspect of the ankle.* (H) *Dorsalis pedis artery on the top of the foot.*

victim's breastbone, with the arms straightened at the elbows (Fig. 9).

3. Using a stiff-arm technique, the breastbone is compressed 1½–2 inches and then released (Fig. 10). Using a smooth motion, the compression phase should equal the relaxation phase, with a rate of 60 compressions per minute.

4. If two rescuers are working together, the second rescuer should give the victim mouth-to-mouth resuscitation, forcing a

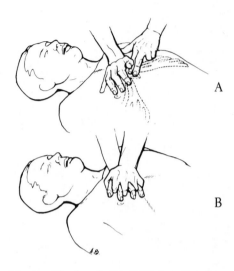

FIGURE 8. *Positioning the hands for CPR (cardiopulmonary resuscitation). (A) The heel of the first hand is placed two fingerbreadths above the bottom edge of the breastbone. (B) The second hand is placed over the first and the fingers are interlocked.*

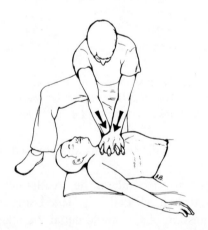

FIGURE 9. *Proper arm and body position for CPR. The rescuer compresses the victim's chest by keeping the arms straight and dropping his upper-body weight directly over the victim.*

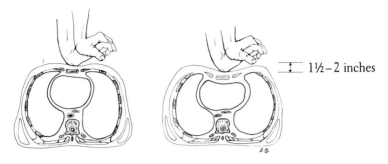

1½–2 inches

FIGURE 10. *Compression of the chest during CPR. With proper technique, the adult breastbone should be compressed 1½–2 inches, with 50–60 compressions per minute.*

breath into him with every 5 chest compressions. The artificial breath does not have to be positioned precisely between compressions. If a single person is performing the rescue, he should alternate 10 chest compressions with two breaths.

Chest compressions in infants and small children can be performed with a stabilizing hand on the back, and the compressing hand (or fingers) on the chest (Fig. 11). Care should be taken to provide a firm compression without separating the ribs from the breastbone. The rate of chest compressions for a child is 80–100 per minute, with 20–25 breaths per minute.

One should continue to administer artificial respiration and chest compressions until help arrives or the rescuer becomes too tired to continue. Miraculous survivals have been reported in victims of prolonged cardiac arrest from cold-water submersion or lightning strike. During a resuscitation, the rescuer(s) should check every few minutes for return of a pulse or spontaneous breathing.

The Condition of Death

CPR in a wilderness setting is rarely successful. Unfortunately, the best efforts at resuscitation may be to no avail, and the victim

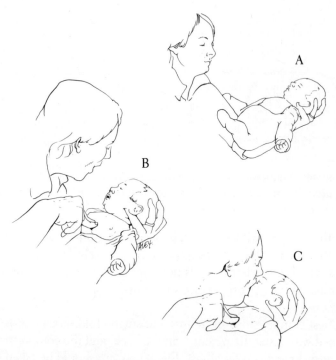

FIGURE 11. *Infant CPR. (A) Positioning the small infant on the forearm. (B) With the forearm for a back support, two fingers of the opposite hand are used to compress the breastbone. (C) The mouth and nose of the infant are covered by the rescuer's mouth for artificial breathing.*

will die. Signs of death include no movement or response to pain; no detectable pulse; absent breathing; dilated pupils that do not contract when exposed to bright light; pale or blue-gray skin, fingernails, and lips; penile erection, uncontrolled urination or bowel movement; and cool body temperature. After a period of an hour or so, the muscles become stiff, the skin mottles, and blood settles visibly in dependent fashion due to gravity, causing large discolored blotches on the victim's back, buttocks, and legs (if he is kept supine). *However, it is absolutely essential to remem-*

ber that hypothermic individuals, who are extremely cold, may appear to be dead (see page 221). Therefore, if hypothermia is suspected, "no one is dead until he is warm and dead." In such cases, resuscitative efforts should be carried out until the victim is revived, his rescuers become exhausted, or a health care professional can pronounce death. This is also true for victims of lightning strike and cold-water drowning, and for children. If a victim is dead, the body should be decently covered and kept in a cool location until extrication is possible. If foul play is suspected, the body should not be moved.

PROTECT THE CERVICAL SPINE

If a victim has fallen, is unconscious, and/or has a significant face or head injury, he may have a fracture of the cervical spine (neck). The rescuer must immediately immobilize the head and neck. This may be done by taping the head to a backboard or stretcher, by applying a rigid collar, or by placing sandbags or their equivalent on either side of the head (Fig. 12). In general,

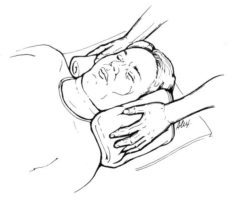

FIGURE 12. *Immobilization of the neck using rolled towels. The rescuer's hands may be replaced with a strap or tape across the forehead to prevent movement.*

the most dangerous direction of motion for a neck (spinal cord)-injured person is chin to chest (flexed). Circumferential neck collars that prevent flexion may be purchased preformed, or fashioned from cardboard, Ensolite sleeping pad material, foam-

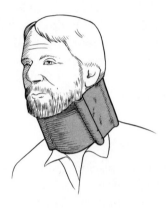

FIGURE 13. *Cervical collar fashioned from a SAM Splint. The malleable foam-covered aluminum allows construction of rigid pillars.*

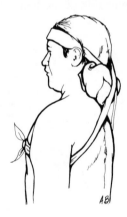

FIGURE 14. *Immobilization of the neck. A rolled towel or shirt is secured behind the neck with a firmly wrapped cravat or cloth. This technique should be used only for an alert and cooperative victim. It provides only enough support to remind the victim not to move his head and neck.*

covered aluminum (SAM Splint) (Fig. 13) or other semirigid materials. If no other equipment is available and if the victim is conscious and cooperative, a thick pad (rolled towel, jacket, etc.) may be placed at the base of the neck. This is secured by wrapping tape or cloth around the forehead, then crossing it over the pad, and bringing it back out under the armpits to be tied across the chest (Fig. 14). Remember, this technique does not guarantee immobilization in a combative victim. NEVER MOVE THE NECK TO REPOSITION IT.

If the patient becomes uncooperative or agitated, the head must be held by the rescuer until it can be firmly immobilized and the victim restrained from motion (Figs. 12 and 15). All of this is necessary to avoid injury to the spinal cord. If the patient must be moved or turned on his side (most commonly, to allow vomiting or to place insulation under the victim), the head should be held fixed between the rescuer's forearms, while the shoulders are held with the hands. In this way, the patient may be "logrolled," using as many rescuers as possible to avoid unnecessary motion.

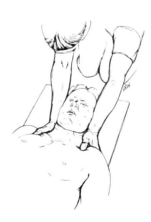

FIGURE 15. *Immobilization of the neck. The rescuer grasps the victim's shoulders and controls the head between his forearms.*

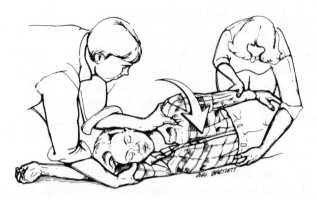

FIGURE 16. *Logrolling the victim. The rescuer at the head immobilizes the neck with his forearms and the victim's extended arm, while an assistant helps to turn the body.*

LOGROLLING THE VICTIM (Fig. 16)

There is little doubt that the best way to carry and immobilize a person who may have an injured spine is to use a scoop stretcher or to slide a backboard underneath the victim. However, when these are not available and a spine-injured person must be turned, logrolling is the best alternative.

1. The first rescuer approaches the victim from the head, and keeps the head and shoulders in a fixed position (no neck movement).

2. The second rescuer extends the victim's arm (on the side over which the patient is to be rolled) above the victim's head. The first rescuer takes this arm and uses it to help support the head in proper position.

3. All rescuers work together to roll the victim, without moving the neck.

Chest Injury

BROKEN RIBS

Direct force applied to the chest wall can break the ribs, causing extreme pain with breathing and/or collapse of a lung (pneumothorax). If the right lower ribs are broken, be alert to the possibility of a bruised or cracked liver, which lies directly below; if the left lower ribs are broken, the underlying spleen may be injured.

FLAIL CHEST

If a number of ribs are broken or detached in series, so that the affected section of the chest wall cannot expand and contract in synchrony with the rest of the chest, then a "flail chest" is present (Fig. 17). Depending on the size of the flail segment, this can cause severe respiratory compromise. Occasionally, the flail segment visibly moves with breathing in a direction opposite to the rest of the chest wall.

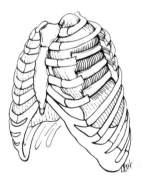

FIGURE 17. *Flail chest. A section of detached (broken) ribs may seriously impede the mechanics of breathing.*

PNEUMOTHORAX

A pneumothorax is a collapsed lung, created when there is an air leak (from the lung or from a penetrating wound of the chest) into the space between the lung and the inside of the chest wall (pleural space). In the normal situation, the pleural space is undetectable and filled with negative pressure, which allows the lung to expand and collapse with chest wall movement. When air is allowed to leak into the pleural space, either from a lung injury or from a hole in the chest wall, the lung collapses, and may be increasingly compressed if air accumulates in the pleural space under pressure (Fig. 18). A collapsed lung is recognized by diminished or absent breath sounds on the affected side, accompanied by chest pain, shortness of breath, and difficulty breathing. If air accumulates under pressure in the affected pleural space, this is called a "tension" pneumothorax. It is characterized by rapidly progressive difficulty in breathing associated with a pneumothorax, cyanosis (blue skin discoloration), distended neck (jugular) veins, and shift of the windpipe away from the affected side.

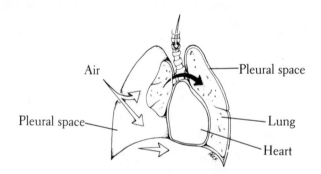

FIGURE 18. *Pneumothorax. Air enters the pleural space lining the lung through the chest wall or from a lung leak, which causes the lung to collapse. A tension pneumothorax occurs when air in the pleural space accumulates under pressure, forcing the lung, heart, and trachea to the opposite side (dark arrow).*

BRUISED LUNG

A bruised lung can result whenever sufficient force is applied to the chest wall. This injury typically causes increased difficulty with breathing after a delay of minutes to hours, as blood and tissue fluid accumulate in the injured lung. In severe cases, the victim will cough up clots of blood.

TREATMENT FOR CHEST INJURIES

1. Attend to any chest wounds. All open wounds (particularly those with air bubbling in the wound) should be rapidly covered, to avoid "sucking" chest wounds that could cause or continue to worsen a collapsed lung (see page 36). For a dressing, a Vaseline-impregnated gauze, heavy cloth, or adhesive tape (Fig. 19) can be used. The dressing should be sealed to the chest on at least three sides. If the victim develops a tension pneumothorax following a penetrating wound to the chest and deteriorates rapidly (difficulty breathing, cyanosis, distended neck veins, collapse followed by unconsciousness), force a finger through the wound

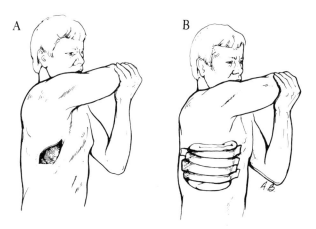

FIGURE 19. *Chest wound dressing. (A) Open chest wound. (B) The dressing is held firmly in place with tape or a cloth wrap.*

into the chest to allow the air under pressure to escape. If your diagnosis is correct, you will hear a hissing noise as the air rushes out. This allows the lung to expand and may save the victim's life. After the release of a tension pneumothorax, cover the wound with a dressing and seal only three sides (to create a flutter valve effect and prevent a recurrence that might come with a complete seal).

2. Administer oxygen. If an oxygen tank is available, oxygen should be administered at a rate of 10 liters per minute by face mask or nasal prongs. Elderly victims who have been heavy cigarette smokers should be watched carefully for signs of decreasing consciousness whenever oxygen is administered. If this occurs (in the absence of head trauma or shock), the supplementary oxygen should be discontinued.

3. Assess the rate and adequacy of breathing. Watch for adequate chest rise, feel and listen to the chest, place a hand near the nose and mouth to check for air movement, and observe skin

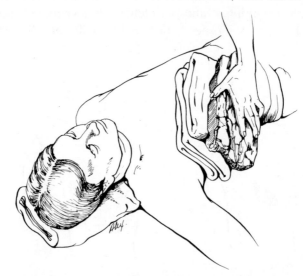

FIGURE 20. *Method of cushioning a flail chest wall segment by applying firm pressure with a blanket and section of tree bark.*

color. If necessary, assist breathing. This may be done with mouth-to-mouth breathing (see page 24) or with a mask device. IF THE VICTIM IS NOT BREATHING, CHECK FOR PULSES AND ASSESS THE NEED FOR CARDIOPULMO-NARY RESUSCITATION (CPR) (see page 25).

4. Anyone who has a significant flail chest will be unable to coordinate the muscular act of breathing, and will need early assistance. The flail segment should be cushioned firmly with pillows, sandbags, or their equivalent (Fig. 20). This prevents movement (pain) and eases the act of breathing.

5. Broken ribs are best managed with cushioning in the position of comfort, and frequent reevaluation of the ability to breathe. Do not tape or tightly wrap the ribs to prevent expansion of the chest (lung) with inspiration. Wrapping predisposes the patient to shallow, inadequate breathing and pneumonia. Encourage the victim to take at least one deep breath or give one good cough each hour.

6. Evacuate the victim as soon as possible. If the chest is injured on one side, transport the victim on his side with the injured side down. This allows better expansion of the good lung and more complete oxygenation of the blood.

Serious Lung Disorders

ASTHMA

Asthma is a disease of the lungs that involves episodes of coughing, shortness of breath, wheezing, and increased secretions in the bronchi. Generally, most people will know that they are prone to asthma attacks; however, first-time episodes may occur in persons exposed to cold, emotional stress, drugs, exertion, or, most classically, during an allergic reaction. In most cases, the mechanism is the same: narrowing and spasm of the small airways, with increased mucus production.

On physical examination, the victim will have difficulty breathing, and have audible wheezing on exhalation (most common) and/or inhalation. Coughing is a major feature, and the patient will be quite anxious. Severe cases lead to extreme respiratory deterioration, cyanosis (blue discoloration of the skin), and the use of accessory muscles of respiration (the victim will sit upright and attempt to move the chest with neck muscles and body movements). When the attack is extreme, wheezing may diminish, as the lungs become so "tight" that there is not enough air movement to create the abnormal sounds.

Treatment for Severe Asthma

1. Administer oxygen by face mask at a rate of 10 liters per minute.

2. Administer an inhalable (aerosol) bronchodilator. Bronchodilators (airway openers) are wonderful drugs which carry the advantages of low side effects and direct delivery to the site of action (the lungs). They are available in metered-dose hand-held nebulizers ("mistometers"), from which the patient inhales therapeutic puffs. Two excellent products for an acute attack are albuterol (Ventolin) and metaproterenol (Alupent). The dose for adults is 2–4 puffs initially, followed by 2 puffs every 3–6 hours. A mild to moderate asthma attack in an adult can frequently be controlled with an inhaled bronchodilator alone. Young children have difficulty using the mechanical device, and therefore require administration of these drugs orally in pill or liquid form. The most effective technique for metered-dose inhalation appears to be to discharge the aerosol into a wide-open mouth while holding the mouthpiece 1–2 inches from the lips. The drug should be released at the beginning of a deep inspiration and the recipient should then attempt to hold his breath for 10 seconds.

3. Administer epinephrine if the victim remains in severe distress after inhalation of a bronchodilator. Epinephrine is a powerful bronchodilator that is injected subcutaneously (see page 352) as an aqueous solution 1:1,000 in a dose of 0.3–0.5 ml for adults and 0.01 ml per kg of weight for children (not to exceed 0.3 ml). For weight estimation, 1 kg equals 2.2 lb. The drug should not be used by untrained persons in the management of patients who are known to have coronary artery heart disease (angina or recent heart attack) or who are older than 45 years of age. Epinephrine is the treatment of choice for a severe asthma attack in a child.

4. Administer a corticosteroid. Patients who have required steroids in the past in order to manage acute asthma attacks should be dosed with prednisone tablets at the earliest possible opportunity, as the onset of action is delayed by 4–6 hours. The dose for adults is 50–80 mg (see Appendix One for instructions on tapering the dose) and for children, 1 mg/kg. If the patient improves greatly after epinephrine and/or an inhaled bronchodilator, steroid administration is not necessary.

Patients with asthma who are in more than minimal distress or who do not have great improvement with these basic pharmacologic maneuvers should be transported rapidly to the nearest medical facility. Great care should be taken to keep the patient well supplied with oxygen and as exertion-free as possible.

PULMONARY EMBOLISM

A pulmonary embolus is a blood clot that has traveled from a vein somewhere in the body to lodge in the circulation of the lungs. Such clots obstruct the flow of blood through the lungs and prevent portions of the circulating blood volume from receiving oxygen.

The most common sources of the original blood clots are the veins of the pelvis or legs ("thrombophlebitis": inflammation of the veins with blood clots). Predisposing factors to thrombophlebitis include dehydration, underlying disease of the veins (such as varicose veins), injuries, cancer, medications (such as birth control pills), cigarette smoking, and prolonged immobility (see page 209).

Symptoms of pulmonary embolism include sudden sharp chest pain (occasionally worse with deep breathing), cough (occasionally with blood), shortness of breath, increased rate of breathing, and increased heart rate. In some cases, the patient will develop a fever. It is often hard to distinguish this presentation from that of pneumonia (see page 44). If the clot is very large, the victim may collapse and expire rapidly.

If a person develops symptoms that may represent pulmonary embolism, he should be rushed to medical attention. If oxygen is available, it should be administered by face mask at 10 liters per minute.

HEART FAILURE

Failure of the heart muscle to pump blood effectively may occur suddenly (usually with a large heart attack) or start gradually and worsen with time (after a heart attack, with infections of the heart muscle, from prolonged cocaine/anabolic steroid/alcohol abuse, from chronic anemia, etc.). The symptoms include shortness of breath (particularly with exertion), swollen feet and ankles (fluid retention), bubbling noises in the lungs (fluid in the lungs), wheezing, and blue skin discoloration (cyanosis) noted under the fingernails, around the lips, and at the ear lobes. Frequently, victims of heart failure cannot lie flat to sleep (because fluid collects in their lungs), so they wake up at night short of breath.

If a victim with known heart failure suddenly worsens, or if a previously healthy individual develops signs of heart failure (which may represent a new heart attack), the person should be kept sitting up, unless he is more comfortable lying on his back. Administer oxygen by face mask, 10 liters per minute, and immediately carry the victim to medical attention. If the patient must travel under his own power, all exertion should be kept to a minimum.

CHRONIC OBSTRUCTIVE PULMONARY DISEASE (COPD)

COPD refers to a number of diseases suffered by those who have exposed their lungs to long-term insults, particularly cigarette smoke. Chronic bronchitis (infection, inflammation, and/or bronchospasm) (see page 160) or emphysema (scarring that leads to lack of elasticity, overinflation, and/or lung collapse) are the two greatest subsets of the disorder. People with COPD have poor respiratory reserve and cannot tolerate extremes of exercise or environment. Victims of COPD suffer attacks of shortness of breath and coughing similar to asthma, but can get into serious trouble much faster because of their underlying debilitation. The earliest signs of respiratory fatigue should be heeded, and evacuation to a restful situation and physician evaluation is of the highest priority.

With the exception of epinephrine, the drugs utilized for the management of asthma can be administered if a patient with COPD experiences shortness of breath. However, it must be noted that the administration of high-flow oxygen (greater than 1.5–2 liters per minute by nasal cannula) carries some risk, as correction of the low blood oxygen level (hypoxia) in some individuals with COPD will cause them to stop breathing. This is because they have lost sensitivity to high carbon dioxide levels in the blood as a stimulus for breathing (they always have a relatively high level of carbon dioxide in the blood), and administration of oxygen removes the remaining stimulus (which is hypoxia) for breathing. Therefore, any patient with COPD who is administered oxygen should be watched closely. If the rate of breathing becomes dangerously slow, or if the patient becomes confused or sleepy, the oxygen flow rate should be lessened. If necessary, the patient may require mechanical assistance with breathing. In general, true shortness of breath is a serious symptom that requires prompt physician interpretation.

PNEUMONIA

Pneumonia is a bacterial infection of the lung that is characterized by combinations of fever, shaking chills (often with chattering teeth), cough, painful and difficult breathing, chest pain, weakness, and the expectoration of discolored (red, green, brown) phlegm. Pneumonia may evolve from bronchitis (see page 160) or arise independently.

Treatment for Pneumonia

1. If respiratory difficulty is extreme, administer oxygen, 5–10 liters per minute, by face mask.
2. Administer antibiotics. Although many different bacteria, viruses, fungi, and other agents can cause pneumonia, the most common organism is the bacterium S. *pneumoniae,* which is sensitive to penicillin or erythromycin (250 mg by mouth 4 times a day). Patients over the age of 50 or debilitated individuals should be treated with ampicillin or erythromycin. Alternatives are trimethoprim-sulfamethoxazole or ciprofloxacin.
3. Evacuate the victim.

Serious lung problems related to specific environmental conditions are discussed in the sections on altitude illness (see page 244), drowning (see page 293), and smoke inhalation (see page 95).

Chest Pain

C HEST pain may be a manifestation of a variety of disorders, ranging from the harmless chest cold to a life-threatening heart attack. It is important to question the patient about the nature of the chest pain, in order to proceed with appropriate therapy:

1. Where is the pain?
2. What is the nature of the pain?
3. How severe is the pain?
4. How long have you had the pain?
5. Does the pain extend into the arm, neck, jaw, or abdomen?

ANGINA

Angina is caused by narrowing or obstruction (spasm or actual occlusion) of the coronary arteries, which supply the heart muscle. The pain most often is described as "heavy" and pressurelike (squeezing, like a weight on the chest), classically located beneath the breastbone, with radiation to the jaw, back (between the shoulder blades), and left arm. Associated symptoms include nausea, sweating, shortness of breath, anxiety, and weakness. It is commonly associated with exertion or lack of oxygen (as at high altitudes). "Atypical angina" is pain that occurs at rest or that awakens the victim from sleep.

The patient who suffers from angina should be kept at absolute rest (sitting or supine) until the pain subsides. If he is carrying his medications, he should place a nitroglycerin tablet 0.4 mg under his tongue (the tablet dissolves) or use sublingual nitroglycerin spray. This may be repeated after 5–10 minutes (not to exceed 3 tablets or spray applications) until there is relief. After the episode is over, the victim should be transported with minimum exertion to an appropriate medical facility. If no relief is obtained, the victim may be suffering a heart attack.

HEART ATTACK (ACUTE MYOCARDIAL INFARCTION)

This is a severe emergency, because it frequently leads to complete cardiac arrest (standstill). A person who is suffering a heart attack will usually show some or all of the following symptoms: crushing substernal (under the breastbone) chest pain that may extend into the back, left arm, and/or neck; shortness of breath; profound weakness; nausea or vomiting; pale, moist, and cool skin; sweating; agitation; and collapse. Typically, the chest discomfort does not subside with the administration of nitroglycerin. When cardiac arrest occurs, the victim stops breathing and has no heartbeat. Any elderly person with chest pain requires prompt physician evaluation.

Treatment for a Heart Attack

1. Send someone for help.
2. If the patient has a pulse and is breathing, he should be kept at absolute rest and arrangements should be made for IMMEDIATE transport to a medical facility. If oxygen is available, it should be administered by face mask at 5–10 liters per minute.
3. If the patient collapses, ASSESS THE NEED FOR CARDIOPULMONARY RESUSCITATION (CPR) by feeling for a pulse (see page 25) and checking for breathing (see page 9). If these are absent, begin CPR (see pages 24, 26).

NONCARDIAC CAUSES OF CHEST PAIN

Infection

Chest pain may be caused by lung infections, such as pneumonia, bronchitis, or pleuritis. Typically, these are characterized by pain that is sharp in nature, and associated with fever, cough, weakness, and production of colored (nonwhite) sputum. Deep breathing usually makes the pain worse. The treatment of these disorders is discussed in other sections. Consult the index.

Heartburn

The pain of gastrointestinal upset (in particular, reflux of food and acid from the stomach into the esophagus) may closely mimic angina. Typically, it occurs after a large meal, particularly when the victim immediately lies down. Foods that are troublesome include alcoholic and carbonated beverages, coffee, chocolate, and fats. The discomfort radiates sharply from the stomach through the breastbone and into the throat. Pain, belching, and a sour taste in the mouth often indicate a hiatal hernia, which allows esophageal reflux. Treatment for heartburn is discussed on page 173. If there is any suggestion that angina (see page 45) is present, seek medical attention. Because the symptoms of a heart attack can be easily confused with heartburn, all elderly persons with chest or abdominal pain require prompt physical evaluation.

Muscle Injuries

Many recreationists are unaccustomed to heavy physical exertion and suffer from overuse syndromes. The pain is related to muscle motion, and is accompanied by pain with motion and soreness to the touch. Treatment for these injuries is discussed on page 205.

Costochondritis

Costochondritis is an irritation of the cartilagenous ends of the ribs where they join the sternum (Fig. 21). The pain is sharp and well localized to the breastbone and adjacent rib ends. It is worsened considerably by pressing on the area or by deep breathing.

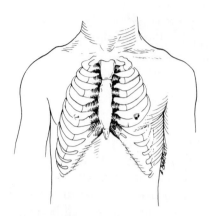

FIGURE 21. *Costochondritis. The attachments of the ribs to the breastbone are inflamed and exquisitely tender to pressure.*

Occasionally, slight painful swellings of the rib ends can be felt. The treatment is administration of aspirin or a nonsteroidal anti-inflammatory drug (e.g., ibuprofen or naproxen).

Bleeding

WHILE perhaps the most visually distressing, bleeding can be one of the easiest problems to manage, because the treatment options are so straightforward. The severity of the injury determines the rate of blood loss and what measures need to be taken to control the blood loss. The following considerations must be evaluated by the rescuer:

1. Where is the bleeding? It is important to consider and identify internal bleeding as well as external. Considerable blood loss is associated with blunt (nonpenetrating) abdominal injury (liver, spleen), as well as long bone or pelvic fractures (2 liters of

blood can rapidly accumulate in the thigh following a broken femur). *Examine the whole patient!*

2. Is the bleeding from an artery or from a vein? Because arterial blood is under higher pressure, blood loss tends to be more rapid from a severed artery than from a vein. Arterial bleeding can be recognized by its spurting nature and rapid outflow. All blood exposed to air, in the absence of unusual drug intoxications, turns red immediately, so that color cannot be relied upon to indicate origin.

ALMOST ALL EXTERNAL BLEEDING STOPS WITH FIRM DIRECT PRESSURE. This should be applied directly to the wound with the heel of the hand, using the cleanest available thick (e.g., four or five thicknesses of a 4″ x 4″ sterile gauze pad) bandage or cloth compress (Fig. 22). Pressure should be maintained for a minimum of 10 minutes, to allow severed vessels to close by spasm (arteries contain small amounts of muscle tissue in their walls) and to allow early blood clot formation. Peeking at the wound under the compress interrupts the process and prolongs active bleeding. The application of cold packs or ice over the compress (*not* under the compress) may hasten the process by initiating spasm and closure of cut blood vessels. It is also useful

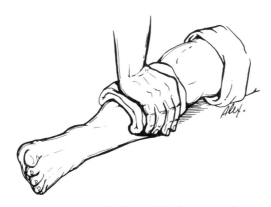

FIGURE 22. *Firm pressure applied to a bleeding wound.*

to have the victim lie down and to elevate the bleeding part above the level of the heart. Scalp wounds tend to bleed freely, and may require prolonged pressure or wound closure for control (see page 57).

If direct pressure to the wound does not stop the bleeding, apply a pressure dressing by covering the wound with a thick wad of sterile gauze pads or the cleanest dressing available and wrapping the area firmly with a rolled gauze or elastic bandage. Do not apply the dressing so tightly that circulation beyond the dressing is compromised (as indicated by blue fingertips or toes, or by numbness and tingling). Watch the dressing closely for blood soaking and dripping, which indicates continuous bleeding, often caused by misplaced pressure. If a pressure dressing soaks through, check to be certain you have positioned it properly and reapply a new dressing if necessary. Simply piling on more bandages will not solve the problem if you are applying pressure in the wrong spot.

Some important things to be aware of with serious wounds are:

1. A victim who has lost 25–30% of his blood volume may suffer from shock. Treatment is discussed on page 53.

2. Prolonged uncontrollable bleeding is rare unless a major blood vessel or more than one is disrupted. In such a case, further intervention would be considered lifesaving. The application of extreme compression to "pressure points," such as the radial, brachial, and femoral arteries, is both difficult and of considerable risk. TOURNIQUETS ARE EXTREMELY HAZARDOUS AND INDICATED ONLY IN A LIFE-THREATENING SITUATION, PROPERLY APPLIED BY EXPERIENCED PERSONS. Only in the case of torrential bleeding is a tourniquet more advantageous than continuous pressure. The decision to apply a tourniquet is one in which a limb is sacrificed to save a life. A tourniquet should be applied to the limb between the bleeding site and the heart, as close to the injury as possible, and tightened just to the point where the bleeding can be controlled with direct pressure over the wound. If possible, it should be

released briefly every 10–15 minutes to see if it is still necessary.

3. If the victim has suffered a large laceration (cut) through which internal organs (e.g., loops of bowel) or bones (see page 62) are protruding, *do not attempt to push these back inside.* Cover them with continually moistened bandages (pads of gauze or cloth), held in place without excess pressure (Fig. 23). Seek immediate help.

4. If the victim has suffered a severe cut in the neck, you must take special care not to disturb the wound, to avoid removing any blood clots that are controlling the bleeding from large blood vessels. Apply a firm pressure dressing (don't choke the victim with the bandage) and seek immediate medical attention.

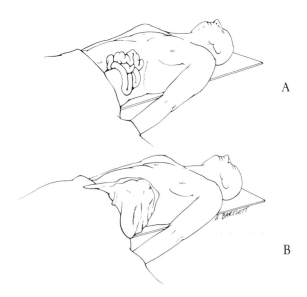

A

B

FIGURE 23. *(A) Loops of bowel protrude from a laceration in the abdomen. (B) These should be covered gently with a moistened bandage or cloth. Do not try to push them back into the abdomen unless necessary for evacuation (e.g., if the victim must walk out under his own power and such activity is forcing more bowel out of the wound).*

5. Bleeding can be quite brisk from a ruptured or torn varicose (dilated) vein in the leg. This can usually be managed with direct pressure, followed by a pressure dressing. Elevate the leg.

6. If a foreign object (knife, tree limb, arrow) is found deeply embedded in the body, do not attempt to remove it. Any attempt at removal may create more damage than already exists, which includes increasing the bleeding. Bandage the wound around the object, which may be cut to a shorter length (e.g., break off the shaft of the arrow) if necessary.

7. Gunshot wounds may cause severe internal damage that is not readily visible from the surface wound. Any victim who has suffered a gunshot wound should be brought to immediate medical attention, no matter how minor the external appearance.

8. After the bleeding is stopped, immobilize the injury. Check all dressings regularly to be certain that swelling has not made them too tight.

INTERNAL BLEEDING

If bleeding is internal, such as from a bleeding ulcer, broken bone, injured spleen or liver, leaking abdominal aneurysm, or lung cancer, the victim may suffer from shock. Symptoms of internal (undetected) bleeding are the same as those of external bleeding, except that you don't see the blood. They include rapid heartbeat, shortness of breath, general weakness, dizziness or fainting when arising from a supine position, pale color (particularly in the fingernail beds and conjunctivas), and cool clammy skin. Other signs include increasing pain and firmness of the abdomen after an injury, vomiting blood or "coffee grounds," blood in the urine or feces, or large bruises over the flank or abdomen. Because it is difficult to predict the rate of internal blood loss and because the only effective treatment for many causes of severe internal bleeding is surgery, medical help should be sought immediately.

Shock

S HOCK is a condition in which the blood supply to various organs of the body is insufficient to meet the metabolic demands. The signs and symptoms are low blood pressure, weak and rapid (thready) pulse, altered mental status (restlessness, anxiety, confusion), moist and cool (clammy) skin, rapid shallow breathing, inability to control urination and bowel movements, nausea, and profound weakness. It is a life-threatening condition and may follow a large number of inciting events. Causes of shock include severe internal or external bleeding, overwhelming infection, burns, dehydration, heart attack or disease, hormonal insufficiency, hypoglycemia, hypothermia, hyperthermia, allergic reaction, drug overdose, and spinal cord injury.

Shock is a true emergency. Unfortunately, there is little that the rescuer can do in the field. The management of shock includes doing the following:

1. Position the patient on his back, with the legs elevated about 30 degrees, in order to encourage blood in the leg veins to return to the central circulation (heart) and head (brain) (Fig. 24). Do not elevate the legs if the victim has a severe head injury (see page 54), difficulty breathing, a broken leg, neck or back injury, or if such a maneuver causes any pain. If the victim is short of breath because of heart failure (see page 42), he may be more comfortable in the sitting position.

2. Keep the victim covered and warm. Remove him from harsh weather conditions. Remember to insulate the victim from below. If insufficient bundling is available, lie next to the victim to share body heat. Take special care to keep the head, neck, and hands covered.

3. Administer oxygen, 10 liters per minute, by mask.

4. Control any obvious sources of external bleeding (see page 48). Splint all broken bones.

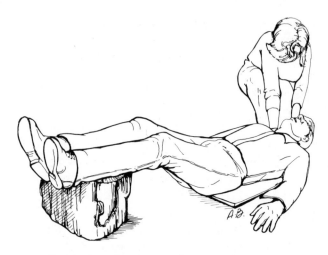

FIGURE 24. *Positioning the victim who is in shock. Elevate the legs, cushion the back, protect the airway, and keep the victim warm.*

5. If the patient is diabetic, consider a hypoglycemic reaction (see page 118). If the patient is conscious and can purposefully swallow, administer a sugar-sweetened liquid by mouth in small sips. Otherwise, do not give the victim anything to eat or drink unless he is alert and thirsty or hungry.

6. If the patient has been stung by an insect, treat the allergic reaction (see page 58).

7. Transport the victim to a hospital as rapidly as possible.

Head Injury

I NJURIES to the head are common, and may be quite serious, depending upon whether or not the brain is involved. Victims can be divided into two groups, according to whether or not they have lost consciousness. Always remember that the dazed or unconscious victim cannot protect his airway, so that you must be vigilant in your observation. The most common complication of head injury is obstruction of the airway with the tongue, blood, or vomit.

LOSS OF CONSCIOUSNESS

If a person has been struck in the head and has lost consciousness, by definition he has suffered a concussion. What you do depends on the subsequent behavior of the victim.

1. PROTECT THE AIRWAY (see page 18) AND CERVICAL SPINE (see page 31).

2. If the patient wakes up after a minute or two, and gradually regains his normal mental status and physical abilities, he has probably suffered a minor injury. If you are exploring in an uninhabited region, no vigorous activity should be undertaken and the victim should be kept under close observation for a period of at least 24 hours. Normal sleep should be interrupted every 2–3 hours to briefly insure that the victim has not deteriorated. Confusion or amnesia for the event that caused the blackout is not uncommon and is not serious, so long as it does not persist for more than 30–45 minutes. Because a serious brain injury may not become apparent for hours, the wilderness traveler who has been knocked out should not venture farther from civilization for 24 hours. If headache and/or nausea persist beyond 2–3 hours, the victim should begin to make his way (assisted by his rescuers) to medical care.

3. If the victim wakes up and is at first completely normal, only to become drowsy or disoriented, or lapse back into unconsciousness (typically, after 30–60 minutes of normalcy), he should be evacuated and rushed to a hospital. This may indicate bleeding from an artery inside the skull, causing an expanding blood clot that compresses the brain (epidural hematoma). Frequently, the unconscious victim will be noted to have one pupil significantly larger than the other (Fig. 25).

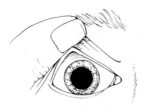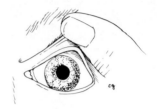

FIGURE 25. *Unequal pupils.*

4. If the patient awakens but has a severe headache, bleeding from the ears or nose with no obvious external injury to those organs, clear fluid draining from the ear or nose, unequal-sized or poorly reactive (do not constrict promptly upon exposure to bright light) pupils, weakness, bruising behind the ears or under the eyes, vomiting, or persistent drowsiness, he might have a skull fracture. Such signs mandate immediate evacuation to a medical facility.

5. If the patient suffers a seizure (see page 59) after a head injury, no matter how brief, he should be transported to a medical facility.

6. If the victim does not wake up promptly after a head injury (unconscious for more than 10 minutes), has bleeding from an ear, unequal or unreactive (do not constrict to bright light) pupils, clear fluid from the nose, has a profound headache, is weak in an arm or leg, is disoriented, has a fluctuating level of consciousness (normal one minute, drowsy the next), he may have suffered a significant brain injury and should be immediately rushed to a medical facility. Because there is a high incidence of associated neck injuries, any person with a serious head injury should have his cervical spine immobilized (see page 31). Remember, head injuries often cause vomiting, and the rescuer must be prepared to turn the victim on his side, so that he doesn't choke (see page 33).

NO LOSS OF CONSCIOUSNESS

If a person has been struck upon the head but was never knocked out, he will rarely incur a serious injury to the brain. The scalp should be inspected for cuts, which generally bleed freely and require considerable pressure to stop the bleeding (see below). If the patient seems normal (answers questions appropriately; knows his name, location, date; walks normally; appears coordinated; has normal muscle strength), there is probably no need to perform a hurried evacuation. If the patient is in any way abnormal, he should be rapidly transported to a medical facility. Small children who have been struck on the head and begin to vomit, refuse to eat, become drowsy, seem apathetic, or generally appear abnormal should be examined by a physician as soon as possible.

LACERATIONS OF THE SCALP

Cuts of the scalp tend to bleed freely, because the blood vessels are positioned in the thick skin in such a way that they cannot go into spasm and seal off after they are severed. For this reason, it is important to apply prolonged firm pressure to any head wound, and to seek care as soon as possible. If you do not have any bandages, and the wound is large, the edges may be brought together by tying hair taken from opposite sides of the wound. If possible, this should be preceded by a quick vigorous rinse of the wound to remove any large pieces of dirt, gravel, or other debris.

Allergic Reaction

A SEVERE allergic reaction (anaphylaxis) can be life threatening if rapidly progressive, and must be handled decisively. It is caused by exposure to animal venoms (e.g., bee stings), plant products, medications, or any other agent to which the victim's immune system has been previously sensitized.

Symptoms include low blood pressure (shock); difficulty breathing (severe asthma) with wheezing; swelling of the lips, tongue, throat, and vocal cords (leading to airway obstruction); seizures; abnormal heart rhythms; itching; hives (red, raised skin welts that may occur singly or in large patches); nausea and vomiting; diarrhea; and abdominal pain. Any or all of these symptoms may be present in varying severity. The most common life-threatening problem is respiratory distress. Facial swelling indicates that the airway may soon become involved. *One must be ready at all times to protect and support the airway.*

TREATMENT FOR AN ALLERGIC REACTION

1. Administer aqueous epinephrine (adrenaline) 1:1,000 in a subcutaneous injection (see page 352). The adult dose is 0.3–0.5 ml and the pediatric dose is 0.01 ml per kg of weight, not to exceed a total dose of 0.3 ml. For weight estimation, 1 kg equals 2.2 lb. The drug is available in preloaded syringes in a number of allergy kits, which include the Ana-Kit (Hollister-Stier) and the EpiPen and EpiPen Jr. (Center Laboratories). Instructions for use accompany the kits. The EpiPen products are generally easier for laypersons to use. Take particular care to handle preloaded syringes properly, to avoid inadvertent injection into a finger or toe.

2. Administer diphenhydramine (Benadryl) by mouth. Milder reactions that do not require epinephrine or corticosteroids may

be managed with diphenhydramine alone. The adult dose is 50–75 mg every 4–6 hours; the pediatric dose is 1 mg/kg. The major side effect of this medication is drowsiness.

3. Administer corticosteroids for a severe reaction. Prednisone tablets in a dose of 50–80 mg should be given to adults; the pediatric dose is 1 mg/kg. The onset of action of steroids is delayed for 4–6 hours; therefore, this drug should be given early in the course of therapy.

4. If the patient is wheezing, administer an inhaled bronchodilator in an initial dose of 2–4 puffs, followed by 2 puffs every 1–3 hours as needed. Use a cartridge-loaded mechanical metered-dose inhaler ("mistometer") containing albuterol (Ventolin) or metaproterenol (Alupent).

5. Transport the victim for medical evaluation.

Allergic reactions to specific agents (e.g., bee stings, plant contact, hay fever) are discussed elsewhere. Consult the index.

Seizures

SEIZURES (epilepsy) represent vigorous involuntary muscle activity and altered consciousness associated with excessive uncontrolled electrical discharges from the brain. They may be caused by a number of underlying disorders, which include structural abnormalities of the brain (scars, birth defects), injuries, tumors, infections, bleeding (stroke), uncontrolled hypertension, lack of oxygen, abnormal blood chemistries (calcium, sodium, glucose), and "recreational" drug abuse (including drug withdrawal).

Most seizures may be grouped into the following types:

Grand mal ("big illness"): In this type of seizure disorder, the patient classically becomes unconscious, has violent repetitive muscle activity with tongue biting, grunting, eye deviation to one side, difficulty breathing, and occasional loss of bladder and/or bowel control. Following the seizure, the victim will be confused or combative for a period of time (10–60 minutes), as he slowly returns to normal. The victim may sleep for a while after a seizure.

Status epilepticus: This is defined as prolongation of the seizure activity for a period that exceeds 1–2 minutes or as multiple seizures without a return of normal consciousness between fits. Status epilepticus is a true medical emergency.

Petit mal ("little illness"): These are "absence" attacks generally seen in a child, in which he seems to be daydreaming, distracted, or confused. They are not associated with violent abnormal physical behavior.

Psychomotor ("temporal lobe"): These are episodes of patterned abnormal behavior, such as lip smacking, olfactory hallucinations, vulgar speech, or repetitive movements, such as arm waving. The origin of the electrical activity is thought to reside in the temporal lobe of the brain.

TREATMENT FOR SEIZURES

1. Protect the airway (see page 18). If the patient vomits, do your best to clear the mouth and nose of debris. Turn the victim on his side. The victim may suddenly bite down and hold his teeth clenched, so take care not to get your fingers caught in the mouth. A padded object which cannot be bitten through (e.g., leather wallet edge) may be used as a bite block to keep the teeth apart and prevent tongue biting. Do not place a hard object in the mouth which might break the teeth. Take care not to force the tongue backward into the throat. *Never try to pour liquids into the mouth of a seizing victim.*

2. Protect the cervical spine (see page 31).

3. Protect the patient from injuring himself during the sei-

zure. This may be done with cushions, a sleeping bag, or constant repositioning of the victim. If the patient needs to be physically restrained, keep him on his side. Loosen all clothing around the neck.

4. In most cases, the grand mal seizure will be brief (30 seconds to 2 minutes) and self-limited. The victim will be confused for a few minutes to an hour after the seizure, and should be watched closely for recurrence or difficulty in breathing. If the patient continues to seize or does not wake up between seizures (status epilepticus), he must be transported to a medical facility as soon as possible for drug administration. Any victim who does not fully awaken, who awakens but has never previously had a seizure, or who appears weak or feverish after a seizure should be rapidly evacuated.

5. When the victim awakens, determine if he has had seizures before, and whether he is supposed to be taking anticonvulsants. The most common cause of seizures is failure to take antiseizure medications. If the victim has been delinquent, he should take his medicine as soon as possible. For an adult, the most common medications will be diphenylhydantoin (Dilantin) 300–400 mg per day, phenobarbital 30–60 mg 3 times a day, or diazepam (Valium) 5–10 mg 3–4 times a day. Never administer oral medications to anyone unless he is awake and capable of purposeful swallowing.

6. A possible cause of unconsciousness or seizures in people who suffer from diabetes is low blood sugar (hypoglycemia). If a diabetic suffers a seizure, he should be given sugar as soon as possible. This may be difficult to do away from the hospital, as intravenous injection is required if the victim cannot swallow. If a diabetic feels weak, sweaty, dizzy, or nauseated, he should immediately ingest a sugar-containing beverage or food (see page 118). If the victim is unconscious, sugar granules can be placed under the tongue, where they will dissolve and be passively swallowed.

Fractures and Dislocations

A BONE fracture (break) may be simple (one clean break) or comminuted (multiple breaks or shattered) (Fig. 26). Furthermore, it may be closed (skin intact) or open ("compound," with the skin broken, often with the bone visible in the wound). An open fracture is highly prone to infection. All fractures may be associated with injuries to adjacent nerves and blood vessels.

A broken bone or dislocation (displacement of a bone at the joint) should be suspected whenever there has been sufficient force to cause such an injury, if a snap or crack was heard, if the victim cannot move or bear weight upon the body part, or if an injured body part is painful, swollen, discolored, and/or deformed. A broken or dislocated bone should be compared with the normal opposite limb; asymmetry is a key sign of a significant injury. Pain tends to be instantaneous and constant with a broken bone (as opposed to a muscle injury), and worsened considerably with motion, which may create a grating sensation and noise. Small children with a fracture or dislocation will not use the affected body part and will cry vigorously with the slightest manipulations. If you think that a bone may be broken, it is best to treat it as a break until an X ray can be obtained or the situation shows obvious marked improvement (which usually requires a period of 4–6 days).

Because of the force necessary to break a bone, any person with a fracture should be examined carefully for other injuries. All fractures cause a certain amount of bleeding, which can be significant with the larger bones (femur, pelvis). Be prepared to treat the victim for shock (see page 53). Do not manipulate a broken limb unnecessarily if circulation to the limb seems normal. Excess motion increases the risk of damage to the bones, nerves, and blood vessels. When examining an injury, always work to-

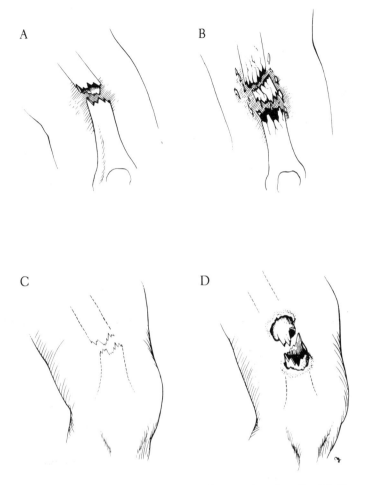

FIGURE 26. *Fractured bones. (A) Simple fracture (one break). (B) Comminuted fracture (multiple breaks). (C) Closed fracture (skin unbroken). (D) Open, or compound, fracture (skin broken).*

ward the injury and manipulate it last. If you mash directly on a broken bone, the victim will not be very appreciative.

If a fracture is open, the skin has been broken in the vicinity of the broken bone. The bone end may or may not be visible through the wound, and bleeding may be minor or major. If the victim has sustained an open fracture, is alert enough to swallow liquids, and is over 6 hours from a medical facility, administer penicillin, erythromycin, or cephalexin 500 mg by mouth every 4 hours. Rinse the wound gently to remove any obvious dirt and cover it with a sterile dressing. Do not vigorously scrub or irrigate the wound. Unless there are signs of loss of circulation (coldness, blue color or paleness, numbness) or it is necessary to realign the limb in order to allow splinting and evacuation, do not try to reposition the injury or to push the bone back under the skin. If you must manipulate the limb, rinse any visible bone with water or disinfectant (e.g., povidone-iodine 10% solution), then allow the bone to slide under the skin without touching it, if at all possible. While holding traction, immediately apply a splint to prevent further motion and damage.

SPLINTS AND SLINGS

A splint should be applied to any broken bone and to bad sprains or severely cut body parts, after gross deformities are corrected, to maintain proper position and immobilize the injured parts, so that they cannot be displaced. This prevents further nerve, blood vessel, and muscle damage, and keeps broken bone ends from grating against each other or from poking through the skin. In addition, pain may be lessened or relieved by eliminating unnecessary motion, allowing more rapid transport.

General guidelines to follow in the application of splints are:

1. Examine every suspected fracture, to see if it is open or closed. Check the circulation below the fracture site by inspecting pulses, skin color, sensation, and movement of fingers and toes. In the arm, check the radial and brachial pulses; in the leg, check the popliteal, dorsalis pedis, and posterior tibial pulses (Fig. 7).

2. Control bleeding (see page 48) and apply a dressing if necessary.

3. If necessary, splint the joint above and below the injury. For instance, to keep the knee from moving, one often needs to prevent motion at the ankle, knee, and hip. There will be times when this is difficult, but do the best you can.

4. If possible, fashion the splint first on an uninjured body part, then transfer it to the injured area. This minimizes pain associated with splinting.

5. Splints may be fashioned from sticks, cardboard, rolled newspapers, pack frames, ski poles, or other similar objects (Fig. 27). The SAM Splint is padded malleable aluminum that can be shaped to splint nearly any injury. A foldable or rollable wire splint can be constructed by cutting a 6″ x 30″ piece of ¼″ wire mesh and covering the sharp edges with tape. Inflatable air splints are less desirable, in that they can only attain one shape and may create circulation problems by exerting too much pressure on injured tissues. If air splints are used, be sure they have zippers (heavier models) rather than nozzles, so that they can be adjusted

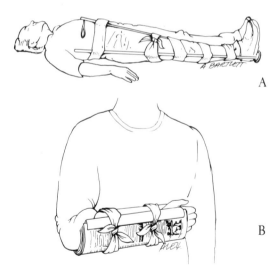

FIGURE 27. *Splints may be fashioned from (A) ski poles or (B) rolled newspaper.*

for changes in air pressure (heat and altitude). Fasteners may include belts, triangular bandages, tape, elastic wraps, shirtsleeves, or blankets. Slings may be fashioned from sheets, ropes, or vines.

6. In general, it is unwise to manipulate an injured limb. If the extremity is deformed, but the circulation is intact (normal pulses, sensation, temperature, and color), do not attempt to straighten it, but splint it in the position in which you have found it ("splint 'em where they lie"). *Unknowledgeable manipulation may result in damage to blood vessels and nerves that is far worse than what you started with.* On the other hand, if the circulation to an extremity is obviously absent (the extremity is numb, cold, and blue or pale), if the victim is in extreme discomfort, or if gross deformity prevents moving the patient out of a dangerous situation or prevents the application of a splint, then an attempt to restore the part to normal position is justified. Early realignment is easier than if it is delayed, may alleviate a major amount of pain, and often allows easier splinting and transport. Be advised, however, that this may be difficult and very painful for the patient. If you are going to realign a limb, it should be done as soon as possible after the injury (preferably, within 3 hours), before swelling and increasing pain and muscle spasm make the maneuver impossible. If there is no deformity, splint the injured body part in the "position of function" (the position it would assume if it were at rest) (Fig. 28).

To attempt to reposition a displaced body part, first apply steady increasing traction (pulling force) to the injury while countertraction is held above the injury. Do not forcefully lever or "snap" bones back into position with quick forceful motions. To gain mobility in a deformed area, it is sometimes necessary to gently rock the body parts or slightly accentuate the deformity while applying continuous traction away from the body. This allows the dislocated part to clear any obstruction and slip back into position. If the part is repositioned, it should be held in place while splinted into position. After such maneuvers, check to see that

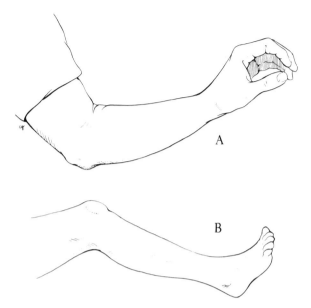

FIGURE 28. *Position of function (normal anatomical resting position). Unless otherwise specified, the upper and lower limbs should be bandaged and/or splinted in these positions. (A) Upper extremity. (B) Lower extremity.*

circulation has been restored. IN NO CIRCUMSTANCE SHOULD A RESCUER EVER TRY TO REPOSITION A SUSPECTED CERVICAL SPINE INJURY.

7. When applying a splint, don't cut off the circulation. Pad all bony prominences and injuries as best possible. This may be done with foam, a sleeping pad, pack material, or clothing.

8. If the injury is closed (skin unbroken) and there are no signs of decreased circulation, apply ice packs intermittently to the swollen area. Do not apply ice directly to the skin.

9. Remove all constrictive jewelry (watches, bracelets, rings, etc.). Left in place, these can become inadvertent tourniquets on swollen limbs and fingers.

10. Administer appropriate pain medication.

11. After a splint is applied, check the limb periodically, to make certain that swelling inside the splint has not cut off the circulation. This is particularly important in cold weather.

12. Elevate the injured body part as much as possible, to minimize swelling.

13. Insist that all victims seek medical evaluation, including X rays, when they return home, to be certain that all bones are properly aligned and that no further intervention is needed.

SPECIFIC INJURIES

Neck

If a fracture of the cervical spine is suspected, because of neck pain, weakness or loss of feeling in the arms or legs, tingling in the arms or legs, or mechanism of injury (for instance, a victim who has fallen, is unconscious, and has a face or head injury), the rescuer must immediately immobilize the head and neck. This may be done by taping the head to a backboard or stretcher, by applying a rigid collar (which may be fashioned from a SAM Splint, as in Fig. 13), or by placing sandbags or their equivalent on either side of the head (Fig. 12). For the ambulatory cooperative victim, if no other equipment is available, a thick pad (rolled towel, jacket, etc.) may be placed posteriorly at the base of the neck. This is secured by wrapping tape or cloth around the forehead, then crossing it over the pad, and bringing it back out under the armpits to be tied across the chest (Fig. 14). Alternatively, a thick removable waistband from a backpack or a rolled Ensolite pad may be used in a horse collar configuration. This technique should not be relied upon to hold the neck immobile; it merely offers gentle support. NEVER MOVE THE NECK TO REPOSITION IT.

If the patient is uncooperative or agitated, the head must be held by the rescuer until it can be firmly immobilized and the victim restrained from motion (Fig. 15). All of this is necessary to avoid injury to the spinal cord. If the patient must be moved or turned on his side (most commonly, to allow vomiting or to place insulation under the victim), the head should be held fixed between the rescuer's forearms, while the shoulders are held with the hands. In this way the patient may be "logrolled," using as many rescuers as possible to avoid unnecessary motion.

Logrolling the Victim (Fig. 16)

1. The first rescuer approaches the victim from the head, and keeps the head and shoulders in a fixed position so that the neck doesn't move.

2. The second rescuer extends the victim's arm (on the side over which the patient is to be rolled) above the victim's head. The first rescuer uses this arm to help hold the victim's head in proper position.

3. All rescuers work together to roll the victim without moving the neck.

IN NO CIRCUMSTANCE SHOULD A RESCUER EVER TRY TO REPOSITION A SUSPECTED CERVICAL SPINE INJURY. An alert victim with a broken neck will usually have enough discomfort from muscle spasm to force him to hold his neck still; however, the victim who has a head injury or who is under the influence of alcohol may feel no pain, and can have an undetected serious injury that will be worsened by motion.

Any victim with a suspected neck fracture should be transported on a firm board if possible.

Skull

See page 55.

Nose

See page 152.

Jaw

A fractured jaw is usually caused by a fall or a blow from a closed fist. The lower bone (mandible) may be broken in one or more places. The victim will complain of pain, swelling, inability to close his mouth, inproper fit of the teeth, and difficulty talking. If the fracture extends into the oral cavity, there may be bleeding from the mouth. Treatment is to wrap a bandage over the top of the head and under the jaw for support (Fig. 29). *It should be easily removable, in case the victim has to vomit.* A liquid diet should be maintained until the victim can reach the hospital.

A dislocated jaw is a distressing affliction that can actually occur with a wide-mouthed yawn or during sleep. The mandible slips loose from its two sockets below the ears and slides forward (Fig. 30A). To replace the jaw, the rescuer must grasp the jaw by placing his thumbs (with cloth or gauze padding for traction) inside the mouth against the lower molars (rear teeth), holding the bone firmly with the remaining fingers. Steady pressure is exerted straight down, until the mandible is felt to "pop" back into place, and the victim says his teeth fit properly (Figs. 30B and 30C). After the jaw is replaced, a bandage should be tied under the chin and over the top of the head, to keep the jaw from

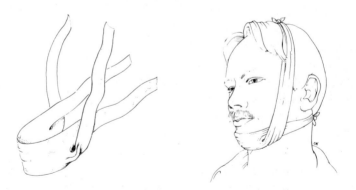

FIGURE 29. *Bandage for a dislocated or fractured jaw. The bandage must be easy to remove, in case the victim needs to vomit.*

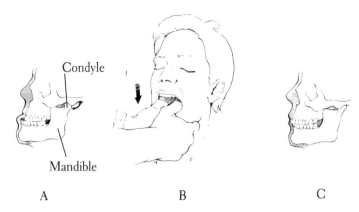

Condyle

Mandible

A   B   C

FIGURE 30. *Dislocated jaw. (A) The condyle of the mandible slips forward out of the joint. The teeth do not fit together properly. (B) The rescuer applies firm downward pressure to relocate the jaw. (C) Normal position is restored, and the teeth fit properly.*

easily dislocating again (Fig. 29). *The bandage must be easily removable, so that a patient can open his mouth to vomit if necessary.*

Wrist, Hand, and Finger

A fracture or dislocation of the hand, wrist, or finger should be positioned and splinted in the normal resting position ("position of function") (Fig. 28A). For a wrist or hand injury, this may be accomplished by allowing the fingers to rest around a padded object in the palm (such as a rolled pair of socks, rolled elastic bandage, or wadded cloth) (Fig. 31), with a circumferential wrap to maintain position (Fig. 32). Every attempt should be made to allow the fingertips to remain uncovered, in order to assess circulation. If the wrist is involved, a rigid splint should be placed to prevent motion (Fig. 33). Fingers may be splinted independently or taped together (with padding in between) for support (Figs. 34 and 35). A sling should be applied to the forearm for support and pain relief (Fig. 36).

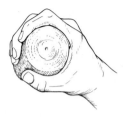

FIGURE 31. *Rolled elastic bandage is gripped gently to maintain the hand in the "position of function."*

If a finger is dislocated at the middle or distal joint, a gentle attempt at relocation should be made by applying steady firm traction to the fingertip (Fig. 34B). Do not try to reposition the joint with a sudden forceful snap. It may be easiest to relocate a finger if the joint is held bent and the distal (overriding) bone is pushed back into position using the rescuer's thumb(s). Do not attempt to reduce a dislocation at the knuckle of the index finger; it is nearly impossible without an operation. After a finger is realigned, it should be taped to one or two adjacent fingers for splinting (Fig. 34C).

If the thumb is dislocated or fractured, it can be taped to prevent further injury, by fixing it with an anchor to the index finger (Fig. 37A) or directly against the hand (Fig. 37B). The anchor technique may be used to hold any two fingers together.

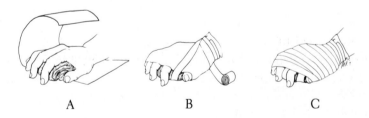

A   B   C

FIGURE 32. *Hand dressing in the "position of function." (A) The fingers hold a pad of cloth in the palm. (B) A circumferential wrap is applied, taking care to pad in between the fingers. (C) The completed wrap exposes the fingertips, which are checked for proper circulation.*

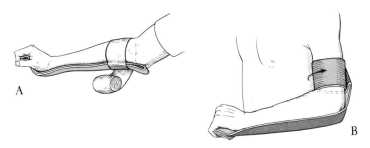

FIGURE 33. *SAM Splint fashioned to stabilize the wrist and forearm. (A) In this method, the elbow is free to bend. (B) The splint can be extended to immobilize the elbow.*

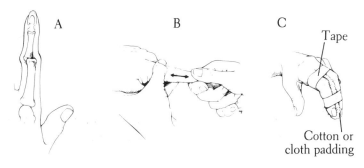

FIGURE 34. *(A) Dislocation of a finger joint. (B) Relocation of the bones with firm steady traction. (C) Buddy-taping method for a finger splint.*

Forearm

A fracture of the forearm should be splinted to immobilize the wrist and bent elbow (Fig. 33B). A sling should be fashioned and attached to the trunk if possible (Fig. 36).

Elbow

A fracture of the elbow should be splinted to include the wrist and shoulder if possible. The elbow should be splinted at an angle of 60–90 degrees. However, if it is painful to move the

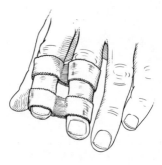

FIGURE 35. A *variation of the buddy-taping method to immobilize a finger. If the fingers are taped together tightly, cotton or cloth should be placed between them for padding.*

elbow, splint it in the position in which it is found. A sling should be fashioned and attached to the trunk if possible. A dislocated elbow should be realigned if necessary to restore circulation to the hand. The arm is held bent 45–90 degrees at the elbow, using a lever motion to pull the bones of the forearm back into posi-

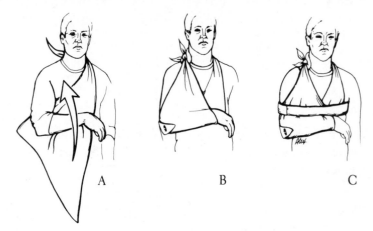

FIGURE 36. *Sling and swath. (A) A cravat is draped under the arm and over the opposite shoulder. (B) The cravat is tied behind the neck and pinned at the elbow. (C) A swath holds the arm against the chest.*

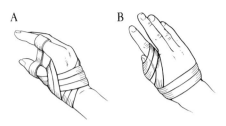

FIGURE 37. *Taping the thumb for immobilization. (A) The buddy-taping method. (B) A "thumb-lock." If possible, padding should be placed between the thumb and the forefinger.*

tion, while the upper arm is held fixed in countertraction (Fig. 38).

Upper Arm

The entire length of the bone of the upper arm can be palpated from the arm's inner aspect. A fracture of the upper arm, particularly if it is close to the shoulder, is often quite difficult to splint.

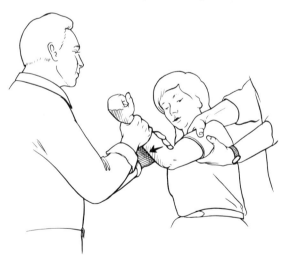

FIGURE 38. *Repositioning a dislocated elbow.*

A "sugar tong" splint can be fashioned using a SAM Splint, by laying the splint along the inner and outer surface of the arm, with the U at the elbow (Fig. 39). If possible, the elbow should be kept bent at 90 degrees and the arm placed in a sling. Attach the sling to the body by using a circumferential (around the chest) swath fashioned from a belt, rope, or long piece of cloth to prevent motion of the arm at the shoulder (Fig. 36).

Collarbone

A fracture of the collarbone is best managed with a sling and swath (Fig. 36) and/or a modified figure-of-eight bandage. The modified figure-of-eight bandage is created by draping a rope, cloth, or cravat behind the neck across the shoulders, then forward over the shoulders and under the arms to be tied in the back (Fig. 40). This will pull the shoulders back in the military position. To provide a tighter fit, the cross-shoulder section may be tied to the lower knot (giving a "figure-of-eight" appearance). After the figure-of-eight bandage is pulled snug, the affected arm may be fixed to the chest using a sling and swath (Fig. 36). If the figure-of-eight bandage cannot be constructed or increases the

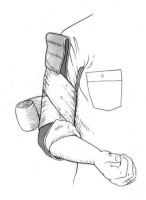

FIGURE 39. *The SAM Splint can be conformed in a "sugar tong" to immobilize the upper arm.*

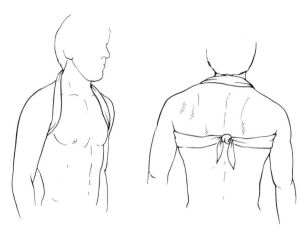

FIGURE 40. *Modified figure-of-eight bandage for a broken collarbone.*

victim's discomfort, a sling and swath may be used alone. Collarbone fractures appear to heal equally well with either technique.

Another alternative is to have the victim wear a properly fitted backpack with shoulder straps and carry approximately 15 pounds of weight in the pack.

Shoulder Dislocation

The long bone (humerus) of the upper arm fits into the shoulder joint with a ball-and-socket mechanism, held in place by a series of muscle attachments (Fig. 41A). When a person falls onto his shoulder, onto the outstretched arm, or has his arm twisted or pulled forcefully, the head of the humerus can dislocate out of the shoulder joint (Fig. 41B). This is usually quite painful and may be associated with a fracture of the humerus or the bone that supplies the shoulder socket. The diagnosis of shoulder dislocation is made by observing and feeling a depression in the shoulder where the bone should be, noting that the victim holds the arm up and away from the body (Fig. 42), and feeling the head of the

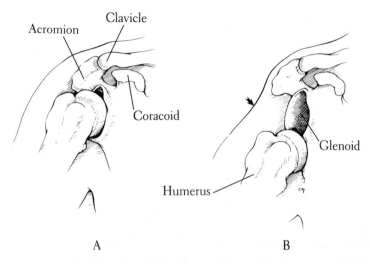

FIGURE 41. *Dislocated shoulder. (A) Normal anatomy. (B) With dislocation, the head of the humerus slips out of the glenoid (socket), and a depression (arrow) is noted in the external appearance of the shoulder.*

humerus as a firm ball 2 or 3 inches below its normal location. This can be compared with the normal shoulder on the opposite side. A person who has suffered a shoulder dislocation previously is often prone to recurrent episodes with lesser forces applied to the joint.

If the injured victim can be transported to a medical facility within 3 to 4 hours, then there is no need to attempt relocation of the arm. Place the arm in a sling, and secure the sling to the victim's chest with a swath to minimize motion and discomfort (Fig. 36).

If more than 3 to 4 hours will elapse before medical help is obtained, if the dislocation is recurrent (has happened to the same shoulder before), or if the victim is suffering intolerable pain, an attempt may be made to reposition the arm bone in order to provide pain relief. *Never attempt relocation if the upper arm or elbow is deformed* (indicating a broken bone). The safest and simplest technique for relocation is to pull with steady forceful traction on the injured arm, directed at a 45–90 degree angle away from the body. At the same time, someone should provide countertraction by holding a sheet or blanket that is wrapped

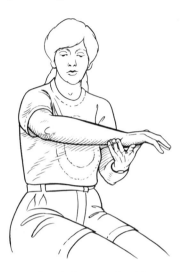

FIGURE 42. *The victim with a dislocated shoulder carries the arm up and away from the body.*

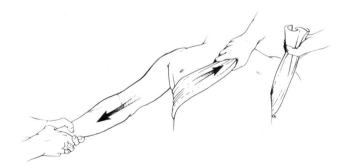

FIGURE 43. *Technique for relocation of shoulder dislocation. One rescuer applies traction at the forearm while another applies countertraction at the chest.*

across the victim's chest and under the affected armpit (Fig. 43). The easiest technique is to tie a sheet, belt, webbed strapping, or avalanche cord around the rescuer's waist and the victim's bent forearm, so that the rescuer (standing or kneeling) can lean back to apply traction, keeping the hands free to guide the head of the humerus back into position (Fig. 44). In all cases, place padding in the armpit and bend of the elbow to prevent a pressure injury to sensitive nerves underneath the skin. A single rescuer may provide countertraction by placing his foot against the victim's chest just below the armpit or fixing the countertraction sheet or rope to a tree or ice ax buried in the ground. *Do not jerk the arm, attempt to twist or lever it into position, or pull with a tugging motion.*

Another technique is to have the victim lie prone so that the injured arm can dangle free. Place a thick pad under the injured shoulder. Attach a 10–20 pound weight to the wrist or forearm

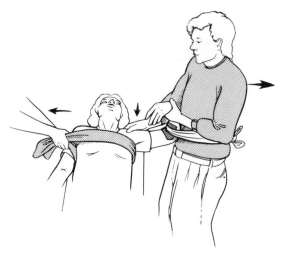

FIGURE 44. *Repositioning a dislocated shoulder. Attached to the victim's forearm with a strap, rope, or sheet, the rescuer uses his body weight to apply traction, leaving his hands free to manipulate the victim's arm. A second rescuer applies countertraction, or the victim can be held motionless by fixing the chest sheet to a tree or ground stake.*

(do not have the victim hold the weight) and allow it to exert steady traction on the arm, using gravity to relocate the humeral head (Fig. 45). Alternately, have the victim bend forward at the waist and pull steadily downward on the arm to simulate the gravity effect, with gentle side-to-side (at the wrist) rotation. If pain medicine is available, the patient should be medicated before relocation is attempted, to allow the greatest possible shoulder and chest muscle relaxation. As the arm bone moves back into proper position (this may require 15 minutes of steady traction), it will "give" in little movements, with a final "pop" back into the socket. Once the bone is back in place, the victim will be able to bring his arm across the chest. If the victim cannot relax the muscles sufficiently to allow motion, if your attempts cause excruciating pain, or if you are otherwise unsuccessful after 15 minutes, leave well enough alone (no one ever died of a dislocated shoulder). Fix the arm near the body in a comfortable position with padding in the armpit and swath bandages, and head for help. The victim who cannot walk should be transported in a sitting (for comfort) position if possible. If the shoulder

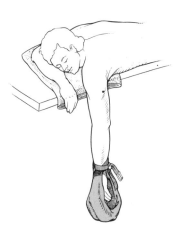

FIGURE 45. A *fanny pack filled with rocks can be used for a weight in the* "dangle" *method of shoulder relocation.*

relocates, it should be placed in a sling and swath to prevent a repeat injury (Fig. 36). A first-time shoulder dislocation that is relocated should be immobilized for three weeks. A recurrent dislocation that is relocated can be exercised gently after 3–5 days.

Rib

A broken rib can be very painful, but there is little that the rescuer can do to improve the situation. Pad the chest wall with blankets or clothing (if the victim needs to be carried out on a stretcher) to restrict unnecessary motion and contact. Never bind the chest tightly; binding discourages deep breathing and prevents full expansion of the lungs, and predisposes the victim to partial lung collapse and pneumonia. Encourage the victim to breathe deeply (sigh) or cough a few times an hour. If there is a segment of detached (flail) ribs (see page 35), attempt to stabilize its position with padding (Figs. 17 and 20). Because of the force necessary to break a rib, anticipate internal bleeding (lungs, liver, and spleen) (see page 52).

Spine (Chest and Lower Back)

Victims who fall a great distance and land on their feet frequently fracture their heels, ankles, and lumbar vertebrae (lower bones of the spine). Symptoms of spinal cord injury include back pain, weakness, numbness or tingling below the injury, loss of bladder or bowel control, or low blood pressure ("spinal shock"). If a fractured spine is suspected, the patient must be completely immobilized to avoid damage to the spinal cord. The victim should be positioned on a firm litter or backboard, and secured so that no motion of the back is possible. If a scoop stretcher or backboard is not available and the patient must be moved, he should be logrolled (see page 34).

Pelvis

If pressing inward on the victim's hips or downward on the pubic bone causes pain, the rescuer should suspect a fracture of the pelvis and immobilize the victim from the waist down. Pelvic fractures are frequently associated with severe internal injuries and bleeding, so rapid evacuation is a high priority. Be prepared to treat the victim for shock (see page 53). Do not allow a patient with a suspected pelvic fracture to walk.

Hip and Thigh

Fractures of the hip socket and femur (the large bone of the upper leg) can be diagnosed by severe pain, inability to bear weight, deformity, and rapid swelling (from bleeding). Often, the affected leg is shortened and the foot is rotated away from the other leg. This injury requires splinting from the hip to the ankle. Because the muscles of the thigh are quite powerful and will tend to force the broken bone ends to overlap, traction is often necessary to control bleeding, maintain position, decrease pain, and prevent further internal muscle and blood vessel damage (Fig. 46). If sufficient rescuers are available, one person should maintain firm traction on the leg at the ankle to oppose the strong muscle contractions of the thigh (Fig. 47). The Kendrick Traction Device is a lightweight, portable field traction apparatus that can easily be carried and applied in wilderness settings (Medix Choice, El Cajon, California). A broken femur can bleed 2 liters of blood into the thigh rapidly, so evacuation is of high priority. Be prepared to treat the victim for shock (see page 53).

If a person (usually elderly) falls with great force directly onto the knee, the large leg bone may be forced backward out of the hip socket, and create a condition known as a posterior dislocation. In such a case, the affected leg appears shorter, is bent at the knee, and the foot and knee are turned inward (toward the other

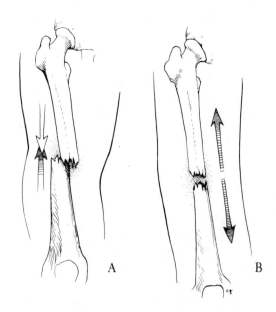

FIGURE 46. *Fracture of the femur. (A) Without traction, strong muscles of the thigh pull the broken bone ends together, causing pain and deformity. (B) Traction straightens the leg and helps to control bleeding and pain.*

leg). This is a serious condition, as the blood supply to the head of the femur (the ball of this ball-and-socket joint) is disrupted. If medical attention cannot be reached within one hour, an attempt should be made at relocation. *This should not be attempted if there is a deformity of the upper leg or knee (indicating a fracture).* The rescuer holds firmly to the leg and knee of the victim, and exerts forceful traction directly down toward the victim's feet, in an attempt to slide the head of the femur back into the hip socket. If successful, a "give" will be felt, and the leg, knee, and foot will regain proper alignment (compared with the opposite, normal leg). Because of the force necessary to perform this maneuver, it is generally necessary to have a second rescuer provide counter-

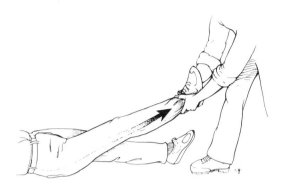

FIGURE 47. *Technique for traction applied to the lower leg.*

traction to the victim's upper body. The two-rescuer method is for the first rescuer to straddle the supine victim directly over his hips, facing toward the victim's head and holding the victim's bent leg between his knees. The second rescuer holds the victim's pelvis to the ground while the first lifts upward on the dislocated femur (Fig. 48). If relocation is successful, the hip should be firmly splinted by securing the legs together slightly flexed with padding in between, and the victim should be promptly evacuated to an orthopedic surgeon. The victim should not attempt to walk.

Knee and Kneecap

A fracture of the knee or kneecap should be splinted from hip to ankle. If there is such great deformity that the foot becomes numb and turns blue or pale and cold (usually seen with a severe dislocation of the knee joint) and pulses cannot be felt, use traction to attempt to realign the leg in a position of function (with the knee bent at a 15–30 degree angle (Fig. 28B) in order to reestablish circulation.

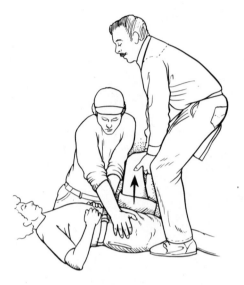

FIGURE 48. *Two-rescuer method for repositioning a dislocated hip.*

If the kneecap becomes dislocated, gently straighten the leg while pushing the kneecap from the lateral side back into place; occasionally, the kneecap will pop back into position. If the maneuver is painful or not easily accomplished, do not apply force. After the kneecap is repositioned, splint the leg straight or at a 15 degree bend (knee) using an Ensolite or foam pad and an elastic bandage(s).

If the knee has been dislocated or fractured, the victim must be carried; if the kneecap dislocation is the only injury, successful treatment will allow the victim to walk, using an ice ax, ski pole, or other object as a crutch.

Lower Leg

A fracture of the lower leg should be splinted from knee to ankle. If necessary, the legs can be attached side by side, with padding in between. If the knee is not involved, keep it bent at 15–30 degrees.

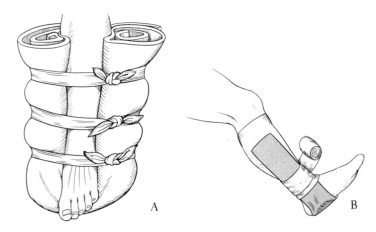

FIGURE 49. *Methods of foot and ankle immobilization. (A) A piece of rolled foam can be used as a "stirrup" to hold the foot and ankle motionless. (B) The SAM Splint is easily configured in a similar fashion.*

Ankle

A fracture of the ankle should be stirrup-splinted or wrapped to prevent movement. This can be accomplished using a SAM Splint, parka, or piece of rolled foam taped or wrapped into place (Figs. 49 and 50). Remove or loosen the boot or shoe, to avoid entrapment due to swelling, which could impair circulation. However, if the victim must walk out under his own power, replace footwear as soon as possible, before swelling makes this impossible.

Toes

A fractured toe may be splinted by buddy-taping. This is performed by placing some padding (cloth or cotton) between the toes, and taping the injured toe to a healthy adjacent toe for support.

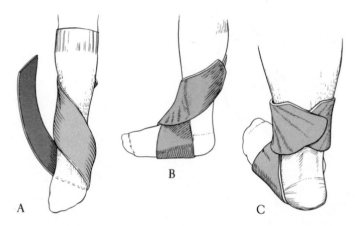

FIGURE 50. *Ankle fixation with the SAM Splint. (A) The splint is wrapped in a figure-of-eight over the top of the ankle. (B) The aluminum is molded to fit snugly against the foot and lower leg. (C) Rear view of completed splint.*

Amputations

AMPUTATION is a loss of a body part, such as an ear, finger, or foot. It is usually associated with a serious force or crushing injury. The immediate threats to life are bleeding and shock (see page 53).

If a body part is detached, apply firm pressure to the site of the bleeding where the tissue loss has occurred. Manage any serious bleeding (see page 48). Cover the wound with the cleanest available bandage, and then wrap tightly. *Do not attempt to reattach the detached body part.* If a digit is hanging on by a small piece of skin or muscle, attempt to bandage it without completing the separation

If the body part can be easily recovered, and the victim can be brought to a hospital within six hours of the injury, do the following:

1. Quickly and gently rinse the body part if the cut end is obviously contaminated with dirt.

2. Wrap the body part in clean cloth or gauze, and keep it moist. The ideal solution is saline (NOT ocean water because of infection risk), if that is available; if not, fresh water will do. Do not immerse the part in a bag of water, but merely keep it moist. To avoid a frostbite injury, *do not apply ice directly to the body part or put it in ice water,* but keep it cool by placing it on ice after wrapping it securely in a bandage, cloth, or towel. Bring the body part with the victim to the hospital.

The application of a tourniquet to stop bleeding is essentially a decision to sacrifice the limb in order to preserve life. If any salvageable part of the limb is still significantly attached, do not apply a tourniquet to stop the bleeding until you have exhausted all pressure techniques (see page 49). If the limb is completely severed, the muscular walls of the arteries will generally contract after a few minutes of direct pressure. However, if an arm or leg is lost and uncontrollable bleeding threatens life, a tourniquet can be justified. This is applied with a cloth or rope circumferentially an inch or two above the wound and tightened just enough to allow direct pressure to stop the bleeding. After 5–10 minutes, it should be loosened briefly to see if the bleeding can be controlled with pressure techniques alone.

Burns

BURNS may be divided into different severities according to the depth of burn and the body surface area involved. First aid and the decision to seek sophisticated medical aid are based on the severity of the burn.

DEFINITIONS *(Fig. 51)*

FIRST-DEGREE BURN: This is a burn that involves the outermost layer of skin, the epidermis. It is often quite painful. The skin is reddened, but there is no blister formation. When a large surface area is involved, as with a severe sunburn, the victim may become quite ill, with fever, weakness, chills, and vomiting.

SECOND-DEGREE BURN: This is a burn that involves the epidermis and portions of the next deeper layer of the skin, the dermis, which contains the sweat glands, hair follicles, and small blood

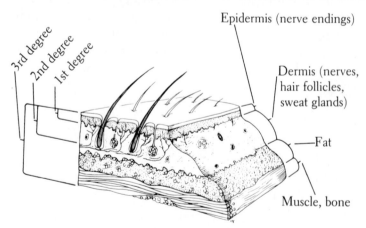

FIGURE 51. *Burn wound. Note that third-degree (full-thickness) burns completely destroy nerves and are painless.*

vessels. It is usually more painful than a first-degree burn, and blisters are present. Large areas of second-degree injury impair the body's ability to control temperature and retain moisture. Thus a severely burned victim loses large amounts of fluid and can rapidly become hypothermic in a cold environment.

THIRD-DEGREE BURN: This is a burn that has penetrated the entire thickness of skin, and may involve muscle, bone, etc. It is typically painless, because of nerve destruction. The appearance is dry, hard, leathery, and charred. Occasionally, the skin will appear waxy and white, with small clotted blood vessels visible as small purple or maroon lines below the surface. Because a third-degree burn is usually surrounded by an area of second-degree injury, the edges of the wound may be quite painful. Third-degree burns nearly always require a skin graft for coverage.

PARTIAL-THICKNESS BURN: First- and/or second-degree burn.

FULL-THICKNESS BURN: Third-degree burn.

INHALATION INJURY: This is a burn that involves any portion of the airway, and occurs when a victim is trapped in a fire or is otherwise forced to inhale smoke, steam, and superheated air (see page 95).

TREATMENT FOR BURNS

1. Remove the victim from the source of the burn. If his clothing is on fire, the victim should be rolled on the ground or into a blanket to extinguish the flames. If the victim has been burned with chemicals, *gallons* of water should be used to wash off the harmful agents. If the eyes are involved, they should be irrigated copiously. Phosphorus ignites upon contact with air, so any phosphorus in contact with the skin must be kept covered with water. Do not attempt to neutralize acid burns with alkaline

solutions and vice versa (e.g., do not apply baking soda to acid burns, etc.); such attempts may cause a reaction that *creates* heat and increases the injury. Stick to irrigation with water.

2. Evaluate the airway. Look for evidence of an inhalation injury: burns of the face and mouth, singed nasal hairs, soot in the mouth, swollen tongue, drooling and difficulty in swallowing saliva, muffled voice, coarse or difficult breathing, coughing and wheezing. If it appears that an inhalation injury has occurred, administer oxygen by face mask, 5–10 liters per minute, and transport the victim to a hospital as rapidly as possible.

3. Examine the patient for other injuries. Unless the airway is involved or the patient is horribly burned, the burn injury will not be immediately life threatening. In your rush to treat the burn, don't overlook a serious injury such as a broken neck. Control all bleeding and attend to broken bones before applying burn dressings.

4. Treat the burn. The following guidelines are designed to allow management until an appropriate facility can be reached.

First-degree. First-degree burns, such as a mild to moderate sunburn, may be treated with cool wet compresses. If the burn is acquired suddenly (as when a child grabs a hot object), the immediate application of very cold water (not solid ice) may help to limit the extent of the tissue damage. The oral administration of anti-inflammatory drugs, such as aspirin (650 mg every 6–8 hours) or ibuprofen (Motrin) 600–800 mg by mouth every 8 hours may provide considerable relief. For severe sunburn ("lobster body"), the administration of oral prednisone in a rapid taper (60 mg the first day, 40 mg the second, 20 mg the third, 10 mg the fourth and fifth days) is indicated. Topical corticosteroid creams are of no benefit. Anesthetic sprays that contain benzocaine may induce allergic reactions and should be used sparingly, if at all. If no blisters are present, a moisturizing cream (such as Vaseline Intensive Care) will help to soothe the skin. Aloe vera lotion or gel seems to work well to promote rapid resolution of extensive first-degree burns.

Second-degree. Second-degree burns should be irrigated gently to remove all loose dirt and skin. This should be done with the cleanest cool water available. *Never apply ice directly to a burn.* The application of ice may cause more extensive tissue damage. Cool compresses may be used for pain relief.

After the wound is clean and dry, cover it with a soft bulky dressing made of gauze or cloth bandages, taking care to keep it snug but not tight. If antiseptic cream such as silver sulfadiazine (Silvadene) is available, it may be applied under the dressing. Another excellent covering is Spenco 2nd Skin underneath an absorbent sterile dressing. Do not apply butter, lanolin, vitamin E cream, or steroid cream preparations to a burn. These all may inhibit wound healing and may cause infections with increased scarring. Dressings should be changed each day to readjust for swelling and to check for early signs of infection. Be certain to keep burned arms and legs elevated as best possible, to minimize swelling and pain.

Blisters should not be opened, unless they are obviously infected and contain pus (this will not occur for 24–48 hours after the injury). If they remain filled with clear fluid, they are an excellent covering for the wound and will minimize fluid loss and infection. There is no rush to remove charred skin from a burn wound; after the injury is properly cleaned, the decisions about trimming can be made by a physician. Victims with large areas of second-degree burns may need to be treated for shock (see page 53).

Third-degree. Third-degree burns should be irrigated gently and covered with antiseptic cream or Spenco 2nd Skin and a dry sterile dressing.

If a first-degree burn involves greater than 20% of the body surface area and the victim suffers from fever, chills, or vomiting, a physician evaluation is required as soon as possible. If a second-degree burn wound involves a significant portion of the face, eyes, hands, or genitals, or an area greater than 5% of the body surface, the victim should be transported to a physician or burn center as rapidly as possible. Body surface area can be estimated using the "palm of hand" rule, where the surface area of the victim's palm and fingers is approximately 1–1.5% of his total body surface area. All third-degree burn wounds are serious and must be seen promptly by a physician. Because an improperly evaluated and treated burn can result in deformity, unsightly scarring, and disability, all but the most minor burn wounds should be seen by a physician.

Wet Versus Dry Dressings

If the burn surface area is small (no greater than 10% of total body surface area), then cool moist dressings (NOT ICE) may be used to cover the burn wound. These often provide greater pain relief than do dry dressings. If the surface area involved is large, however, dry nonadherent dressings should be used, in order to avoid overcooling of the victim and the introduction of hypothermia (see page 221). Because the skin is the major thermoregulatory organ of the body, it is difficult for a severely burned patient to control his body temperature, and great care must be taken when wetting down such a person. If the victim begins to shiver, then cooling is too extreme.

Antibiotics

Antibiotics are not necessary for burns unless they become infected. This is indicated by the presence of pus, foul odor, cloudy blisters, increasing redness and swelling in the normal skin that surrounds the burn, and fever greater than 101° F (38.3° C). If a burn becomes infected, administer dicloxacillin, cephalexin, or erythromycin, and be certain to change all dressings daily. If a person sustains a serious burn that becomes infected after exposure to ocean water, administer ciprofloxacin or trimethoprim-sulfamethoxazole in addition to the other antibiotic chosen (above). Blisters that appear infected should be unroofed and drained, then covered properly.

TAR BURNS

If a victim is splashed with hot roofing tar or paving asphalt, immediately immerse the affected area in cool water to solidify the tar and to limit the burn. If a large surface area is involved (greater than 5% of the total body surface area), leave the tar on the skin and seek medical attention immediately. If only a few small areas are covered with tar, and you cannot reach a physician, the tar may be removed by gently rubbing it with repeated coatings of bacitracin ointment or mayonnaise, which will turn brown as the tar dissolves into it. Do not injure the skin by attempting to peel off the tar. After the tar is removed, treat the burn as described above. If you cannot remove the tar, cover the wound with bacitracin ointment and a clean dressing. Seek immediate medical attention.

Inhalation Injuries

INHALATION injuries include thermal (heat) and chemical (smoke, noxious gas) inhalations. A third type of inhalation injury is that of aspiration (inhalation) of ocean water, stomach contents, and/or blood into the lungs. The severity of each injury is determined by the chemical nature of the substance (acid or caustic), temperature, volume, toxicity (e.g., carbon monoxide or cyanide), and underlying health of the victim.

Most rescuers are concerned with the acute effects of the injury (airway obstruction, inability to breathe [drowning], lack of oxygen, poisoning) rather than with the chronic sequelae (infections, scarring, emphysema). In all cases, the rescuer must have a high index of suspicion for an inhalation injury, as prompt extrication and first aid will frequently be lifesaving. In-water drowning is discussed on page 298.

THERMAL INJURY

In thermal inhalation, the airway is injured by the introduction of superheated air or steam. Such injuries almost always occur in enclosed spaces, although occasional mishaps occur in association with wildland fires (see page 243). Because water conducts heat approximately 30 times as efficiently as air, the risk of injury is far greater with steam than with dry superheated air.

The heat injures the inside of the mouth and nose, throat, vocal cords, trachea, bronchi, and occasionally even the lungs. The damage is essentially a burn wound, and may be serious enough to be a rapid threat to life. External signs of an inhalation injury include burns about the face and mouth, singed nasal hairs, and soot in the mouth and nose. Symptoms include shortness of breath; wheezing; coughing (particularly of carbonaceous black sputum); raspy coarse breathing (stridor) noted most often on inspiration, with a barking quality that seems to originate in the neck; muffled voice; drooling; difficulty in swallowing; swollen tongue; and agitation.

Once the burn injury has occurred, there is no effective way to limit its progress, so THE VICTIM SHOULD BE TRANS-PORTED AS RAPIDLY AS POSSIBLE TO AN EMERGENCY FACILITY. If oxygen is available, it should be administered at 5–10 liters per minute by face mask. If the victim's condition deteriorates rapidly because the airway becomes swollen and obstructed, the only hope for survival is the placement of a tube directly through the vocal cords and into the trachea (endotracheal intubation) or the surgical creation of an air passage in the neck (tracheostomy). These surgical procedures need to be performed by skilled health care personnel.

SMOKE (CHEMICAL) INJURY

Most smoke is composed of soot and various chemicals. Although each specific substance causes its own variation on the basic lung injury, the differences do not justify separate discussions here. The immediate therapy for a suspected toxic chemical inhalation is removal of the victim from the offending agent, and the IMMEDIATE ADMINISTRATION OF OXYGEN. If the victim is having difficulty breathing or is without respiration, he should be supported with mouth-to-mouth breathing (see page 24). Difficulty in breathing may be delayed for a few hours after a chemical inhalation, so all victims should seek immediate medical attention even if they feel fine initially.

The utmost caution must be exercised in removing a victim from the source of suspected toxic gases, so as not to create additional victims. Rescuers should wear gas masks, if they are available. Carbon monoxide intoxication is discussed on page 244.

ASPIRATION INJURY

Vomiting and inhalation of stomach contents is the most common complication of hypothermia or drug overdose. The key factor is altered mental status, as a person who has a depressed level of consciousness does not protect his airway. In any situation where a victim is unconscious and prone to vomit, and WHEN THE NECK IS KNOWN TO BE UNINJURED, the victim should be placed on his side, so that vomit and blood will drain from the mouth, rather than into the lungs. If a neck injury is suspected, and the victim must be kept on his back with the neck immobilized, a rescuer must keep constant watch for vomiting. If the victim vomits, he must be quickly turned on a stretcher or backboard or logrolled (see page 34) and the mouth cleared of debris. This is an unpleasant task, but essential.

Abdominal Pain

T HE causes of abdominal pain are myriad, but may be broken down by classical symptom complexes. As with any other disorder, there are serious causes of abdominal pain and there are minor disturbances. The purpose of taking the patient's history and performing a physical examination is to determine the urgency of the situation, in order to plan for evacuation if necessary. Because differentiation between various diseases is often difficult, the recommendations that follow are ultraconservative. Any person with severe abdominal pain should be seen by a physician as soon as possible.

GENERAL EVALUATION

The following history must be obtained:

1. *Nature of the pain.* Is the pain sharp (knifelike), aching (constant), colicky (intermittent and severe), or cramplike (squeezing)? Has the victim ever suffered a similar episode?

2. *Location of the pain.* Is the pain well localized to one particular area, or does it radiate to another region (e.g., back or groin)? Did the pain begin in one region and move to another?

3. *Mode of onset of the pain.* Did the pain occur suddenly, or has it gradually increased in intensity? How long has the victim been in pain?

4. *Associated symptoms.* Is the patient short of breath, nauseated, vomiting, suffering from diarrhea or constipation, or dizzy? Is the patient vomiting blood or bile (green liquid produced by the gallbladder)?

5. *Relief of pain.* Is there a position that the victim can assume that provides lessening of the pain? Does the victim feel better in a quiet position, or is he agitated and constantly moving around?

6. *Menstrual history.* In the female patient, it is important to

determine if there is any chance that the abdominal pain is related to a disorder of pregnancy.

PHYSICAL EXAMINATION

The following physical examination should be performed:
1. Observe the patient. Note whether he is active or avoids movement. If possible, note the severity of distress when the patient has his attention diverted (and he is not focusing all of his attention on your examination).
2. Note the patient's color, pulse rate and strength, rate of respirations, ease of breathing, mental status, and temperature. Abnormalities of any of these heighten the possibility of a serious problem.
3. Examine the abdomen. This is best done by having the victim lie quietly on his back, with knees drawn up. Gently press on the abdomen, *proceeding from the area of least discomfort to the area of greatest discomfort.* For the purposes of examination, the abdomen can be divided by lines through the navel into four quadrants: right upper, left upper, right lower, and left lower (Fig. 52A). The epigastrium is the area of the abdomen directly below the breastbone in the midline. Note where the patient complains of pain, and whether it is affected by your examination. If the patient has increased sharp pain when the hands are suddenly released from the abdomen after a pressing maneuver, this may indicate "rebound" pain associated with general inflammation of the lining of the abdominal cavity (peritonitis). Rebound pain may be caused by severe infections, stomach acid, or blood that has leaked into the abdominal cavity, or other problems that are generally quite serious.

When a specific area of the abdomen is tender, there are certain disorders to consider:

Epigastrium: heart attack, ulcer, gastroenteritis, heartburn, pancreatitis.

A

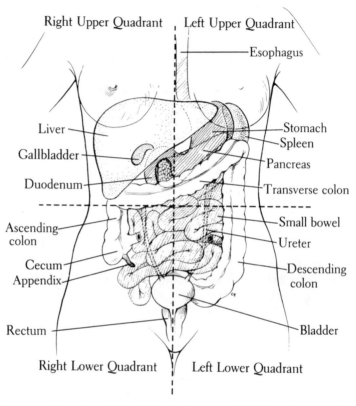

Right Upper Quadrant | Left Upper Quadrant

Esophagus

Liver

Gallbladder

Duodenum

Stomach
Spleen
Pancreas
Transverse colon

Ascending colon

Cecum
Appendix

Small bowel
Ureter

Descending colon

Rectum

Bladder

Right Lower Quadrant | Left Lower Quadrant

FIGURE 52. *Location of the abdominal organs. (A) View from the front, with the abdomen divided into four quadrants.*

Right upper quadrant: injured liver, hepatitis, gallstones, pneumonia.

Left upper quadrant: injured spleen, gastroenteritis, pancreatitis, pneumonia.

Right lower quadrant: appendicitis, kidney stone, ovarian infection, colitis, bowel obstruction, hernia.

Left lower quadrant: diverticulitis, colitis, kidney stone, ovarian infection, bowel obstruction, hernia.

B

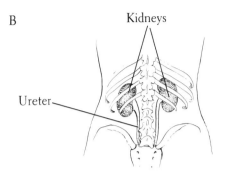

Kidneys

Ureter

FIGURE 52 (CONT.). *(B) The kidneys are located posteriorly in the abdomen, and may be the cause of flank or back pain.*

Lower abdomen (central): abdominal aortic aneurysm, ovarian infection, ovulation disorder, bladder infection, colitis, bowel obstruction.

Flank: abdominal aortic aneurysm, kidney stones, kidney infection.

By quadrant, brief descriptions of and treatments for these disorders follow below.

EPIGASTRIUM

Heart Attack

The symptoms of a heart attack can include pain that is located in the epigastrium, rather than in the chest. If the patient has a history of heart disease, has dull epigastric pain, nausea, shortness of breath, and weakness, the possibility of a heart attack should be considered (see page 46). If a heart attack is suspected, even minimally, plan for immediate rescue or evacuation.

Ulcer

An ulcer is an erosion in the lining of the stomach (gastric ulcer) or duodenum (peptic ulcer) that penetrates the protective mu-

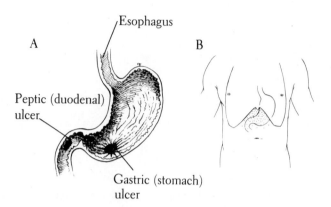

A

Esophagus

B

Peptic (duodenal)
ulcer

Gastric (stomach)
ulcer

FIGURE 53. *Ulcers. (A) Location of ulcer craters in the duodenum and stomach. (B) Epigastric region of the stomach, where ulcer pain is often noted.*

cous layer and allows acid and digestive juices to erode deeper into the tissues (Fig. 53). This causes extreme pain and can lead to bleeding from leaking blood vessels in the ulcer crater. Symptoms include constant burning pain in the epigastrium that is made worse by pressing and is often associated with nausea and/ or belching. In minor cases, the pain is relieved by meals. In severe cases, when the ulcer has eroded into a blood vessel or has perforated the wall of the stomach or bowel, the victim will vomit red blood or dark brown clotted blood ("coffee grounds"), and complain of pain that can radiate to the back. Rebound tenderness and peritonitis may be present. Dark black tarry bowel movements (melena) are caused by blood that has made its transit through the bowel. Bright red blood or blood clots with a bowel movement can be caused by brisk bleeding from an ulcer. Mild bleeding from an ulcer may actually decrease the pain, as blood acts as an antacid.

In minor cases of ulcer disease, the pain may be relieved by antacids (2–3 tablespoons 30 minutes after meals, at bedtime, and as needed). Liquids appear to be more effective than tablets. A number of other medications are used to decrease acid secretion, decrease bowel activity and cramping, and to line the wall of the stomach and bowel (see page 371). Solid food and milk are no longer recommended as antacids. While they may decrease the pain briefly, they actually stimulate the secretion of acid a few hours after ingestion. If the victim has an understanding of his disease, and can control his pain readily with his medications, the journey can continue. Cigarette smoking and alcohol ingestion are strictly prohibited. If pain is not immediately controlled, or if there is any suggestion of bleeding or perforation, rapid transport to a hospital is indicated.

Gastroenteritis

Gastroenteritis is the "stomach flu" that strikes at the most inopportune moments (see the discussion about diarrhea on page 162). Symptoms include waves of crampy upper and/or lower abdominal pain, followed by loose bowel movements. Nausea and vomiting may be present. Occasionally, the victim has symptoms of an upper respiratory infection, with cough, runny nose, sore throat, headache, and fever. The treatment of gastroenteritis is rarely very satisfying; it includes a clear liquid diet, antacids, and medicine for intolerable vomiting (see page 173). When a victim vomits green bile, this should be taken as a sign that the problem is more serious than straightforward gastroenteritis.

Heartburn

See page 172.

Pancreatitis

The pancreas is an organ situated in the posterior upper abdomen that secretes a number of enzymes used to digest food. These travel through a duct, where they are released through a small opening into the duodenum (the first portion of the bowel after the stomach). In addition, the pancreas synthesizes hormones such as insulin, which regulate the storage and use of sugar in the body. If the pancreas becomes inflamed, either by alcohol abuse (binge drinking is far and away the most common cause), viral infection, or blockage of the main secretory duct by a gallstone, severe epigastric pain is the rule. This is accompanied by nausea and vomiting (which may contain bile). The diagnosis of pancreatitis (as distinct from gastroenteritis) requires some medical sophistication. A person with pancreatitis needs to be hospitalized, because the only effective treatment is to eliminate oral intake for a period of time (to decrease stimulation of the pancreas). Out of the hospital, allow the victim clear liquids and antacids only, and pain medicine if pills can be kept down. Seek immediate physician care.

RIGHT UPPER QUADRANT

Injured Liver

If a fall or blow to the abdomen, right flank, or right lower chest is followed by abdominal pain that is worsened by pressing on the right upper quadrant, a torn or bruised liver should be considered. The victim is at risk for severe internal bleeding and should be observed for signs of shock (see page 53). Evacuate the victim as soon as possible.

Hepatitis

See page 175.

Gallstones (Cholecystitis)

Gallstones are formed in the gallbladder, which lies under the liver in the right upper quadrant of the abdomen and stores the bile (manufactured in the liver) that is released into the duode-

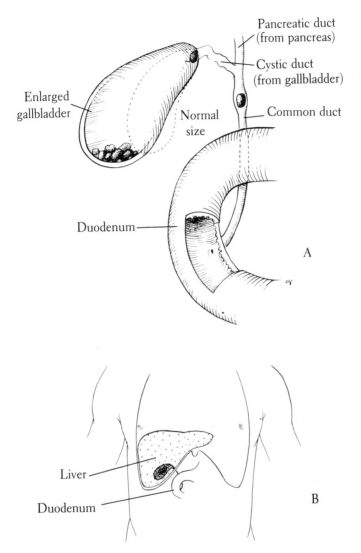

Pancreatic duct (from pancreas)

Cystic duct (from gallbladder)

Common duct

Enlarged gallbladder

Normal size

Duodenum

A

Liver

Duodenum

B

FIGURE 54. *Gallbladder with gallstones. (A) The stones are formed in the gallbladder and travel through a narrow passageway (cystic and common ducts), which is easily blocked. (B) Location of the gallbladder adjacent to the liver in the right upper quadrant of the abdomen.*

num to aid in digestion following each meal (Fig. 54). An attack of cholecystitis occurs when the outlet from the gallbladder or the main bile duct into the duodenum becomes obstructed (usually by a stone) and the gallbladder cannot empty. This causes stretching of the gallbladder, inflammation, and painful contraction against an impenetrable passage.

A typical attack occurs immediately after a meal, and is sudden in onset. The pain is colicky and located in the right upper quadrant or epigastrium. It may be associated with nausea, vomiting, and fever. Occasionally, it radiates to the back or right shoulder. Examination of the abdomen demonstrates tenderness in the right upper quadrant. Occasionally, one can feel a tennis-ball-sized tender mass (the swollen gallbladder).

The definitive treatment for cholecystitis is removal of the gallbladder, although some surgeons prefer to quiet down the situation first with antibiotics and intravenous fluids. The victim of a gallbladder attack should be transported to a hospital for evaluation. Pain medicines can be given safely, although certain narcotics may increase spasm of the bile passage and, paradoxically, briefly worsen pain. Solid foods (particularly fats) are prohibited during an attack. Maintain the victim on clear liquids and begin ampicillin if pills can be kept down. Transport the victim to a hospital.

Pneumonia

See page 44.

LEFT UPPER QUADRANT

Injured Spleen

If a fall or blow to the abdomen, left flank, or left lower chest is followed by abdominal pain that is worsened by pressing on the left upper quadrant, a torn or bruised spleen should be considered. The victim is at risk for severe internal bleeding and should be observed for signs of shock (see page 53). Evacuate the victim as soon as possible.

Gastroenteritis

See page 103.

Pancreatitis

See page 103.

Pneumonia

See page 44.

RIGHT LOWER QUADRANT

Appendicitis

The appendix is a small sausage-shaped bowel appendage, with no modern function, that is located near the transition point where the small bowel becomes the large bowel (colon) (Fig. 55). When it becomes infected or obstructed (acute appendicitis), the patient typically has a history of crampy pain that begins in the center of the stomach, and moves over the course of hours to become constant in the right lower quadrant. The patient may have associated constipation or diarrhea, vomiting, fever, and weakness. Examination demonstrates tenderness on pressing the right lower quadrant. Frequently, the patient will resist any movement of the body or legs, as such movement causes abdominal pain. Rebound tenderness is associated with a swollen appendix that is ready to burst or has already ruptured. If the appendix ruptures, the pain may diminish considerably for a few days until an abscess forms. If appendicitis is suspected, the patient should

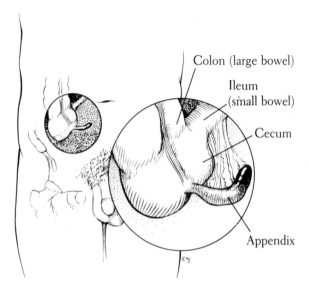

Colon (large bowel)

Ileum
(small bowel)

Cecum

Appendix

FIGURE 55. *Appendicitis. Pain is felt in the right lower quadrant of the abdomen.*

be transported to a hospital for surgical evaluation. Unless there is a real risk of dehydration due to prolonged (greater than 24 hours) transport, do not give the victim anything by mouth. Antibiotics (penicillin or ampicillin) should be administered only if no hospital can be reached within 48 hours.

Kidney Stone

See page 116.

Ovarian Infection (and Other Disorders of the Female Reproductive System)

See page 113.

Colitis

See page 170.

Bowel Obstruction

If the intestine becomes obstructed, either by scar tissue, injury, or waste products, the victim rapidly becomes quite ill. Symptoms include nausea and vomiting, frequently of green bile or feculent (feces-like) material. The patient has waves of cramping pain that are associated with waves of bowel motion that may be visible through the abdominal wall, which is frequently distended by the dilated loops of bowel. Occasionally, the victim will have small squirting loose bowel movements, as a little liquid slips past the obstruction. If a bowel obstruction is suspected, the victim should be immediately evacuated to a hospital. Do not attempt to manage potentially seriously ill persons without a physician unless you are forced to do so.

Hernia

If the intestine slips through the muscles of the abdominal wall, usually in the groin or around the umbilicus (navel), a hernia is formed (Fig. 56). Symptoms include a visible bulge, abdominal pain, and pain at the site of the hernia. The victim should be made to lie quietly on his back with knees drawn up, and cold packs should be placed on the hernia. Pain medicine is given to control the discomfort. If reasonable relaxation is obtained, the hernia may slip back through the wall and the bulge will disappear. Afterward, the victim should wear a support (truss or belt) to prevent recurrence until the problem can be corrected surgically.

If a victim has a painless hernia (bulge) that cannot be corrected, he should avoid straining, and seek the aid of a physician.

If the intestine will not slip back through, the hernia is incar-

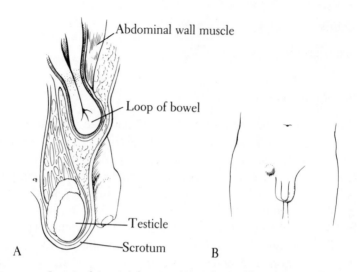

FIGURE 56. *Inguinal (groin) hernia. (A) A loop of bowel bulges through a defect in the lower abdominal wall. (B) Location of external bulge. In some cases, the swelling extends into the scrotum.*

cerated (caught). This is an emergency, because if the blood supply to the bowel is pinched off, the tissue can be severely damaged or die, and/or a bowel obstruction (see page 109) can be created. An incarcerated hernia is extremely painful, and if the bowel is injured, the overlying skin frequently becomes reddened or dusky in appearance. Because the aforementioned maneuvers for reduction of a hernia will not be successful and pain will increase, the victim should be rapidly evacuated to a hospital.

LEFT LOWER QUADRANT

Diverticulitis

Diverticuli are small outpouchings that develop at weak points along the wall of the colon (large bowel), probably because of high pressures associated with muscle contractions in the passage of stool. When these sacs become obstructed and/or inflamed (most frequently in middle-aged or elderly individuals), they enlarge and create pain and fever. Usually, the left lower quadrant is involved, because diverticuli tend to form in the left side of the colon (descending colon) more frequently than the right (ascending colon). A ruptured diverticulum can cause a clinical picture much like that of a ruptured appendix (see page 107), with pain in the left abdomen instead of the right. The victim should seek medical attention, and be limited to clear liquids. Antibiotics (ampicillin or penicillin) should be administered only if help is greater than 48 hours away.

Colitis
See page 170.

Kidney Stone
See page 116.

Ovarian Infection (and Other Disorders of the Female Reproductive System)
See page 113.

Bowel Obstruction
See page 109.

Hernia
See page 109.

LOWER ABDOMEN (CENTRAL)

Abdominal Aortic Aneurysm

An aneurysm is a dilated blood vessel that has been weakened by the ravages of age, high blood pressure, and atherosclerosis (Fig. 57). At a certain point, the wear and tear become too much, and the blood vessel rips, causing either a slow leak or rapid massive bleeding that leads to sudden collapse and death. This generally occurs spontaneously only in the elderly; traumatic tears of the aorta can occur in any age group.

The aorta is the large artery that carries blood from the left ventricle of the heart to the body. The symptoms of a ruptured abdominal aortic aneurysm are intense unrelenting ripping pain in the abdomen that may radiate to the back or chest, weakness, dis-

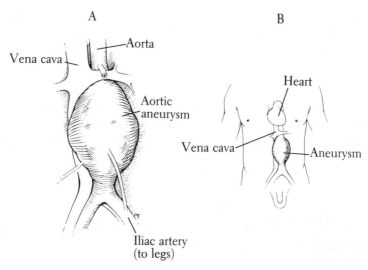

FIGURE 57. *Abdominal aortic aneurysm. (A) The dilated aorta is ravaged by age, high blood pressure, and disease. (B) Location of the aorta in the abdomen. Leaking or rupture causes pain in the abdomen, back, and flank.*

coloration of the legs with mottling, and rapid collapse. Gentle examination of the abdomen may demonstrate a pulsating expanding mass. Rigidity is due to the rapid accumulation of blood. ANY ELDERLY PERSON WHO SUDDENLY DEVELOPS ABDOMINAL PAIN OR BACK PAIN ASSOCIATED WITH WEAKNESS, A FAINTING SPELL, DECREASED SENSATION AND/OR ABNORMAL COLOR IN THE LEGS AND FEET, OR SHORTNESS OF BREATH SHOULD BE IMMEDIATELY RUSHED TO A HOSPITAL. In the best of circumstances, this is a highly critical situation. Be prepared to treat the victim for shock (see page 53).

Ovarian Infection

The ovaries and the fallopian tubes, which carry eggs from the ovary to the uterus, may become infected, commonly with the bacteria that cause gonorrhea (a form of venereal disease) or by other infectious agents (such as *Chlamydia trachomatis*) (Fig. 58). Symptoms include abdominal pain in the lower quadrants

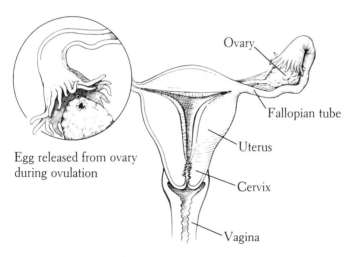

Ovary

Fallopian tube

Uterus

Egg released from ovary
during ovulation

Cervix

Vagina

FIGURE 58. *Female reproductive tract.*

(greatest on the side of the affected ovary), fever, shaking chills, nausea, vomiting, and weakness. Occasionally, the victim will complain of a yellow-greenish vaginal discharge. If such an infection is suspected, the victim should be taken to a hospital immediately. If more than 24 hours will pass before a doctor can be reached, the patient should be started on tetracycline 500 mg 4 times a day. An alternative drug is metronidazole 250 mg 3 times a day.

Ovulation, Ovarian Cyst, and Torsed Ovary

Some women suffer intense sudden abdominal pain at the time of ovulation (when the egg is released from the ovary) (Fig. 58). This is caused by a small amount of blood and ovarian fluid that irritates the lining of the abdomen. Symptoms include pain that suddenly develops in the right or left lower quadrant, and is worsened by movement or deep palpation of the area. Treatment is pain medicine and rest. A ruptured ovarian cyst (which releases tissue fluid or blood) or torsed (twisted) ovary causes similar but much more severe symptoms, which may include excruciating pain, nausea and vomiting, and a rigid (to the pressing hand) abdomen. Any of these conditions may be difficult to distinguish from appendicitis (see page 107) if the right ovary is involved. Treatment often requires surgery. If appendicitis, ruptured ovarian cyst, ovarian infection, or torsed ovary is suspected, a physician should be consulted immediately. *Any sudden abdominal discomfort in a woman of childbearing age should be promptly evaluated by a doctor.*

Bleeding from the Vagina

If bleeding from the vagina accompanied by abdominal pain is not clearly part of a normal menstrual period, a woman should seek prompt medical attention. If the bleeding is clearly part of a normal menstrual period, and the pain is unquestionably due to menstrual cramps, then the victim may benefit from the administration of ibuprofen (Motrin) 400–600 mg every 6 hours.

If abnormal pain and/or bleeding (in amount or character) occurs during or between menstrual periods, the cause should be determined by a physician. Until the evaluation is performed, exertion should be kept to a minimum. If periods have been missed (or if the patient is known to be pregnant) and copious vaginal bleeding develops, the victim should be placed at rest and transported rapidly by litter if possible to a physician. If the bleeding is spotty, the victim may walk with assistance. A ruptured tubal (ectopic) pregnancy can rapidly become life threatening.

Vaginitis

Vaginitis is a condition of irritation and inflammation of the vagina, commonly noted as a secondary infection that follows administration of a common antibiotic, such as ampicillin, to a woman. The antibiotic alters the normal bacterial population of the vagina and allows overgrowth of the culprit agents, which are often yeast. With a yeast (candidiasis or moniliasis) infection, the victim notes a white and creamy ("cottage cheese") discharge, vulvar and vaginal itching, and burning pain on urination. The victim should use clotrimazole (Gyne-Lotrimin) vaginal tablets (7 days) or cream (14 days). An alternative drug is miconazole nitrate (Monistat) vaginal suppositories or cream. If the infection is due to trichomoniasis, the victim will have a frothy white-gray discharge and may also have abdominal pain and fever. In such a case, the antibiotic of choice is metronidazole 250 mg 3 times a day for 5–7 days.

Bladder Infection

See page 212.

Colitis

See page 170.

Bowel Obstruction

See page 109.

FLANK

Abdominal Aortic Aneurysm

See page 112.

Kidney Stones

Kidney stones originate in the urine-collecting system of the kidney, and most commonly cause pain when they travel down the ureters to the bladder (Fig. 59). Once in the bladder, they may enter the urethra, and continue to wreak havoc.

The pain of a kidney stone is often intolerable, and usually is sudden in onset. The location of the pain is related to the location of the stone. If the stone is high in the ureter, the pain is in the back (on the affected side), with some radiation to the abdomen. Lightly tapping over the flank and lower ribs on the back of a patient with a kidney stone will often cause extreme pain. If the stone is passing through the lower ureter, the patient will have extreme pain in the back, abdomen, and genitals. When the stone is not moving, the pain may disappear as quickly as it came on.

A patient who is passing a kidney stone finds no relief from remaining still, and will appear quite agitated, constantly changing positions. Associated symptoms include nausea, vomiting, bloody urine, pain on urination, and sweating.

If the diagnosis of a kidney stone appears relatively certain, the patient should be given the strongest pain medicine that is safely available, and encouraged to drink copious amounts of liquid.

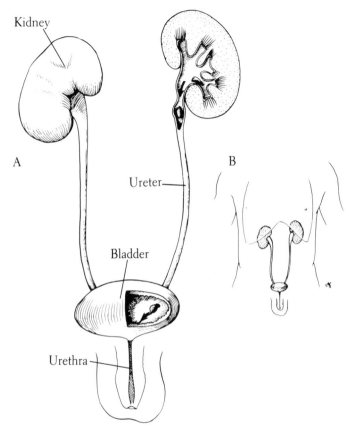

Kidney

A

Ureter

Bladder

B

Urethra

FIGURE 59. *Kidney with kidney stones. (A) The stones are formed in the kidney and travel through the ureter, bladder, and urethra before they are passed in the urine. (B) Location of the genitourinary (urogenital) system.*

Seek physician evaluation as soon as possible. IF THE PATIENT IS ELDERLY, CONSIDER THE DIAGNOSIS OF RUPTURED AORTIC ANEURYSM (see page 112). If there is any suspicion that the patient might have an aneurysm, evacuate the victim immediately.

Kidney Infection

See page 213.

Diabetes

DIABETES mellitus is a disorder in which the pancreas cannot create sufficient insulin hormone and/or in which available insulin is not totally effective. Insulin allows the body to utilize and store sugar; in the diabetic state, the victim suffers from high blood sugar. Many diabetics need to take insulin by injection to manage the disease; others can control their blood sugar by diet and/or oral medications.

The most common dangerous situation incurred by diabetics is a hypoglycemic reaction (low blood sugar) induced by an inadvertent overdose of insulin or after a normal dose of insulin accompanied by extraordinary exercise or insufficient food intake. The manifestations of an insulin reaction are weakness, sweating, hunger, abdominal pain, and altered mental status (which may include confusion, belligerent behavior, fainting, seizures, or coma). The solution is to administer sugar as rapidly as possible. If the patient is unconscious, it is generally prohibited to administer anything by mouth, because of the danger of choking and aspiration of food or fluid into the lungs. However, sugar granules can be placed under the tongue, where they will dissolve and be passively swallowed. Otherwise, sterile glucose solution must be injected intravenously, a process that requires a trained medical professional. If the patient is awake and capable of swallowing, a naturally sweetened solution (apple or orange juice, sugar-containing soft drink), banana, or candy bar (chocolate, sugar cube) should be administered by mouth. As soon as the patient is fully alert, a meal should be eaten, in order to avoid a recurrence.

It is important for anyone who suffers from diabetes to wear appropriate medical identification, in case he requires assistance. No person who is insulin-dependent should attempt physical exertion in a dangerous environment without adequate glucose intake.

If the blood sugar gets dangerously high, the diabetic may become very ill, as the blood becomes acidotic with the by-products of metabolism, dehydration increases, and body chemistries become unbalanced. Such a patient is confused, combative, or comatose. The breathing rate increases, breathing becomes shallow, and exhaled breaths have a fruity or acetone (like fingernail polish remover) odor. Because of dehydration, the skin is very dry and there is little sweating (dry armpits). Such a picture calls for immediate transport of the victim to the hospital. If he can drink, he should be encouraged to force unsweetened fluids. The definitive treatment is an injection of insulin, which must be dosed according to the measured blood sugar level.

If you cannot differentiate between an insulin reaction (low blood sugar) and altered mental status due to high excessive blood sugar, you should err on the side of predicting a hypoglycemic episode, and give the victim something sweet to eat or drink. If you have guessed correctly, the improvement will be dramatic; if your diagnosis was wrong, the extra sugar will not cause any significant harm. If a diabetic person carries a blood glucose monitor (e.g., Tracer Micro-monitor or Accu-Chek II blood glucose monitor), be sure you are instructed in its proper use.

Stroke

A STROKE is caused by a blood clot that blocks an artery which supplies part of the brain, or by bleeding into the brain. It occurs suddenly and can be minor or major, depending on the area and amount of the brain involved. If it involves the brainstem, it may affect the breathing center and cause rapid death.

Symptoms include sudden headache, nausea, vomiting, blurred or double vision, weakness or paralysis of the arms and/or legs, difficulty speaking or understanding speech, difficulty walking, confusion, loss of consciousness, coma, seizures, and collapse.

Once a stroke has occurred, there is little anyone can do to reverse it or to prevent the progression of illness, unless it is related to an air embolism associated with a scuba diving accident (see page 293). If someone has stroke symptoms that last for a few minutes to an hour and then gradually resolve, he has received a warning that he may soon have a stroke. In this case, he should immediately seek the attention of a doctor.

If someone develops the symptoms of a stroke, he should be placed at absolute rest with the upper body and head elevated by an angle of at least 30 degrees. If his level of consciousness declines, pay attention to the airway (see page 18), so that the victim does not vomit and choke. Seek immediate medical attention. Remember that low blood sugar may cause symptoms that mimic a stroke. If the victim can swallow purposely without choking, a sweetened liquid should be administered (see page 118).

Infectious Diseases

FOREIGN travel is increasingly a component of the wilderness experience, and thus American travelers are increasingly exposed to numerous diseases that are usually not indigenous to the United States. For instance, approximately 2 million to 3 million Americans travel to malarious regions each year. In addition, domestic outdoor activities expose persons directly to the natural vectors (carriers, such as mosquitoes or ticks) of microorganisms that generate diseases such as Eastern equine encephalitis, Rocky Mountain spotted fever, and Lyme disease. This section addresses some of the more common, worrisome infectious diseases associated with outdoor activities; immunizations are discussed on pages 334–340.

MALARIA

Malaria is caused by infection by one of four microscopic parasites: *Plasmodium falciparum, P. vivax, P. malariae,* or *P. ovale.* These are transmitted in the wild by the bite of an infected female *Anopheles* mosquito. Most cases of malaria acquired by U.S. citizens are contracted in sub-Saharan Africa, with most of the remainder linked to travel to Southeast Asia, Central and South America, the Indian subcontinent, the Middle East, and Oceania.

When an infected mosquito bites a human, it releases malaria sporozoites (an immature form of the parasite), which mature in the liver and then within red blood cells. From these locations, the organisms can invade the vital organs, such as the brain, lungs, liver, and kidneys. The incubation period between acquisition of the parasites and onset of symptoms is 8–28 days, depending on the species. Typical symptoms include a flulike illness, with headache, chills, fatigue, loss of appetite, muscle aches, nausea, and vomiting. This is soon followed by episodes of headache, intense chills, high fever, and sweating. Jaundice and anemia may occur. The episodes last 1–8 hours and are separated by 2–3 days. Persons infected with falciparum malaria may be significantly more ill, with episodes of fever and chills at closer intervals lasting for more than 30 hours. Severe malaria can be fatal or lead to anemia, heart and kidney failure, and/or coma; untreated infections can cause recurrent illness for years.

Identification of the specific plasmodium is accomplished by observing the parasites under the microscope in blood smears. Persons infected with P. *falciparum* are treated with quinine sulfate in combination with pyrimethamine-sulfadoxine (Fansidar) or tetracycline. Persons infected with P. *vivax*, P. *malariae*, or P. *ovale* are treated with chloroquine and primaquine phosphate.

Unfortunately, there is not yet a useful vaccine against malaria. Avoidance of mosquito bites is key to prevention. Because the *Anopheles* mosquito tends to feed during the evening and nighttime, it is particularly important to sleep under nets, spray living quarters (e.g., with a pyrethrum-containing product) and clothing (e.g., with permethrin), and wear adequate clothing and insect repellent (N,N-diethyl-meta-toluamide, called DEET) at these times (see page 288).

If travel is undertaken to a region where P. *falciparum* is resistant to chloroquine and Fansidar (most regions), then prophylaxis can be accomplished with mefloquine. The adult dose is 250 mg weekly. The pediatric dose varies according to the weight of the child, as follows: weight 15–19 kg, 63 mg; weight 20–30 kg, 125 mg; weight 31–45 kg, 188 mg; and over 45 kg, 250 mg. (For estimating purposes, 1 kg equals 2.2 lb.) Mefloquine should be started 1–2 weeks before travel, then administered once a week during travel in malarious areas and for 4 weeks after a person leaves such areas. Mefloquine should not be taken during pregnancy. An alternative drug for travelers who cannot take mefloquine is doxycycline (adult dose, 100 mg a day beginning 1–2 days prior to travel and for 5–6 weeks after; pediatric dose, 2 mg/kg a day, up to adult dose). Doxycycline is not advised for pregnant women or children under the age of 8 years, and may cause increased skin sensitivity to sunlight. A final alternative drug prophylaxis against malaria is accomplished with chloroquine phosphate (adult dose, 300 mg of the base once a week; pediatric dose, 5 mg/kg of the base, up to adult dose, once a week), which should be taken beginning 1–2 weeks before a person enters a malarious region and continued until one month after the journey. Chloroquine is recommended for travelers who cannot take mefloquine or doxycycline, particularly pregnant women and children who weigh less than 15 kg. If a person uses chloroquine for prophylaxis, he should carry 3 tablets of Fansidar to be taken in the event of a flulike illness or otherwise unexplained fever, assuming the absence of an allergy to sulfonamide antibiotics.

Proguanil (Paludrine) is a drug that may be used for antimalarial prophylaxis in areas where *P. falciparum* is resistant to chloroquine. The drug is available without prescription in parts of Europe, Scandinavia, and Africa, but is as yet unavailable in the United States. It is administered in an adult dose of 200 mg daily (pediatric dose: under 2 yrs, 50 mg; age 2–6 yrs, 100 mg; age 7–10 yrs, 150 mg; over 10 yrs, 200 mg), along with weekly chloroquine (the latter to protect against other forms of malaria). It may be used by persons who will spend more than 3 weeks in rural areas of East Africa (particularly Kenya and Tanzania), but does not appear to be useful in Papua New Guinea, West Africa, or Thailand.

Thus, if a person is stricken in an area where the malaria organism(s) is felt to be sensitive to chloroquine, but he has not been taking prophylaxis, begin treatment with chloroquine (adult dose, 600 mg of the base immediately, followed with 300 mg at 6 hours and once a day on days 2 and 3; pediatric dose, 10 mg/kg of the base up to 600 mg immediately, followed with 5 mg/kg at 6 hours and once a day on days 2 and 3). In a region where *P. falciparum* is resistant to chloroquine, administer quinine sulfate (adult dose, 650 mg every 8 hours for 3 days; pediatric dose, 8 mg/kg up to 650 mg every 8 hours for 3 days) PLUS tetracycline (adult dose, 250 mg 4 times a day for 7 days; pediatric dose, 5 mg/kg up to 250 mg 4 times a day for 7 days) or Fansidar (adult dose, 3 tablets; pediatric dose, weight 5–10 kg, ½ tablet; weight 11–20 kg, 1 tablet; weight 21–30 kg, 1½ tablets; weight 31–45 kg, 2 tablets; weight over 45 kg, 3 tablets). *In all cases of suspected malaria, seek the advice of a physician as soon as possible.*

To determine the malaria risk within a specific country and to learn of the most recent recommendations for prophylaxis and drug therapy, you can call the Malaria Hotline sponsored by the Centers for Disease Control (Atlanta) at 404-332-4555.

YELLOW FEVER

Yellow fever is a viral disease transmitted by the *Aedes aegypti* mosquito. "Jungle" yellow fever is seen in forest-savannah zones of tropical Africa, parts of Central America, forested areas of South America, and Trinidad. The "urban" variety is seen in South America and West Africa. The disease has not yet been noted in Asia.

The illness begins 3–6 days after the culprit mosquito bite(s). Symptoms include sudden onset of fever, headache, muscle aching, nausea, and vomiting. Less common are skin rashes and liver and kidney failure. In serious cases, the victim becomes jaundiced (hence, "yellow" fever) and bleeds easily. The disease can be fatal. Treatment is supportive and based upon symptoms.

A live virus vaccine is available. A single injection induces immunity after 10 days that is adequate for 10 years (see page 337).

DENGUE FEVER

Dengue fever is a viral disease that follows the bite(s) of infected *Aedes albopictus* and female *A. aegypti* mosquitoes. As opposed to the night-feeding mosquitoes that transmit malaria, these species tend to feed during daylight hours and to bite below the waist. Dengue fever is seen chiefly in the Caribbean and South America, as well as other tropical and semitropical areas, such as Southeast Asia and Mexico. In the United States, cases have been noted in Texas.

The incubation period following the mosquito bite is 2–8 days. The disease is self-limited (5–7 days) and characterized by sudden onset of severe headache, fever, chills, muscle aches, sore throat, reddened eyes, bone and joint pain ("breakbone fever"), and a fine red, itchy skin rash that typically appears simultaneously with the fever on the proximal arms, legs, and trunk, sparing the face, palms, and soles. Although the fever usually remits spontaneously, an occasional victim will relapse. Children under a year of age are vulnerable to particularly severe forms of dengue virus infection, associated with severe bleeding problems.

Treatment is supportive and based upon symptoms. There is no vaccine available against dengue fever.

SCHISTOSOMIASIS

Schistosomiasis is a term that describes a variety of diseases caused by different species of parasitic flatworms. The intermediate hosts are freshwater snails, which release the immature infective stages into the water; thus, the infections are acquired by persons who bathe or swim in contaminated water. The early symptoms caused by all of the species of worms are similar. When the fork-tailed cercariae (early stages of the immature worm) penetrate the skin, they cause itching and a rash at the site of entry that lasts for 1–2 days. Four to six weeks later, the victim shows loss of appetite, fatigue, night sweating, hives, and late afternoon fever lasting 5–10 days ("snail," "safari," "Katayama," or "Yangtze River" fever). After a few months, the different species cause specific organ damage.

Schistosoma haematobium is prevalent in Africa, the Middle

East, the islands of Madagascar and Mauritius, and in India. The worms reside in the blood vessels of the bladder and genitalia, and induce bloody, painful, and frequent urination. *S. mansoni* is prevalent in Africa, the Arabian peninsula, Madagascar, Brazil, Suriname, Venezuela, and some Caribbean islands. The worms reside in the blood vessels surrounding the large bowel and induce bloody and mucus-laden diarrhea. In late stages of the disease, the liver can be severely damaged. *S. japonicum* is prevalent in China, the Philippines, Japan, and the island of Sulawesi. The worms reside in the blood vessels supplying the small bowel and induce severe bloody and mucus-laden diarrhea. Other schistosomal species are less virulent.

Treatment for schistosomiasis includes the antihelminthic (antiparasitic) drug praziquantel, a prescription drug that kills the parasites.

To prevent schistosomiasis, it is necessary to prevent the entry of cercariae into the body. In a region of high risk, it is unwise to bathe or swim in an untreated pond or stream. Shallow, stagnant water is more contaminated than that in swift-moving currents. Always wear hip boots or waders when passing through streams or swamps. If contact with water occurs, apply rubbing alcohol to the skin and briskly towel off. Boil or disinfect all bathing water, or store it for 3 days (the life span of the cercariae) before using it (be certain it is free of snails). Unfortunately, there is not yet an effective repellent or vaccine against schistosomiasis.

Detailed information regarding world schistosomiasis risk is available from the International Association for Medical Assistance to Travelers (IAMAT) (see page 381).

ROCKY MOUNTAIN SPOTTED FEVER

Rocky Mountain spotted fever is caused by *Rickettsia rickettsii*, a tick-borne parasite. The disease is most commonly noted in the late spring and early summer, when a person is likely to be outside and become a host for the dog tick (*Dermacentor varia-*

bilis) or western wood tick (*Dermacentor andersoni*). Other ticks can also carry the parasite. Most infections are reported in the southeastern states: North Carolina, South Carolina, Texas, Tennessee, Virginia, Maryland, and Georgia. Recent cases have been noted in New York City.

The incubation period is 2–14 (average 7) days after the tick bite, at which time the fever begins abruptly. Two to six days after the onset of fever, the red spotted rash typically begins on the hands (including palms), wrists, feet (including soles), and ankles and spreads toward the trunk. The face is rarely involved. Some patients never develop a rash (Rocky Mountain "spotless" fever). Other symptoms include headache, joint and muscle aching, cough, puffy eyelids and face, swollen hands and feet, reddened eyes, abdominal pain, nausea, and vomiting. Severe cases can cause death.

If a person is thought to suffer from Rocky Mountain spotted fever, a physician's help should be sought immediately. Tetracycline (adult dose, 500 mg 4 times a day; pediatric dose, 10 mg/kg 4 times a day) or doxycycline (adult dose, 100 mg twice a day) should be given for 6 days, or until the victim is without fever for 3 days. Although it is generally not recommended to administer tetracycline to a pregnant woman or to a child less than 6 years of age because of the risk of tooth discoloration or abnormal bone development (the latter in a fetus during pregnancy), in a case of suspected Rocky Mountain spotted fever when a physician is not available to administer an alternative antibiotic (chloramphenicol), tetracycline should be given.

LYME DISEASE

Lyme disease, caused by infection with the spirochete *Borrelia burgdorferi*, is now the most common tick-borne illness in the United States. The most common seasons of occurrence are the summer and early autumn, during peak outdoor activities. The two ticks implicated in transmission of the spirochete are

Ixodes dammini (deer tick) in the Northeast (particularly Connecticut, Massachusetts, New Jersey, New York, Pennsylvania, and Rhode Island) and Midwest (particularly Wisconsin and Minnesota), and *Ixodes pacificus* in the West (particularly California and Oregon). The adult ticks of these species are extremely small, about the size of a sesame seed. Worse yet, the disease can be transmitted by nymphal forms, which may appear only as black specks on the skin. Other potential carriers in the United States include the dog tick, wood tick, rabbit tick, and Lone Star tick (*Amblyomma americanum*). Lyme disease has been reported in Canada, the Soviet Union, Australia, Europe (linked to the sheep tick, *Ixodes ricinus*), Scandinavia, and China.

The distinctive skin lesion of Lyme disease, erythema chronicum migrans, appears 3–32 days after the tick bite. It is usually found on the trunk, upper arm, or thigh as a small red spot that expands into a large (up to 30 inches in diameter) and irregular circle or oval with a red raised or flat outer border surrounding paler ("fading," but slightly red) skin in the center. The rash may itch or burn. In some cases, multiple smaller similar red areas appear simultaneously, but never on the palms or soles. These areas clear spontaneously over 1–21 (average 3) weeks. Variations of the rash include diffuse hives or a more measleslike eruption.

Appearing just prior to or coincident with the skin rash(es) are flulike symptoms that include muscle aching (particularly of the calves, thighs, and back), stiff neck, fatigue, low-grade fever, chills, painful joints, loss of appetite, nausea, cough, sore throat, swollen lymph glands, headache, abdominal pain (particularly in the right upper quadrant), irritated eyes (conjunctivitis), swelling around the eyes, and aversion to light. Most of the symptoms disappear in 2–3 weeks (along with the rash), but fatigue and muscle aching may last for months. Pets may also become ill, suffering lameness, swollen joints, lethargy, and loss of appetite.

If Lyme disease is not treated with antibiotics, the disease can progress to severe heart and nervous system disorders weeks to months after the rash disappears. Months or years later, up to

60% of untreated victims will suffer arthritis. The current recommendation for initial antibiotic therapy for adults with Lyme disease at the time of the initial rash or symptoms is tetracycline 250 mg 4 times a day or doxycycline 100 mg twice a day for 10–30 days. Children should be treated with phenoxymethyl penicillin in a dose of 13 mg/kg up to 500 mg 4 times a day or amoxicillin 7 mg/kg up to 250 mg 3 times a day for 10–30 days. The drugs of second choice are: adults — phenoxymethyl penicillin 500 mg or erythromycin 250 mg 4 times a day for 10–30 days; children — erythromycin 8 mg/kg up to 250 mg 4 times a day for 10–30 days. There are occasional treatment failures; such patients generally require hospitalization for intravenous antibiotics.

Prevention is key. Persons should avoid tick bites by wearing proper clothing (light colored for spotting ticks, tightly woven, collared shirts, closed boots, long sleeves and pant legs, hats), impregnated with 0.5% permethrin (Permanone) or N,N-diethyl-meta-toluamide (DEET) repellent in the critical locations. When traveling in tick country, keep shirts and pant cuffs tucked in. All hair-covered areas and warm, moist locations on the skin should be inspected carefully. Any tick found on the skin should be removed promptly and properly (see page 285). Following a tick bite, watch for the characteristic rash and symptoms. It is not yet recommended to administer antibiotics following all tick bites to prevent the occurrence of Lyme disease. In an area where carrier ticks and the disease are frequent, it is not unreasonable to administer an appropriate antibiotic for a week following removal of an embedded or blood-engorged tick.

PART THREE

MINOR MEDICAL PROBLEMS

Although the afflictions discussed in this section are rarely life threatening, they account for the majority of health care problems encountered in a recreational or wilderness setting. For the sake of simplicity, this section is organized by body organ system. Specific disorders can be rapidly located in the index.

Whenever a traveler or expedition member becomes ill, it is necessary to assume that the disorder can become progressively worse. If this is done, unnecessary risks are avoided, while health and safety are preserved. For instance, bronchitis can progress to pneumonia in situations of stress and suboptimal environmental conditions. Therefore, if a member of the party develops bronchitis, he should not remove himself farther from civilization until it is clear that medical management is going to halt progression of the disease.

I have not included disorders that originate from substance abuse (such as alcohol or illicit drugs), or indiscriminate sexual contact (venereal diseases). However, I would like to say that alcohol abuse (drinking to the point of intoxication) is a major contributor to injury and disease and is inexcusable when it places others at risk.

General Symptoms

UNCONSCIOUS (OR SEMICONSCIOUS) VICTIM

As discussed in detail in the section "Major Medical Problems" (see page 17), a proper approach to the unconscious (comatose) victim may make the difference between life and death. On a less immediate level, but with the same degree of concern, one must evaluate the semiconscious (stuporous, dazed, confused, or combative) individual. To discover the cause of an altered mental status, one must be a bit of a detective, while performing those tasks that prevent the victim from hurting himself. Always assume that an unconscious person may be seriously injured.

1. Open and maintain the airway (see page 18). Check for adequacy of the pulse (see page 25).

2. Protect the cervical spine (see page 31). EVERY INJURED PERSON HAS A BROKEN NECK UNTIL PROVEN OTHERWISE.

3. Carefully examine the victim for evidence of an obvious injury, and treat accordingly.

4. Consider low blood sugar, and treat the victim with glucose if he is alert enough to cooperate (see page 118).

Don't:

1. Don't shake a patient vigorously to awaken him, without first protecting the neck. NEVER shake a patient to awaken him if you suspect that hypothermia is present. If you think that the victim is merely intoxicated, snap an ammonia inhalant under his nose, give him a few whiffs, and stand back. If there is any chance of a neck injury, do not perform this maneuver without maintaining the head and neck in a stable position.

2. Don't attempt to carry an unconscious victim or manage a belligerent person if it is going to exhaust you. Send someone for help and stay with the victim until relief arrives.

3. Unless there is no other way to get help, never leave an unconscious or dazed person unattended.

FAINTING

Fainting is defined as sudden brief loss of consciousness not associated with a head injury. There are innumerable causes of fainting, but most episodes are associated with decreased blood flow (oxygen and/or glucose) to the brain. This may be caused by low blood sugar (hypoglycemia), slow heart rate ("vagal" reaction, in which the vagus nerve, which slows the heart rate, is overstimulated: fright, anxiety, stomach irritation, drugs, fatigue), rhythm disturbances of the heart, dehydration, heat exhaustion, anemia, bleeding, and others.

If you witness a fainting episode, or are with someone who is becoming lightheaded (sweating, weak, ashen colored), quickly help the person to lie down, with the legs elevated. This position increases venous blood flow back to the heart, which in turn pumps more blood to the brain. After a fainting episode, examine the victim for any sign of serious illness or injury. If nothing serious is suspected, have him sit for a while, drink cool sweetened liquids, and slowly regain an upright posture. If the victim is elderly, particularly if the pulse is irregular, seek immediate medical attention.

FEVER AND CHILLS

Fever is an elevation in body temperature caused by infection. The causative organism (most commonly, a bacterium or virus) releases into the bloodstream substances that reach the part of the brain which acts as the body thermostat. Thus, body temperature is "reset" at a higher level. This probably helps to fight infection, but the temperature may need to be lowered if the elevation is severe or prolonged.

Normal body temperature is 98.6°F (37°C) measured orally and 99.6°F (37.5°C) measured rectally. Temperature should be measured with a thermometer. To take a temperature, the thermometer should be shaken to pool the mercury or alcohol below 94°F (35°C). If the victim is suspected to be hypothermic, a special thermometer is necessary (see page 221). To take a temperature by mouth, the thermometer is placed under the tongue, the mouth is closed, and a reading is taken after 3–4 minutes. To take a temperature rectally (the most reliable method and the necessary one in a case of suspected hypothermia), the thermometer is *gently* placed, ideally with oil or petroleum jelly lubrication, one inch into the rectum. It is held for 4–5 minutes and read. Never leave a child or confused adult unattended with a thermometer in the mouth or rectum.

Generally, infections will not elevate the core (rectal) body temperature higher than 105°F (40.5°C). Persons who have temperatures measured above that level should be examined for heat illness (see page 232), stroke (see page 120), or drug overdose. Vigorous prolonged muscular activity (seizures or marathon running) can raise the core temperature above 107°F (41.7°C).

If a person has a temperature higher than 100.5°F (38°C), and it is felt to be due to an infection, he will be made more comfortable by the administration of aspirin, ibuprofen, or acetaminophen (Tylenol). To avoid Reye's syndrome (postviral encephalopathy and liver failure), *do not use aspirin to control fever in a child under the age of 17*. Infants and small children with fevers (usually due to ear infections or viral illnesses) should be treated as soon as any elevation of temperature is noted, to prevent febrile seizures (epilepsy caused by fever). An infant (younger than 6 months) with a fever should be rapidly transported to a physician. IF THE VICTIM SUFFERS FROM ENVIRON-MENTAL HEAT-INDUCED ILLNESS (see page 232), HE WILL NOT BENEFIT FROM AND SHOULD NOT BE

GIVEN ASPIRIN OR ACETAMINOPHEN. Ibuprofen is not as dangerous but is clearly *not* helpful.

Chills are caused by the release of bacteria or viruses (or their toxins) into the bloodstream. The victim will suddenly feel very cold, begin to shiver, with teeth chattering, goose bumps, and weakness. The "chill" may actually occur during a fever.

COUGHING BLOOD

If a victim coughs up blood, the problem may originate anywhere from the mouth to the lungs. Causes of coughing blood include:

Sore Throat

The victim will complain of an irritated throat and difficulty swallowing, and will cough up whitish phlegm streaked with specks of blood. If the victim is not short of breath and appears in no real distress, rapid medical attention is not necessary (see page 155). Similarly, if a person has a nosebleed, he may cough and spit a lot of blood (see page 152).

Pneumonia

The patient will complain of fever, chills, chest pain, and shortness of breath, and will cough up green or rust-colored thick sputum (see page 44).

Pulmonary Embolism

The patient will complain of difficult and painful breathing, shortness of breath, agitation, and weakness. Generally, only severely ill persons will cough up small clots of blood (see page 41).

Lung Cancer

The patient will suddenly cough up small pieces of spongy lung tissue or tumor, along with small blood clots. Attend to the airway (see page 18), and seek medical attention.

Lung Injury

If a victim is struck in the chest, particularly if ribs are broken, the underlying lung can be bruised or torn. The victim will cough up small clots of blood or, if the injury is major, mouthfuls of blood. This is extremely serious and requires constant attention to the airway (see pages 18, 36).

DIZZINESS

Dizziness is a feeling of lightheadedness, with or without a sensation of spinning (vertigo). It often precedes a fainting episode (see page 134), or may be the harbinger of a stroke (see page 120), heart attack (see page 46), low blood sugar (see page 118), heat illness (see page 232), ear infection (see page 139), the bends (see page 295), plant poisoning (see page 304), motion sickness (see page 326), and many other disorders. Frequently, dizziness is caused by an infection or disorder of the middle ear, which controls balance. Indeed, if the external ear canals are blocked by wax, this alone can cause dizziness.

If a victim is dizzy, he should lie on his back, and attempt to regain orientation to his surroundings. Examine him for obvious causes, and treat accordingly. If the dizziness does not resolve, particularly if the victim is elderly (in which case it might indicate a stroke), he should be taken to a physician. True vertigo is very distressing to the victim and described by him as "the room spinning around," with nausea and/or vomiting, weakness, ringing in the ears, and occasional slow jerking or fluttering movements of the eyeballs. A viral infection of the middle ear (often associated with a recent cold) is known as labyrinthitis. It is treated with the same medications used for motion sickness (see page 326). This is a diagnosis to be considered by a physician after more serious problems are excluded.

Head (Also Eye, Ear, Nose, Throat, and Mouth)

HEADACHE

Routine *tension or fatigue headaches* are characterized by throbbing pain in the temples, over the eyes, and in the posterior neck and shoulder muscles. They may be treated with rest, sunglasses, and moderate pain medication, such as aspirin or acetaminophen, every 3–4 hours. Sometimes, warm packs or massage applied to the tired muscles relaxes them and helps to decrease the pain.

Migraine headaches are generally more severe, caused by painful dilation or constriction of small arteries in the head. Such headaches are typified by true photophobia (aversion to light), nausea, vomiting, runny nose, and occasionally by weakness of an arm or leg, with difficulty walking. Some people experience an "aura" prior to the headache, in which they may smell strange odors or see flashing lights. Migraines require stronger pain medicine, and may be treated with narcotics (codeine), prochlorperazine with diphenhydramine, or drugs which directly constrict the arteries (the last should *only* be used under the guidance of a physician, as they may worsen the effects of certain types of migraines). If an oxygen tank is available, the victim may find relief by breathing a high concentration (10 liters/minute) by face mask. Elderly persons with a severe migraine, which may be confused with a stroke (see page 120), should seek immediate medical attention.

Sinus headaches are associated with sinus infections (see page 154), and are typified by fever, nasal congestion, production of a foul nasal discharge, and pain produced by tapping over the affected sinuses. They should be treated with oral decongestants (pseudoephedrine), nasal spray (Neo-Synephrine 0.25% or Afrin 0.05%), antibiotics (cefadroxil, ampicillin, or erythromycin) if an infection is present, and warm packs applied over the affected sinuses.

Meningitis is an infection that involves the lining of the brain and spinal cord, and is a true emergency. The headache of meningitis is severe, and often accompanied by nausea, vomiting, photophobia, fever, altered mental status, and weakness. The classic sign of meningitis is a stiff neck, in which the patient demonstrates extreme discomfort when the chin is flexed forward against the chest. It is important to note that infants can suffer meningitis without a stiff neck and may merely present with poor feeding, fever, vomiting, seizures, and extreme lethargy ("floppy baby"). If meningitis is suspected, the patient must be evacuated rapidly.

A headache that is atypically severe or prolonged may be the manifestation of a severe problem, such as a brain tumor, infection, or hemorrhage. The victim of such should be evaluated by a physician at the earliest opportunity. If a person develops a severe headache associated with a fainting spell or stiff neck, or is known to suffer from high blood pressure, keep him as calm as possible, and urgently seek assistance.

EAR

Earache

An earache may be caused by infection, injury, or a foreign body in the ear. For a discussion of ear squeeze (barotitis) that occurs with scuba diving, see page 296.

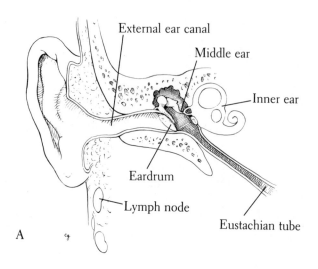

External ear canal

Middle ear

Inner ear

Eardrum

Lymph node

Eustachian tube

A

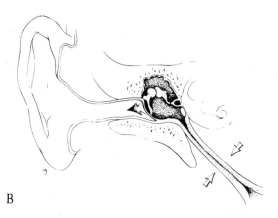

B

FIGURE 60. *Ear infections. (A) Normal ear anatomy. (B) Otitis media (inner ear infection). The eardrum bulges outward as the middle ear fills with fluid. The eustachian tube narrows or closes.*

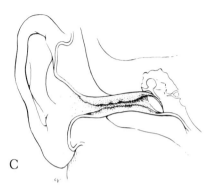

C

FIGURE 60 (CONT.). *(C) Otitis externa (external ear canal infection). The canal becomes swollen and drains pus.*

Ear Infection

Ear infections can be either internal (otitis media) or external (otitis externa) to the eardrum (tympanic membrane) (Fig. 60).

OTITIS MEDIA: Infections may occur that involve the eardrum and cause blood, serum, or pus to collect behind the drum (Fig. 60B). With otitis media, there is no drainage from the external ear (unless the eardrum ruptures, which is quite unusual), the patient has a fever, and often has a sore throat. In many cases, the victim has a history of prior infections. Most often, otitis media occurs in children; when it occurs in adults, it may be associated with sinus infections or functional obstruction to the eustachian tube (the pressure-release mechanism from the middle ear into the throat). Young children can rapidly become severely ill from middle ear infections; infants may develop meningitis (see page 139) following an ear infection.

If otitis media is suspected, the patient should be treated with oral decongestants and antibiotics. Adults should use penicillin, trimethoprim-sulfamethoxazole, or erythromycin; children should be treated with amoxicillin, ampicillin, or trimethoprim with sulfamethoxazole. Aspirin or acetaminophen should be used to control fever. Due to the potential danger of their contracting Reye's syndrome, children younger than 17 should not be given aspirin to control fever.

OTITIS EXTERNA (SWIMMER'S EAR): Infections that develop in the external ear canal (often noted in swimmers and divers who can never keep the canal completely dry) rarely involve the eardrum (Fig. 60C). Symptoms include a white to yellow-green liquid or cheesy discharge from the ear, pain, and decreased hearing. Occasionally, the patient complains of exquisite tenderness when the ear lobe is tugged, and has tender swollen lymph glands in the neck on the affected side. In severe cases, the patient may have a fever and appear quite ill.

If the patient has only a discharge without fever or swollen lymph glands, he may be treated with eardrops, such as 2% nonaqueous acetic acid (Vosol). Household vinegar diluted 1:1 with fresh water or with rubbing alcohol may be used as a substitute in a pinch. These should be administered 4–5 times per day, and may be retained with a cotton or gauze wick gently placed into the external ear canal. Do not attempt to clean out the ear with a cotton swab or similar object, to avoid injuring the eardrum.

If the patient has a discharge with fever and/or swollen lymph nodes, the eardrops should contain hydrocortisone (Vosol HC), and the patient should also be administered oral ciprofloxacin, erythromycin, or penicillin. Aspirin or acetaminophen should be used to control fever, with the precaution to not use aspirin in children under the age of 17 years.

To prevent swimmer's ear, the external ear canal should be irrigated with Vosol or diluted vinegar (described above) after each scuba dive or prolonged swim.

Referred Pain

"Referred" pain is pain that appears in one body region but actually originates in another. This occurs because different body regions are supplied with nerves that share common central pathways. In the case of ear pain, the cause may be a sore throat, tooth infection, or arthritic jaw. The ear pain will not disappear until the real underlying cause is corrected.

Injury to the Eardrum

If something is poked into the ear, a hard blow is struck to the external ear, a diver descends rapidly without equalizing the pressure in the middle ear (see page 296), or a person is subjected to a loud explosive noise, the eardrum may be ruptured. This causes immediate intense pain and loss of hearing, and occasional nausea, vomiting, and dizziness. If the eardrum is ruptured, cover the external ear to prevent the ingress of dirt, and seek the aid of a physician. If debris has entered the ear, start the victim on penicillin or erythromycin by mouth. Do not put liquid medicine into the ear if you suspect that the eardrum is ruptured. If the dizziness is disabling, administer medicine for motion sickness (see page 326). Use appropriate pain medication.

Foreign Body in the Ear

A foreign body in the ear can be incredibly painful, particularly if it is dancing on the eardrum or resting against the sensitive lining of the ear canal. An inanimate foreign body (piece of corn, peanut, foxtail, stone, etc.) may be left in the ear until an ear specialist with special forceps can remove the object. If a live creature (cockroach, bee) enters the external ear canal and causes pain that is intolerable, the ear should be filled with 2–4% liquid lidocaine (topical anesthetic), which will numb the ear and drown the bug at the same time. If lidocaine is not available, mineral oil may be used, with the caution that it will frequently cause the insect to struggle, which may encourage a sting or bite, and incredible temporary pain. Once the animal is dead (a few minutes) a gentle attempt should be made with small tweezers to remove the bug. Removal should not be attempted unless part of the bug can be seen. Don't push the bug in farther, or you might rupture the eardrum.

EYE

Foreign Body Under the Eyelid

If a foreign body lodges on the cornea (without actual penetration of the eyeball), irrigate the eye copiously with water, and see if that removes the object. If this is not successful, have the victim look downward, grasp his upper lid firmly by the eyelashes, and fold it up and inside out over a cotton swab (Fig. 61). If you can see the foreign body on the upper eyelid, gently wipe it off with a piece of moistened cloth or cotton swab. If you do not see the object, check between the lower eyelid and the eyeball. Once

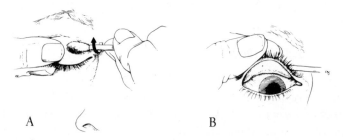

A   B

FIGURE 61. *Eversion of the eyelid to locate a foreign body. (A) The lid is grasped and pulled over a cotton swab or small blunt stick. (B) The underside of the eyelid is inspected for a foreign body while the victim looks downward.*

you have removed the object, if the patient still feels as if something is in the eye, he may have suffered a scratch on the cornea (clear surface of the eye). In this case, patch the eye closed for 24 hours. *Never patch an eye closed if there is an active infection* (pus or discharge). When the patch is removed, if the eye does not feel and look normal, see a doctor as soon as possible.

To patch an eye, a half-inch-thick pad of soft cloth or bandage should be shaped to fit neatly over the eye socket, and affixed snugly to the face with tape or bandages. Prepackaged sterile elliptical eye pads are available. If only tape is available, the eyelids may be taped closed with a single small piece of tape. If an eye shield is necessary, it may be fashioned from a cravat bandage (Fig. 62). If the eye cannot be patched, sunglasses should be worn.

Injured Eyeball

If the eyeball is perforated, there will be a combination of loss of vision (ranging from hazy vision to blindness), pain, excessive tearing, a dilated pupil, and visible blood in the eye. Do not attempt to rinse out the wound vigorously; remove obvious dirt

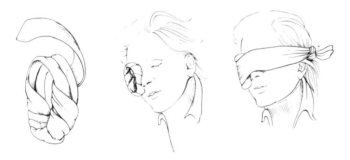

FIGURE 62. *Bandage for the injured eye. A cravat or cloth is rolled and wrapped to make a doughnut-shaped shield, which is fixed in place over the eye.*

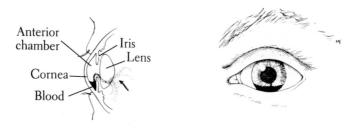

FIGURE 63. *Hyphema. Bleeding into the eye causes an accumulation of blood in the anterior chamber, where it settles into a layer behind the cornea. In severe cases, the pupil is obscured by red blood.*

and debris only. Immediately close the eyelid gently, and cover the eye with a protective shield. This can be fashioned by cutting gauze pads or soft cloth to the proper size, or by fashioning a doughnut-shaped shield with a cloth, cravat bandage, or shirt (Fig. 62). Metal or plastic eye shields are available. Do not exert pressure on the eyeball, as this can increase the damage. If possible, instruct the victim to keep both eyes closed. The patient should be started on penicillin, cephalexin, or erythromycin. Seek immediate medical attention.

Bleeding into the Eye

If the eyeball is struck (not necessarily torn or ruptured), there may be bleeding from small blood vessels within the eye into the clear liquid that fills the space behind the cornea. Such bleeding is called a hyphema. It first appears as diffuse bloody (red) clouding of the fluid behind the cornea, which settles over the course of 6–8 hours into a clearly visible layer of blood (Fig. 63). If such a condition is noted, the victim should have the eye patched closed (see previous section) or wear sunglasses, and should be transported immediately to an eye doctor. If possible, the head should be kept elevated and in an upright position.

Removal of Contact Lenses

If a victim is severely injured, and he is wearing contact lenses, they should be removed. Either soft or hard lenses can be removed by this technique (Fig. 64).

1. Slide the lens off the clear surface of the eye (cornea) over to the white area away from the nose.

2. Place one finger at the outside edge of the lower eyelid, and pull the eyelid taut, while keeping the eye slightly open. This should lift the edge of the lens, so that you can pick it up. If you cannot remove the lens, position it so that as much as possible is over the white (and not on the cornea).

3. Place the lens in a container with contact lens solution or water (if possible, add 1 teaspoon of salt per pint of water).

4. A soft contact lens can often be removed by simply pinching it gently between the thumb and index finger.

Subconjunctival Hemorrhage

Bleeding into the whites of the eyes (subconjunctival hemorrhage) may occur spontaneously or after coughing, strangulation,

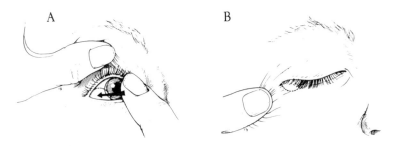

FIGURE 64. *Contact lens removal.* (A) *The lens is pushed gently to the lateral (away from the nose) white portion of the eye.* (B) *A downward and outward pull on the skin at the lateral corner of the eye pops the lens free.*

or vigorous exertion (straining) (Fig. 65). The bleeding is painless, does not interfere with vision (the cornea is not involved), and does not require any therapy. The blood will reabsorb over a period of a few weeks.

Red Eye

The red or pink, itchy eye is usually caused by a viral infection. Other causes include bacterial infection, allergy, foreign body (see page 144), irritation from chemicals or smoke, snow blindness (see below), or injury (see page 145). If the infection is caused by a virus or bacteria, symptoms include itching, tearing, discharge (runny yellow or greenish pus), crusted eyelashes and lids, and swollen lids, which are often stuck together upon awakening in the morning. If the cause is a known allergy or irritation from smoke, use Vasocon or Visine eyedrops. If there is much yellowish discharge, suspect a bacterial infection and administer antibiotic eyedrops (gentamicin or sodium sulamyd 10%), 2 drops every 2 hours while the patient is awake. Never use steroid-containing eyedrops unless directed to do so by an eye doctor.

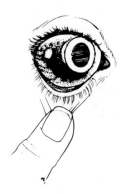

FIGURE 65. *Subconjunctival hemorrhage. The red discoloration does not involve the cornea, which remains clear.*

Snow Blindness

Exposure to ultraviolet light from the sun can lead to a "sunburn" of the cornea (clear surface of the eye). This occurs when proper protection is not taken at high altitudes, where a greater amount of unfiltered (by the atmosphere) ultraviolet light is present, and the exposure may be compounded by reflection from the snow. The intensity of ultraviolet energy increases by a factor of 5–6% for every 1,000-foot increase in altitude above sea level. Smoke can act as an ultraviolet filter, while dust and water increase scatter and may intensify the exposure. Snow reflects 85% of ultraviolet B (the culprit wavelengths that cause snow blindness); dry sand reflects 17%, grass or sandy turf reflects 2.5%. Water may reflect 10–30% of ultraviolet B, depending on the time of day and location.

Symptoms include excessive tearing, pain, redness, swollen eyelids, pain when looking at the light, headache, a gritty sensation in the eyes, and decreased (hazy) vision. Similar symptoms occur when the surface of the eye is physically scratched (corneal abrasion). Treatment consists of patching the eye closed (see page 145), as the surface of the cornea will regenerate spontaneously in 24–48 hours. It is important to check the eye first for a foreign body (see page 144). After patching, the eye must be rechecked in 24 hours. If the eye appears infected with pus, then it should be left unpatched, antibiotics should be administered (see page 148), and the victim should wear sunglasses. Pain medicine should be used as appropriate. If both eyes are involved, then only the more severely affected eye should be patched, so that the victim can continue to make his way.

PROTECTIVE EYEGLASSES (SUNGLASSES): Standards for ultraviolet protection in nonprescription sunglasses are set by the American National Standards Institute. These state that such lenses should block 99.8% of ultraviolet B light. If they are advertised for mountaineering or specifically for ultraviolet protection, they also block out considerable ultraviolet A light.

Sunglasses should be equipped with side protectors and, if necessary, optional nose guards. Frames should be prepared with wraparound temples and retaining straps or lanyards.

In general, amber-brown-rose lenses filter out blue light and increase the perception of contrast. Green and gray lenses soften glare and transmit a spectrum that does not increase contrast. Ambermatic lenses (darker in bright sunlight) contain millions of silver halide crystals, which darken when exposed to ultraviolet light close to the visible spectrum.

Recommended sunglasses that provide excellent protection from ultraviolet light include Bolle Mountain, Rēvo, Corning Serengeti, Ray-Ban (Bausch and Lomb) in the G-15 series, and either of the Nautilux or PX-5000 (Vuarnet). Most recreation supply companies (see page 331) carry their own sunglasses and wraparound goggles which meet ANSI standards.

Injury to the Retina

The retina is the thin inner posterior-surface tissue layer of the eye, the "screen" upon which images are transmitted by light. From the retina, nerves from the eye carry signals to the brain. The retina may be injured by the transmission of unrestricted infrared rays (wavelengths of light beyond the red end of the visible spectrum), as occurs when someone stares at the sun. Usually, this occurs when someone views the sun directly during an eclipse or when a person stares at the sun while under the influence of hallucinogenic drugs. Symptoms include pain and blindness. If such an injury is suspected, sunglasses should be worn or the eye should be patched. The victim should be transported to an eye doctor.

Occasionally, a blow to the eye or the aging process will cause the retina to become separated from the back of the eye (retinal detachment). Early symptoms include flashes of light and persistent floating spots in the field of vision ("floaters"). As the retina peels off further, a person loses vision painlessly, as if a curtain were descending. Retinal detachment is a serious condition and requires surgical repair. The victim should seek immediate medical attention.

Glaucoma

Glaucoma is a condition in which the pressure of the fluid within the eye is elevated. If this happens suddenly, the pressure can injure the nerves within the eye that record vision and blindness can result. Symptoms of an acute attack of glaucoma include severe pain, blurred vision, clouding of the cornea (clear surface of the eye), intense reddening of the white of the eye, a dilated pupil that doesn't react (constrict) to light, nausea, vomiting, and headache. The victim of acute glaucoma is truly miserable. If an attack occurs, the victim should be kept in a sitting or standing position and rushed to an eye doctor.

Injured Eyelid

If the eyelid is injured, wash the eye carefully and then patch the eye closed (see page 145). If the eye cannot be covered with eyelid, apply a thick layer of bacitracin ointment to the eyelid and exposed eyeball and patch the eye. Seek medical attention.

Sty

A sty is a small abscess (see page 188) that develops in one of the glands at the base of an eyelash. The infection causes the eyelid to swell, redden, and become painful. The victim may notice increased tear production and the sensation of a foreign body in the eye. Usually, the sty comes to a head on the outside of the lid, but occasionally it will come to a point on the inside of the eyelid. If a sty begins to develop, the victim should hold warm moist compresses to the eyelid for 30 minutes 4 times a day to soften the abscess. It will either disappear, or it will enlarge and come to a head. *Never squeeze an abscess on the face.* If it enlarges, comes to a head, and is extremely painful or interferes with vision, but will not open spontaneously, it may be carefully lanced with a sharp blade or needle to drain the pus. A physician should perform this procedure, unless the victim is over 48 hours from medical attention and the infection has worsened to the extent that there is progressive swelling of the cheek or forehead. In this event, also administer dicloxacillin, erythromycin, or cephalexin.

NOSE

Nosebleed

Nosebleeds are classified as anterior or posterior, depending on where they originate within the nose. Generally, anterior nosebleeds are less serious, because the victim will drain blood outward (to the external face) from the nostrils. Posterior nosebleeds are more difficult to control, and the victim often drains blood back into the throat, with coughing and potential choking. Because anterior nosebleeds are much more common and can often be managed outside of the hospital, their management will be discussed. IF A POSTERIOR NOSEBLEED IS SUSPECTED (brisk bleeding into the throat, continued bleeding into the throat after the anterior bleeding has been controlled), IMMEDIATELY EVACUATE THE VICTIM TO A HOSPITAL.

To control an anterior nosebleed, attempt simple maneuvers first. Have the patient blow his nose to remove all clots. Keep him upright and calm, and firmly press both nostrils closed against the nasal septum (middle cartilage). Hold this position for 15 minutes without release; letting go prior to this time will only restart the bleeding, as it takes the small blood vessels and scratched surface a while to stop oozing. After 15 minutes, let go and see if the bleeding has stopped. If not, gently but firmly pack both nostrils with a gauze or cotton roll soaked with phenylephrine 0.25% (Neo-Synephrine ¼%) and repeat the pinching maneuver for 20 minutes. Generally, this does the trick; if it doesn't, repeat the packing without the phenylephrine. After the bleeding has stopped, leave the packing in place for 2 hours and then gently remove it. Cold compresses applied to the bridge of the nose or a roll of gauze or cotton placed beneath the upper lip are of limited usefulness when dealing with a brisk nosebleed. A useful device for packing the nose to stop a nosebleed is the Rhino-Rocket (Denver Splint Co., Inc., see page 332), which is a compressed medical-grade foam sponge with applicator (syringe). The syringe is used to guide the foam into place, where it swells on contact with moisture (blood) to 8–10 times its compressed size. A string is attached to the sponge so that it can be easily removed.

Broken Nose

A fractured nose may or may not be deformed. If the nose is obviously depressed or deformed to one side, and the patient is having difficulty breathing through his mouth, the nose can be relocated, but this is quite painful. Grasp the bridge of the nose firmly, and crunch it upward and back over to the midline. In the wilderness, application of an external split is cumbersome and unnecessary. Treat any nosebleed as previously discussed. *Remember, the only reason to relocate the injury is to improve breathing if mouth breathing is inadequate.* The nasal bones won't really begin to set solid for 5 days; cosmetic manipulation can easily be performed after such a delay. If the skin is cut deeply over a broken nose, begin the victim on an antibiotic (penicillin, cephalexin, or erythromycin).

Another risk from a broken nose is the formation of a blood clot under the skin that lies over the nasal septum (cartilage). If such a clot is not promptly drained, it can cause collapse of the cartilage, infection, or erosion through the septum, leaving a problematic hole in the middle of the nose. Anyone who has suffered a broken nose needs to be examined by a physician within 3–5 days of the injury, in order to avoid erosion of the nasal septum by a blood clot.

Sinusitis

The sinuses are spaces filled with air and lined with mucus-producing tissues found in the front of the skull and in the bones of the face (Fig. 66). Sinusitis is a blockage and infection of the sinuses, usually caused by bacteria, and characterized by headache, fever, tenderness in and over the involved sinus, with or without foul yellow or green discharge from the nose. Occasionally, the pain will radiate to the eyes, bridge of the nose, and upper molars. A patient with sinusitis can become quite ill and suffer from nausea and vomiting. Treatment involves the administration of antibiotics (cefadroxil, ampicillin, or erythromycin) and decongestants (nasal sprays and oral antihistamines), as well as warm packs over the affected area. Topical decongestants should not be used for more than 3 or 4 consecutive days, to avoid "rebound" swelling of the inside of the nasal passages from chemical irritation and sensitization to the drugs. Patients who suffer from sinusitis should avoid rapid changes in altitude (as in scuba diving or air travel in unpressurized aircraft).

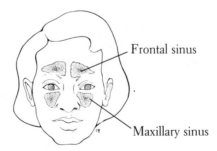

FIGURE 66. *Location of the sinuses.*

THROAT

Sore Throat and Tonsillitis

Sore throat (pharyngitis) is a common complication of viral infections (the common cold, infectious mononucleosis), breathing dry air ("altitude throat"), or primary bacterial throat infections ("strep throat"). Symptoms of an infection include pain with swallowing, fever, swollen lymph nodes ("swollen glands") in the anterior neck, red throat, swollen tonsils, and pus over the tonsils and throat (Fig. 67).

Because the symptoms of a viral throat and tonsil infection and a bacterial strep throat are frequently identical, it is hard to make the differentiation without a throat swab culture. Because the potential complications (kidney or heart disease) of an untreated strep throat in a young person outweigh the complications of antibiotic use, it is advisable to treat with penicillin or erythromycin for a full 10-day course anyone on a journey who may have a strep throat. Even if the victim improves after 2–3 days, the antibiotic should be taken for 10 days.

Adjuncts to care include saltwater gargles (½ teaspoon salt in 1 cup warm water), throat lozenges (Cepacol or Sucrets), warm fluids (to moisten and soothe the throat), and aspirin or acetaminophen to control fever. Do not administer aspirin to children under the age of 17 years.

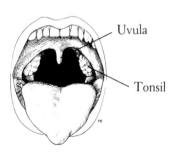

FIGURE 67. *Inflamed tonsils.*

If a person with a sore throat is examined and found to have a high fever associated with difficult or noisy breathing, muffled voice ("like talking with a potato in his mouth"), drooling, stiff neck, or any visible swelling (bulging) in the back of the throat, he should be made as comfortable as possible and transported immediately to a hospital. Such a condition may indicate an abscess (see page 188) in the back of the throat or next to the tonsils, which can rapidly expand and obstruct the airway.

If a person develops tender swelling under the tongue and/or under the chin, particularly associated with swollen lymph glands in the neck, fever, difficulty swallowing and foul breath, this may indicate an infection in the floor of the mouth. Treat the victim with antibiotics as for a strep throat and seek immediate physician consultation.

Infectious Mononucleosis

Mononucleosis ("mono") is a viral disease characterized by low-grade (less than 101°F [38.3°C]) fever, sore throat, swollen lymph glands (mostly in the neck, but occasionally in the armpits or in the groin), headache, fatigue, and occasionally, skin rash, dark urine, muscle aching, and an enlarged spleen. Treatment consists of increased rest (sometimes requiring weeks) and elimination of any physical activity that requires heavy exertion or risks abdominal injury (and rupture of the spleen). The diagnosis is confirmed by a blood test; until that can be performed, the patient should be treated for a possible strep throat (see page 155). Because the disease can be spread in saliva, infected persons should avoid sharing eating utensils and towels.

Common Cold

See page 151.

MOUTH

Fever Blisters (Cold Sores)

Crops of blisters on the face, mouth, and lips that break out in times of stress (viral illness, emotional crisis, sun exposure) are often caused by reactivated herpes simplex virus. The blisters often weep, and may become infected (see page 188). Unfortunately, there is little to do for these when they first appear except to keep them clean and dry. If the skin cracks and becomes painful, the blisters may be lubricated with bacitracin ointment. Anesthetic ointments can be used if they are helpful. Further sun exposure should be prevented with an adequate lip sunscreen (see pages 180–181). Untreated, the lesions will disappear spontaneously in 10–15 days. All herpes viruses are contagious. During times of visible blisters, eating and drinking utensils should not be shared. To maximize prevention, fever blister–sensitive persons should apply sunscreen or lip balm with a high (greater than 20) sun protection factor and consider taking acyclovir (400 mg twice daily) the day before and during intense ultraviolet light exposure.

Canker Sores

These painful white patches form inside the mouth and may be associated with viral infections. Usually they are a chronic problem, and recur with unfortunate regularity. They may be treated with topical application of anesthetic lidocaine ointment 2.5% for a minute or two prior to eating, in order to kill the pain temporarily. One authority recommends application of a pinch of powdered alum (as in a styptic pencil) to initiate a cure. A physician might prescribe triamcinolone dental paste. The inside of the mouth should be rinsed thoroughly after eating to prevent food from becoming trapped in the sores. Any new sore in the mouth of an elderly person or frequent user of tobacco should be seen by a physician.

Toothaches and Tooth Infections

Toothaches occur in teeth that are decayed. Symptoms of tooth infection include pain in the tooth and jaw that occasionally travels into the neck and ear, pain on contact with cold or hot liquids, and headache. If an abscess (pocket of infection) develops in the root of the tooth or in the gum, there may be associated fever, swelling of the gum and jaw, and swollen lymph glands under the jaw and in the neck.

The patient should be started on penicillin, metronidazole, or erythromycin, and given appropriate pain medication. A remedy that may help to control pain is application of a cotton pad moistened with oil of cloves to the tooth cavity. Take care to keep the oil off the gums, lips, and inside surfaces of the cheeks. Alternately, Anbesol may be applied to the gums. The patient needs to be taken to a dentist to have the tooth repaired or removed.

Broken or Lost Tooth

If a tooth is cracked (with the root still present and in place), there is little for the victim to do other than to keep the mouth clean and to avoid contact with extremes of temperature. If air coming in contact with an exposed nerve causes intolerable pain, a temporary cap (shield) can be created by mixing melted paraffin (candle wax) with a few strands of cotton. When the mixture begins to harden but can still be easily molded, a wad can be pressed onto the tooth, using the teeth on either side as anchors.

If a tooth is knocked cleanly out of the socket, it can sometimes be replaced successfully if the victim can reach a dentist within the first hour. After 2 hours, there is little hope for salvage of that particular tooth. The best treatment for a tooth that has been out of the socket for 15 minutes or less is to gently rinse it clean (*do not* scrub the root of the tooth) and reinsert it with firm pressure into the socket to the level of the adjacent tooth. Otherwise, or if the tooth has been out of the socket for more than 15 minutes, it should be rinsed and carried by the patient in the space between his lower lip and lower gum (taking care not to swallow the tooth!). Alternately, the tooth may be placed in a container and covered with a small amount of cool, pasteurized whole milk (*not* yogurt, low-fat milk, or powdered milk) for transport. Do not carry the tooth on a dry cloth or paper; do not soak the tooth in tap water. *Do not place a tooth back into the socket unless transport to a dentist will be within 24–48 hours, so that positioning can be corrected, antibiotics administered to avoid an infection, and tetanus toxoid given if necessary.*

Upper Respiratory Disorders

COMMON COLD

Most "colds" are upper respiratory tract infections caused by any of a host (at least 200) of viruses. It is not true that exposure to a cold climate ("catching a chill") causes a cold. Symptoms include runny nose, cough, sore throat, headache, muscle aches, fever, fatigue, weakness, and occasional nausea with vomiting and/or diarrhea. Unfortunately, even though some intranasal sprays of a substance called interferon show promise in preventing colds caused by rhinoviruses, there is no cure for the common cold. The best medicine is rest, increased fluid intake to prevent dehydration, and aspirin or acetaminophen for fever. Keep the victim warm and dry. Treat nasal congestion with mild decongestants. Persons who breathe steam (which has *not* been proven to improve a common cold) must be careful to avoid burns. There is no scientific evidence to support the use of megavitamins (specifically, vitamin C) in the prevention or amelioration of viral illnesses. Clearly, the most important factor in rehabilitation is adequate rest. *Do not attempt to "sweat out" a cold with vigorous exercise.* Such harmful behavior causes worsened fever, debilitation, and dehydration. It is a method guaranteed to convert a common cold into pneumonia. A person with a cold should see a doctor if he is ill for more than 2 weeks, his temperature exceeds 102°F, the victim develops a cough productive of yellow-green or darkened phlegm, or the victim develops chest pain with breathing, shaking chills, a severe earache, or a headache with a stiff neck. Since colds are spread by contact, take particular care to wash hands after contact with an infected person.

INFLUENZA

The influenza virus is responsible for seasonal epidemics of the flu, a predominately respiratory disease that waylays many a wilderness traveler. The illness is recognized by sudden high fever, sore throat, cough, headache, muscle aches, weakness, and occasional nausea with vomiting and/or diarrhea (in other words, a severe cold). Elderly or infirm individuals are at greatest risk for becoming severely debilitated or developing complications such as influenza pneumonia. The general therapy is the same as that for a cold: namely rest, adequate nutrition, increased fluid intake, and medicine for fever. Vaccines are prepared each year that are effective in the prevention of both types A and B influenza (see page 340). During epidemics, elderly or infirm persons may benefit from the administration of the oral drug amantadine hydrochloride, which is available by prescription for the prevention and treatment of type A influenza (it is ineffective against type B).

BRONCHITIS

Bronchitis is an infection of the air passages (bronchi), characterized by cough, the production of sputum (yellow or green phlegm), fever, and fatigue. Pneumonia is much more severe than bronchitis, and involves severe progressive pulmonary deterioration; bronchitis is a less debilitating infection. Cigarette smokers are prone to recurrent bouts of bronchitis, because they suffer from scarred lungs and constantly paralyze the defense mechanisms of the nose, throat, and lungs with cigarette smoke. Treatment consists of oral antibiotics (trimethoprim-sulfamethoxazole or erythromycin), vigorous fluid intake, inhalation of humidified warm air (taking care to avoid steam burns) in order to loosen secretions and ease coughing, and aspirin or acetaminophen for fever. It is best to allow the patient to cough up the copious amounts of secretions he will produce; however, if coughing fits become intolerable, cough medicines (see Appendix One) should be used. If pneumonia is suspected (page 44), treat appropriately and seek immediate medical attention.

HAY FEVER

Hay fever ("rose fever," "catarrh") is an allergic reaction, often seasonal, to dust, animal dander, plant (usually ragweed, sage, trees, and grasses) pollens, or other compounds found in the air. The victim suffers from red, itchy, and watery eyes, a runny nose with large amounts of clear mucus, sneezing, and general misery. In severe cases, victims may suffer asthma, sinusitis, loss of smell, and fatigue. In most cases, the symptoms can be relieved by taking antihistamine tablets, such as Actifed, but these have side effects, the most troublesome of which is drowsiness. Newer prescription antihistamines, such as terfenadine (Seldane) or astemizole (Hismanal), cause much less or no sedation. Unfortunately, what the sufferer needs most is to change environments, which occasionally means giving up the trip. Nasal decongestants, such as Afrin or Neo-Synephrine, will clear out the nose, but do not halt the allergic reaction. An allergy doctor can be consulted to evaluate the victim with skin tests for desensitization injections. If allergies are debilitating and a change in environment is impossible, the victim will almost certainly benefit from a tapering dose of prednisone (see Appendix One). Cromalyn sodium nasal spray (Nasalcrom) is recommended by some allergists as another useful adjunct.

PLEURITIS

The lining of the lung, the pleura, is two layers of tissue that are separated by a thin film of lubricating fluid, which allows the lung to expand with a gliding motion when the chest wall moves outward during inhalation. When the pleura is irritated by an infection, most often caused by a virus, the inflammation may allow fluid to accumulate in this space and cause pain with breathing, localized to the area of irritation. The pain is sharp and worsened by a cough or deep breath. The treatment for viral pleuritis is rest and aspirin. The patient should be encouraged to breathe deeply. If he is weak or has a high fever, a physician should examine the patient to be certain that the infection is not part of pneumonia (see page 44).

Disorders of the Gastrointestinal Tract

DIARRHEA

Although diarrhea is included in the "minor problems" section, we all know that severe diarrhea can be devastating. Diarrhea can be due to a number of causes, which include anxiety, food poisoning, viral infection, bacterial infection, and infection with protozoa. It is not always easy to determine the cause of loose bowel movements, but I will attempt to describe the most common presentations and their management.

In all cases of diarrhea, a common discomfort is the irritated anus (particularly one that has been wiped with leaves or newspaper!). Every traveler should carry a roll of toilet paper and a small container (1 ounce) of 1% hydrocortisone lotion or ointment for an irritated bottom.

General Therapy for Diarrhea

The following is a reasonable approach to dealing with "the runs":

DIET: If nausea and vomiting do not prevent eating, adjust the diet as follows:

1. When diarrhea is severe, stick to clear fluids such as mineral water, carbonated soda, Kool-Aid, or broth. Apple and grape juice are good, but orange, tomato, pineapple, and grapefruit juice may irritate the stomach. Avoid milk products, tea, coffee, fruits and vegetables and fatty foods. Do not take aspirin.

2. As soon as there is improvement (less frequent bowel movements, decreased cramping, increased appetite), begin solid foods, starting with broth, crackers, toast, gelatin, and hard-boiled eggs.

3. As the diarrhea subsides, add applesauce, mashed bananas, rice, boiled or baked potatoes, and noodles.

4. When stools begin to harden, add cooked lean meat, cooked vegetables, yogurt, and cottage cheese. Avoid alcohol, spicy foods, and stewed fruit.

FLUID REPLACEMENT: If fluid losses are significant (more than 5 bowel movements per day), begin to replace liquids as soon as you can.

1. Mild diarrhea/dehydration: Drink soda water (bottles), clear juices (apple), tea, broth, and Gatorade.

2. Moderate diarrhea/dehydration: Drink diluted (by ½ with water) Gatorade, mineral water (bottled), or homemade solutions (one quart of disinfected water plus ½–1 teaspoon sodium chloride [table salt], ½ teaspoon sodium bicarbonate [baking soda], ¼ teaspoon potassium chloride [salt substitute], and glucose [6–8 teaspoons table sugar or 1–2 tablespoons honey]). Take care not to oversweeten (exceed 2–2.5% glucose) the solution with sugar, because this may actually worsen the diarrhea. The latter should be supplemented (alternated) with ½–1 liter of plain disinfected water. Oral Rehydration Salts that meet World Health Organization standards are available in a dry mix, 1 packet per quart of water. If premeasured salts are not available, you can alternate glasses of the following two fluids: glass one — 8 ounces of fruit juice (apple, orange, etc.) with a pinch of salt and ½ teaspoon honey or corn syrup; glass two — 8 ounces of boiled or disinfected water with ¼ teaspoon baking soda.

3. Severe diarrhea/dehydration: Same as moderate. See a physician.

ANTIMOTILITY (DECREASED BOWEL ACTIVITY) AGENTS: If fever, severe cramping, and bloody diarrhea are *absent*, the following drugs are safe to use. They should be immediately discontinued if diarrhea lasts for longer than 48 hours. (If diarrhea lasts longer than 3 days, if the patient has a temperature greater than 101°F (38.3°C), if the patient cannot keep liquids down because of vomiting, if there is blood in the stool, if the abdomen becomes swollen, or if there is no significant pain relief after 24 hours, a physician should be sought immediately.)

1. Lomotil, loperamide, or Pro-Banthine (see Appendix One). Of these, loperamide (Imodium) is probably the safest.

2. Pepto-Bismol (see Appendix One).

ANTIBIOTICS: These should be used if the diarrhea is moderate to severe (more than 8 bowel movements per day), particularly if it is bloody and associated with severe cramping, vomiting, and fever.

1. Administer ciprofloxacin (Cipro) 500 mg twice a day or trimethoprim with sulfamethoxazole (Bactrim or Septra DS), 1 pill twice a day for 3 days. These will treat *E. coli* and *Shigella*, may be of use for *Salmonella*, and will not adversely affect the course of viral, *Staphylococcus*, or *Campylobacter* infections. Enteric fever caused by *S. typhi* (typhoid fever) is best treated with ciprofloxacin in adults.

An alternative drug is doxycycline (Vibramycin) 100 mg twice a day. Children younger than 12 years of age should not be given doxycycline, as it may cause permanent discoloration of the teeth. Because ciprofloxacin may affect bone growth in children, it should only be given to adults.

2. If the clinical picture clearly points to *Giardia lamblia* (see page 168), administer Flagyl 250 mg 3 times a day for 7 days. (A woman who is possibly pregnant should not use this drug except under the advice of her physician.)

Viral Diarrhea

Viral gastroenteritis includes diarrhea as a symptom. It is often associated with nausea and vomiting, fever, stomach cramps, copious rectal gas, and a flulike syndrome. The diarrhea is typically watery, frequent (up to 20 movements per day), and often foul smelling, discolored (green to greenish brown), and without significant mucus or blood. Generally, the victim will have cyclic waves of lower abdominal cramps, relieved by bowel movements.

Therapy requires continuous oral hydration with clear liquids such as tea, apple juice, or broth. If available, electrolyte-sugar solutions such as Gatorade are excellent for fluid replacement. It is crucial to keep the patient from becoming dehydrated. What comes out below should be replaced from above.

The cramps can be controlled with propantheline bromide (Pro-Banthine), loperamide (Imodium), or diphenoxylate (Lomotil), which will also help to limit the diarrhea. It should be noted, however, that these drugs will slow down the activity of the bowel and allow any toxins that are in the gut to remain in contact with the bowel wall. With certain bacterial infections, these drugs may prolong the carrier state and actually increase the severity and duration of the disease. Therefore, it is prudent to avoid the use of Lomotil or Imodium unless the intake of fluids cannot keep pace with the diarrhea, and dehydration has become debilitating. NEVER GIVE THESE AGENTS TO INFANTS OR CHILDREN.

Food Poisoning

Food poisoning is caused by toxins that are produced by a number of bacteria, with the most common being *Staphylococcus*. Improper preservation (generally, lack of refrigeration) of food allows bacterial proliferation, which is not corrected by cooking. Typically, the symptoms occur 2–6 hours after eating, and consist of severe abdominal cramps, with nausea and vomiting. Diarrhea may be delayed by an hour or two, or may occur simultaneously with the nausea and vomiting. The diarrhea is often "explosive." As with viral gastroenteritis, the bowel movements may be foul and blood tinged. The disease is self-limited, and generally subsides after 6–12 hours. Treatment consists of rehydration with clear liquids, and plenty of moral support. Antimotility drugs such as Lomotil may prolong the disorder, and should not be used unless the victim cannot replenish the fluid losses.

Traveler's Diarrhea

Traveler's diarrhea ("turista") is caused by toxins most commonly (80%) produced by forms of the bacterium *Escherichia coli*, which is introduced into the diet as a fecal contaminant in water or on food. Symptoms usually occur 12–36 hours after ingesting the bacteria, and include the gradual or sudden onset of frequent

(4–5 per day) loose or watery bowel movements, rarely explosive, and far less violent than diarrhea associated with classic food poisoning. Fever, bloating, fatigue, and abdominal pain are of minor to moderate severity. Nausea and vomiting are less frequently found than with viral gastroenteritis.

The affliction will resolve spontaneously in 2–5 days if untreated, but may be hastened to a conclusion if antibiotics are administered. The current recommendation is to treat with ciprofloxacin (Cipro) 500 mg 2 times a day for 3 days or trimethoprim with sulfamethoxazole (Septra or Bactrim) 1 double-strength tablet 2 times a day for a 3-day course. For known traveler's diarrhea, the addition of loperamide to an antibiotic regimen can have dramatic benefit, with the precaution that it should be used *only* in the absence of high fever or bloody diarrhea. Alternately, the diarrhea can be treated with bismuth subsalicylate (Pepto-Bismol). However, to be effective, it must be given in large quantities (see Appendix One).

To prevent traveler's diarrhea, persons who are traveling to high-risk regions with questionable hygiene and water disinfection standards (developing countries of Latin America, Africa, the Middle East, and Asia) can take prophylactic trimethoprim and sulfamethoxazole (1 double-strength tablet once a day) or ciprofloxacin 500 mg once a day during the journey. Southern Europe (Spain, Greece, Italy, Turkey) and parts of the Caribbean pose a lesser risk. Another drug that can be used is doxycycline hyclate (Vibramycin) 100 mg once a day. This should only be done under the guidance of a physician, who will explain the risks (allergic reactions, blood disorders, antibiotic-associated colitis, vaginal yeast infection, skin rashes, photosensitivity) versus benefits (particularly for persons who are prone to infectious diarrhea or who would suffer unduly from an episode of severe diarrhea). Alternately, it has been recommended that a person can drink 4 tablespoons of Pepto-Bismol 4 times a day (this necessitates carrying one 8-ounce bottle for each day). The tablets (2 tablets 4 times a day) are less palatable. However, this prophylaxis is not intended to substitute for dietary discretion. In addition, large doses of bismuth subsalicylate may be toxic, particularly to persons who regularly use aspirin. In general, it is safe to brush your teeth with foreign or mountain water, so long as you spit and don't swallow. Salads, raw vegetables, raw meat, raw seafood, unpeeled fruits and vegetables, cold sauces, ice cream, tap water, and ice are risky business. Water disinfection is discussed on page 323. Stick to boiled water, hot (steamed) meals, dry foods (bread), bottled carbonated beverages, and reputable food establishments.

Giardia Lamblia

Giardia lamblia is a flagellate protozoan (one-celled organism) that has become a worldwide problem, particularly in wilderness settings in the western United States, Nepal, and the Soviet Union. It is transmitted as cysts in the feces of many animals, which include men, elk, beavers, deer, cows, dogs, and sheep. Dormant *Giardia* cysts enter the water, where they are ingested by humans. If more than 25–50 cysts are swallowed, the organisms establish residence in the duodenum and jejunum (first parts of the small bowel), and after an incubation period of 7–20 days emerge in another form (trophozoite) to cause stomach cramps, flatulence, swollen lower abdomen, often explosive and foul-smelling watery ("floating") diarrhea, and nausea. Fever and vomiting are unusual except in the first few days of illness. Because of the delay in onset after ingestion of the cysts, many a backpacker develops the illness after he returns to civilization, and he does not make the mental connection to his recent journey. The diagnosis is made by a physician who recognizes microscopic cysts in the stool of the victim, takes a sample of mucus from the duodenum, or is confident with a clinical diagnosis.

Therapy for *Giardia* infestation is the administration of metronidazole (Flagyl) 250 mg 3 times a day for 7 days. An alternative prescription drug is quinacrine hydrochloride (Atabrine). A good drug that is available in Nepal and some other foreign countries is tinidazole, which is taken in one or two 2 gm doses. Particularly when an expedition will not reach civilization for 3–4 weeks, there is no reason to withhold treatment awaiting physician input. If the diagnosis is correct, in most cases drug therapy will cause dramatic relief from symptoms within 3 days. There is no prophylactic drug that is recommended to prevent infestation.

Other Infectious Diarrheas

Diarrhea can be caused by a number of parasites and other infectious agents, which include *Campylobacter, Shigella, Salmonella, Yersinia, Vibrio,* and *Entamoeba histolytica.* Each pathogen may cause a constellation of fever, chills, nausea, vomiting, diarrhea (with or without mucus and blood), weakness, and abdominal pain. Because the clinical picture can be similar with infection from all of these organisms, the differentiation frequently relies on examination of the stool under the microscope by a physician and/or a culture of the stool to identify the offending organism. For the sake of the brief expedition, the treatment is the same: rehydration with copious amounts of balanced electrolyte solutions, and antimotility agents only when essential for survival. If the victim suffers from high fever with shaking chills, has persistent bloody or mucus-laden bowel movements, or is debilitated by dehydration, he should seek the care of a physician. Meanwhile, the administration of Bactrim or Septra DS (trimethoprim with sulfamethoxazole) or Cipro (ciprofloxacin) will treat *E. coli* and *Shigella,* may eradicate *Salmonella,* and will not adversely affect other infections. As soon as the victim of persistent diarrhea returns to civilization, he should visit a physician for a thorough evaluation.

Emotional Diarrhea (Colitis)

Emotional diarrhea, or "irritable colon," is a manifestation of anxiety, often otherwise unrecognized, that is characterized by abdominal distention, the passage of flatus, cramping, and mucus-laden diarrhea, which can be debilitating. Occasionally, the sufferer will also complain intermittently of constipation. Many victims know that they suffer from this disorder, and carry their own medication, such as clidinium bromide with chlordiazepoxide (Librax). Irritable colon is a diagnosis of exclusion which should be made by a physician. If a person is known to suffer from irritable colon, he should be encouraged to eat adequate fiber (bran, steamed vegetables) and to avoid coffee.

CONSTIPATION

If a person becomes constipated (difficult bowel movements with hard stools), the discomfort can ruin an otherwise halcyon expedition. The approach to constipation is twofold: prevention and treatment.

The greatest contributing factors to constipation are dehydration and lack of exercise. During outdoor exercise, care should be taken to drink fluids at regular intervals. In addition, sufficient fiber (bran, whole grain cereals, vegetables, fruits) must be maintained in the diet. The "city backpacker" diet of chocolate bars, peanuts, and cheese sandwiches will turn the most irascible bowels into mortar. A dose of a stool softener such as dioctyl sodium sulfosuccinate (Colace), or bulking agent such as psyllium seed hydrophilic mucilloid (Metamucil) must be ingested with at least two glasses of water in order to be effective.

In order to relieve the victim of constipation, the following measures should be taken:
1. Force fluids.
2. Adjust the diet (prevention).

3. Consider the use of stool softeners (mineral oil, Colace, Metamucil) or gentle laxatives (prune juice, milk of magnesia, mineral oil). In general, it is best to avoid the use of enemas or potent laxatives, as they can cause large fluid losses and have significant abuse potential.

4. If a victim becomes hopelessly impacted (has not had a bowel movement for 5–10 days due to constipation), you may have to perform the physical removal of stool from the rectum, using an enema or a gloved finger. This should be done gently, to prevent injury to the anus and walls of the rectum. In many cases, the threat of these manipulations will induce a bowel movement. An elderly person with any significant change in bowel habits should see a physician.

HEMORRHOIDS

Hemorrhoids are enlarged veins that are found outside (external) or inside (internal) the anal opening (Fig. 68). They cause problems that range from minor itching and skin irritation to excru-

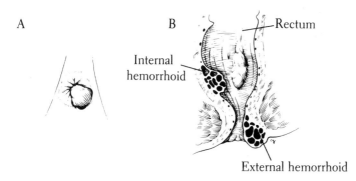

A   B   Rectum

Internal hemorrhoid

External hemorrhoid

FIGURE 68. *Hemorrhoids. (A) External view of the anus with an enlarged external hemorrhoid. (B) A cross-sectional view of the anus and rectum shows dilated veins that protrude into the rectum (internal hemorrhoids) and externally from the anus.*

ciating pain, inflammation, and bleeding. The bleeding is noticed as bright red blood either on the outside of the stool (not mixed in with the excrement), in the toilet water, or on the toilet paper. Bleeding is usually sporadic, associated with difficult bowel movements (constipation) with straining and the passage of hard stools. To avoid problems, the traveler should keep the stools soft. If hemorrhoids flare, the treatment is sitz ("sitting") baths in warm water for 30 minutes 3 times a day, and the application of medication in the form of cream or suppositories (Anusol or Anusol HC with hydrocortisone). Unless bleeding is severe, it can be managed with sterile pads and gentle pressure.

A thrombosed hemorrhoid is one in which the blood has clotted and formed a visible and palpable enlarged, hardened, and dark blue knot. Pain is generally severe, and the victim may be unable to have a bowel movement. The treatment usually involves incision and removal of the clot; until the victim can be transported to a physician, warm soaks may ease the discomfort. Generally, all elderly persons with rectal bleeding should be fully evaluated by a physician, to be sure that there is not a second, more serious cause.

FLATUS

The rectal passage of bowel gas offers relief and occasional embarrassment. If stomach cramps are due to excessive gas production, the drug of choice is simethicone (Mylicon or Mylicon-80), which causes the dissolution of large gas collections and eases the passage of flatus. Because intestinal gas (methane) can be flammable, one should not attempt to ignite rectal gas or direct the stream of gas into a campfire. Backflashes and minor burns are a real risk.

HEARTBURN

Heartburn is a manifestation of esophageal reflux, where stomach contents containing acid and food travel backward from the stomach into the esophagus. This causes irritation and pain, which is typically sharp or burning and located under the breastbone and/or in the upper abdomen. It may be associated with belching, a sour taste in the mouth, and/or near-vomiting. When severe, the pain may be confused with angina (see page 45). Heartburn is best managed with antacids, particularly Gaviscon, which forms a "foam" that floats upon the stomach contents and protects the esophagus from refluxed acid. Metoclopramide hydrochloride (Reglan) is a newer drug that helps to control muscle tone at the sphincter (junction) between the stomach and esophagus, and thus helps prevent reflux. Meals should be kept small, and should not be eaten immediately prior to reclining (i.e., no bedtime snacks). Known gastric irritants (alcohol, cigarettes, pepperoni sandwiches, etc.) should be avoided. If possible, one should sleep with the head of the bed or sleeping bag elevated; occasionally, it is necessary to sleep in the sitting position, to counteract the simple forces of gravity.

NAUSEA AND VOMITING

Nausea and vomiting may be from causes as simple as anxiety, or may represent serious illnesses such as appendicitis, ingestion of a poisonous plant, or a response to head injury. When vomiting is secondary to a serious underlying disorder, the basic problem must be remedied. Any victim with nausea and vomiting who suffers from altered mental status, uncontrollable high fever, extreme abdominal pain, chest pain that might represent heart disease, or who is either very young or very old, should be evacuated promptly. Anyone who vomits blood should be taken to a hospital immediately.

If nausea and vomiting due to gastroenteritis become excessive, they can be managed with antiemetics. The drug of choice is prochlorperazine, which can be administered orally or as a suppository. An alternative is promethazine, which comes in suppository form. If the patient is so ill that he cannot keep anything in his stomach, it makes no sense to administer an oral medication, and it should be given as a suppository. A person who requires medication to control vomiting should see a physician.

VOMITING BLOOD

Bleeding from the gastrointestinal tract can cause the victim to vomit blood (either bright red or dark brown "coffee grounds"). If the blood is not vomited, it passes through the bowels and emerges as dark black tarry stools (melena) or occasionally as maroon clots or bright red blood. Brisk bleeding in the stomach or bowels may be painless; any bleeding should be considered serious. Even if the bleeding episode is brief (except that clearly from known hemorrhoids), the victim should be evacuated immediately to a hospital. If the patient is known to have ulcer disease and ceases vomiting, antacids should be given by mouth.

Persistent retching can cause the stomach wall to tear and begin to bleed. For this reason, persistent nausea and vomiting should be controlled with medications if possible.

ULCER DISEASE

A gastric ulcer is an erosion into the stomach; a peptic ulcer is an erosion into the duodenum (first portion of the small bowel) that is caused by the effect of gastric acid (Fig. 53). The major symptom of ulcer disease is burning, sharp, or aching pain in the upper abdomen that is usually relieved by the ingestion of food or antacids. Classically, the pain occurs when the stomach is empty, particularly during times of emotional stress. Because the greatest amounts of acid are secreted following meals and during the hours of midnight and 3 A.M., these are times when pain is most frequent.

Therapy

1. *Antacids.* These are the traditional mainstay of therapy and should be taken 1 and 3 hours after meals, at bedtime, and as necessary for pain.
2. *Drugs to inhibit the secretion of acid.* These are relatively new, and include cimetidine (Tagamet) and ranitidine (Zantac). Occasionally, these drugs are given in combination with antacids.
3. *Drugs to line the stomach.* Sucralfate (Carafate) is a drug that binds with the ulcer and protects the bowel lining from further erosion. Because it requires the presence of acid in the ulcer crater to be activated, it should not be given at the same time as antacids.
4. *Avoidance of alcohol, tea, coffee, cigarettes, and known gastric irritants.*
5. *Do not use household baking soda to neutralize acid in the stomach.* Baking soda (bicarbonate) reacts with the acid to create heat and gas. Make every attempt to keep on a regular meal schedule and to take medication properly during waking hours.

HEPATITIS

Hepatitis is a damaging inflammation of the liver that is commonly caused by viral infection or parasitic infestation, drugs, toxic chemicals, or alcohol abuse. Type A hepatitis (short-incubation infectious hepatitis) is the more commonly encountered viral form. The virus is excreted in urine and feces and contaminates drinking water and food products (such as raw shellfish). Type B hepatitis (long-incubation serum hepatitis) is caused by a virus that is found in many body fluids (blood, saliva, semen) and is spread by direct person-to-person contact. Type C hepatitis (formerly non-A, non-B hepatitis) is caused by at least one virus and most commonly associated with blood transfusion. Hepatitis causes the victim to have a constellation of signs and symptoms which include yellow discoloration of the skin and eyes (jaundice, from the buildup of bilirubin pigment which the diseased liver cannot process properly), nausea and vomiting, fatigue, weakness, fever, chills, darkened urine, diarrhea, and pale-colored bowel movements (which may precede the onset of jaundice by 1–3 days), abdominal pain (particularly in the right upper quadrant over the swollen and tender liver), loss of appetite, joint pain, muscle aching, itching, and red skin rash. Young children may suffer from type A infection yet show only a mild flulike illness.

Anyone suspected of having hepatitis should be placed at maximum rest and immediately transported to a physician. Drug and alcohol ingestion should be avoided, because the metabolism of drugs is altered in the victim with a diseased liver. The patient should be encouraged to avoid dehydration and should maintain adequate food intake. If the cause of hepatitis is viral, the patient's disease may be contagious for the first two weeks of illness; eating utensils or washrags should not be shared by other members of the party. Body secretions (saliva and waste products) frequently carry the virus; therefore, strict attention should be paid to handwashing. Sexual contact should be avoided during the infectious period. In no case should a needle used for injection of medicine into one person be reused for another individual.

Protection against hepatitis is best accomplished by prevention of virus transmission through good hygiene. In countries of high hepatitis incidence (poor sanitation, infested water or food), pooled immune serum globulin (ISG, or gamma globulin) injections are advised (see page 338) to protect against hepatitis A and to diminish the symptoms in infected persons. Hepatitis B vaccine is intended for health care workers or persons who will reside for prolonged periods in regions of high endemicity. It is of little benefit to protect against hepatitis A. There is not yet a specific vaccine on the market directed against hepatitis A.

Skin Disorders

R ASHES, infections, and allergic reactions can rapidly progress
from nuisance severity to major health hazards. Because
most skin disorders can be easily managed (if they are properly
diagnosed, which isn't always easy), they don't have to ruin the
trip.

SUNBURN

Sunburn is a cutaneous photosensitivity reaction caused by exposure of the skin to ultraviolet radiation (UVR) from the sun.
Ultraviolet exposure varies with the time of day (greatest between
10 A.M. and 3 P.M.), season (greater in the summer), altitude (4%
increase per each 1,000 feet of elevation above sea level), time of
day (greater at noon with increased proximity and decreased angle of light rays), location (greater near the equator), and weather
(greater in the wind). Snow or ice reflects 85% of UVR, dry sand
17%, and grass 2.5%. Water may reflect 10–30% of UVR, depending upon the time of day, location, and surface. Most clothes
reflect (light-colored) or absorb (dark-colored) UVR. However, it
is important to note that wet cotton of any color probably transmits considerable UVR.

If the skin is not conditioned with gradual doses of UVR (tanning), then a burn can be created. A person's sensitivity to UVR
depends on his skin type and thickness, pigment (melanin) in the
skin, and weather conditions. Depending upon the exposure, the
injury can range from mild redness to blistering and disablement.
The red of sunburn is caused by dilatation of superficial blood
vessels. Wind appears to augment the injury, as do heat, atmospheric moisture, and immersion in water. ("Windburn" is not
possible without UVR or abrasive sand.)

People may be more sensitive to UVR after they have ingested certain drugs (such as tetracycline, doxycycline, vitamin A derivatives, nonsteroidal anti-inflammatories, sulfa derivatives, thiazide diuretics, and barbiturates) or have been exposed to certain plants (such as lime, citron, bitter orange, lemon, celery, parsnip, fennel, dill, wild carrot, fig, buttercup, mustard, milfoil, agrimony, rue, hogweed, Queen Anne's lace, and stinking mayweed).

For a mild sunburn, where no blistering is present, the patient may be treated with cool liquid compresses, nonsensitizing skin moisturizers (such as Vaseline Intensive Care), and aspirin to decrease the pain and inflammation. Topical anesthetic sprays, many of which contain benzocaine, should be avoided, as they can cause sensitization and allergic reactions. If the victim is deep red ("lobster") without blisters, then a stronger oral anti-inflammatory drug, such as ibuprofen, may be given. A five-day course of prednisone (50 mg on the first day; 40 mg the second; 30 mg the third; 20 mg on the fourth and 10 mg on the fifth) works wonders to decrease the discomfort of sunburn. This should be given under the guidance of a physician. Topical steroid creams, such as pramoxine with hydrocortisone (Pramosone cream or lotion), may be used if blisters are not present. However, if steroid creams are applied to blistered skin, wound healing is delayed and infection is more likely. On the other hand, aloe vera lotion or gel may be soothing and promote healing. Vitamin E is an antioxidant that, when mixed with aloe vera, may soothe the skin; however, this hasn't been proven.

For a severe sunburn, in which blistering is present, the victim should be taken to a medical facility, for he has in fact suffered a second-degree burn and needs to be managed for such (see page 93). Gently clean the burned areas and cover with a sterile dressing. Encourage fluid intake and use pain medicines appropriate for the situation.

SUNSCREENS

Ultraviolet light (beyond the violet end of the visible spectrum with a wavelength shorter than that of visible light) represents 10% of the radiation that reaches the earth from the sun. It is composed of ultraviolet A (wavelength 320–400 nanometers), ultraviolet B (wavelength 290–320 nm), and ultraviolet C (wavelength 200–290 nm). Ozone in the atmosphere filters out ultraviolet C. Ultraviolet B is the culprit in the creation of sunburn; ultraviolet A is of less immediate danger but is a serious cause of skin aging, drug-related photosensitivity, and skin cancer. Sunscreens (available as lotions or creams) either absorb light of a particular wavelength, act as barriers, or reflect light. Travelers should choose sunscreens based on the estimated exposure and on their own propensity to tan or burn. Dermatologists classify sun-reactive skin types (based on the first 45–60 minutes of sun exposure after winter or prolonged period of no sun exposure) as follows:

Type I — always burns easily, never tans
Type II — always burns easily, tans minimally
Type III — burns moderately, tans gradually and uniformly (light brown)
Type IV — burns minimally, always tans well (moderate brown)
Type V — rarely burns, tans profusely (dark brown)
Type VI — never burns, is deeply pigmented (black skin)

In all cases it is wisest to overestimate the protection necessary and carry a strong sunscreen. To protect hair from sun damage, wear a hat.

Para-aminobenzoic acid (PABA) is a sunscreen that absorbs ultraviolet light B (*not* ultraviolet A) and that accumulates in the skin with repeated application. The most effective method of application is to moisturize the skin (shower or bathe), and then apply the sunscreen. For maximal effect, this should be done at least 15–30 minutes prior to exposure, and the skin should be kept dry for at least 2 hours after sunscreen application. A recommended preparation is 5–10% PABA in 50–70% alcohol. Sunscreens come in different concentrations (e.g., PreSun "8" or "15") (see Appendix One). A higher sun protection factor (SPF) number (range 2 to 50) indicates a greater degree of protection. In general, a sunscreen with an SPF number of 8 or less will allow tanning. Persons with sensitive or unconditioned skin should use a screen with an SPF number of 10 or greater. Fair-skinned persons who never tan or tan poorly (types I, II, and III) or mountain climbers (there is more ultraviolet exposure at higher altitudes and more is reflected off snow) should always use a screen with an SPF number of 15 or greater. Sunscreens should be reapplied liberally after swimming or heavy perspiration. Bald-headed men should protect their domes. All children should be adequately protected; however, avoid PABA products in children less than 6 months old. Lesser concentrations of PABA still allow tanning, probably by ultraviolet A light exposure. Persons sensitive to PABA may use Piz-Buin, Ti-Screen, Uval, and Solbar products. Eating PABA does not protect the skin.

Substantivity refers to the ability of a sunscreen to resist water washoff. Good waterproof choices include Vaseline 15, PreSun 29, Sundown 30, BullFrog 36, Solbar 50, and Aloegator 40. Layering sunscreens doesn't work well, as the last layer applied usually washes off.

Benzophenones are sunscreens that are more effective against ultraviolet light A. These should be used in 6–10% concentration. Because they are not well absorbed by the skin, they require frequent reapplication. Photoplex broad-spectrum sunscreen lotion contains a PABA-ester combined with a potent ultraviolet A absorber, Parsol 1789. This is an excellent sunscreen for sensitive persons, particularly those at risk for drug-induced photosensitivity.

For total protection against ultraviolet and visible light, a sunscreen (sunblock) can be prepared from a mixture of titanium dioxide, talc, zinc oxide, kaolin, red ferric oxide, and a benzophenone. This preparation or a similar commercial product ("glacier cream") is used for lip and nose protection.

Substances that are ineffective as sunscreens and may in fact increase the propensity to burn include baby oil, cocoa butter, and mineral oil.

Although "tanning tablets" or "bronzers" induce a pigmentary change in the skin that resembles a suntan, they provide minimal, if any, true protection from ultraviolet exposure. Like the sun, tanning machines may induce skin changes that lead to premature skin aging and cancer.

Aspirin or ibuprofen taken every six hours for three doses prior to sun exposure may help to protect the sun-sensitive person.

Many effective sunscreens, particularly those advertised to "stay on in the water" (e.g., BullFrog Sunblock) are extremely irritating to the eyes, so one should take care when applying these to the forehead and nose. Near the eyes, avoid sunscreens with an alcohol or propylene glycol base; instead, use a sunscreen cream.

POISON IVY, POISON SUMAC, AND POISON OAK

The rashes of poison ivy, poison sumac, and poison oak are caused by a resin (urushiol) found in the resin canals of leaves, stems, berries, and roots (Fig. 69). The potency of the sap does not vary with the seasons. Because the plant parts have to be injured to leak the resin, most cases are reported in the spring, when the leaves are most fragile. Dried leaves are less toxic; however, smoke from burning plants carries the resin in small particles and can cause a severe reaction on the skin and in the nose, mouth, throat, and lungs. Other plants or parts of plants that contain urushiol include the India ink tree, mango rind, cashew nut shell, and the Japanese lacquer tree. Because the resin is long-lived, it may be spread by contact with tents, clothing, and pet fur.

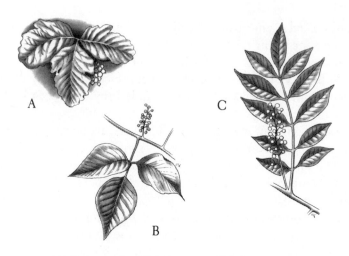

FIGURE 69. *(A) Poison oak. (B) Poison ivy. (C) Poison sumac.*

Sensitivity to the resin varies with the individual (a skin test for urushiol sensitivity may soon be available to the public). The first exposure produces a rash in 6–25 days. Later exposures can cause a rash in 8 hours to 10 days, with a 2–3 day interval most common. Unless the resin is removed from the skin within 10 minutes of exposure, a reaction is inevitable. There are few commercially available topical chemical preparations that act as effective barriers, although it appears that activated charcoal, aluminum oxide, and silica gel may work. Ivy Shield (Interpro, Haverhill, Massachusetts) is an excellent protective agent for sensitive persons. It should be applied over any sunscreen, and must be washed off carefully after use according to instructions. After exposure, there is nothing significantly better to remove the resin than soap and cool water. Technu poison oak and ivy wash (alkane/alcohol) works quite well when applied shortly after exposure, rubbed in for 2 minutes, and rinsed off, with a repeat of the entire sequence.

Everyone has a favorite treatment for poison ivy, and so it is with this author. Shake lotions such as calamine are soothing and drying, and they control itching. A good nonsensitizing topical anesthetic is pramoxine HCl 1% (Prax cream or lotion). Avoid *topical* diphenhydramine, benzocaine, and tetracaine. Antihistamines (such as Benadryl) control itching and act as sedatives. Nonsedating antihistamines, such as terfenadine (Seldane), may also diminish itching. A soothing bath in tepid (not hot) water with baking soda or oilated Aveeno (1 packet) is the author's favorite. Topical steroid creams are generally of little value. Alcohol applications are extremely painful.

If the reaction is severe (facial and/or genital involvement or intolerable itching), the patient should be treated with a course of oral prednisone (60 mg the first 4 days; 40 mg the next 4 days, 20 mg the next 4 days; 10 mg the last 4 days).

Once the resin has been removed from the skin, the rash is not contagious. However, if the resin is still present, scratching the involved skin will allow resin to be transferred to other areas. All clothes, sleeping bags, and pets should be washed with soap and water, as the resin can persist for years, particularly on woolen garments and blankets.

Other Irritating Plants

Some plants produce fluids or crystals which act as primary irritants to the skin, in a nonallergic reaction. Some of the plants include buttercup, daisy, mustard, radish, pineapple, lemon, crown-of-thorns, milkbush, candelabra cactus, daffodil, hyacinth, stinging nettle, itch plant, dogwood, barley, millet, prickly pear, snow-on-the-mountain, primrose, geranium, narcissus, oleander, opuntia cactus, mesquite, tulip, mistletoe, and horse nettle.

The therapy for these is the same as for poison ivy rash. The skin should be thoroughly washed with soap and water. The administration of prednisone is rarely necessary. If barbs are embedded in the skin, removal may be easiest by applying the sticky side of adhesive tape to the skin, and peeling the barbs off with the tape. Small cactus spines may be removed by applying facial gel (mask), allowing it to dry, and peeling it off.

SWIMMER'S ITCH

A number of plants and small animals found in the ocean cause skin irritations. The most common of these irritations are:

Seaweed Dermatitis

There are more than 3,000 species of algae, which range in size from 1 micron to 100 meters in length. The blue-green algae, *Microcoleus lyngbyaceus*, is a fine hairlike plant that gets inside the bathing suit of the unwary aquanaut in Hawaiian and Floridian waters, particularly during the summer months. Usually, skin under the suit remains in moist contact with the algae (the other skin dries or is rinsed off), and becomes red and itchy, with occasional blistering and/or weeping. The reaction may start a few minutes to a few hours after leaving the water. Treatment consists of a generous soap-and-water scrub, followed by a rinse with isopropyl (rubbing) alcohol 40–70%, and application of hydrocortisone lotion 1% twice a day. If the reaction is severe, the victim should see a physician, who may administer oral prednisone for a severe allergic skin reaction.

Swimmer's Itch

True swimmer's itch (clamdigger's itch) is caused by skin contact with cercariae, which are the immature larval forms of parasitic schistosomes (flatworms) found throughout the world in both fresh and salt waters. Snails and birds are the intermediate hosts for the flatworms; they release hundreds of fork-tailed microscopic cercariae into the water.

The affliction is contracted as a film of cercariae-infested water dries on the exposed (uncovered by wet clothing) skin. The cercariae penetrate the outer layer of the skin, where itching is noted within minutes. Shortly afterward, the skin becomes reddened and swollen, with a marked rash and occasional hives. Blisters may develop over the next 24–48 hours. If the area is scratched, it may become infected and develop impetigo (see page 188). Untreated, the disorder is self-limited to 1–2 weeks. Persons who have had swimmer's itch previously may be more severely affected on repeated exposures, which suggests that an allergy can be developed.

The disorder can be prevented by briskly rubbing the skin with a towel immediately after leaving the water, to prevent the cercariae from having time to penetrate the skin. Once the reaction has occurred, the skin may be lightly rinsed with isopropyl (rubbing) alcohol and coated with calamine lotion. If the reaction is severe, the patient should be treated as if he suffered from poison ivy (see page 183).

Because the cercariae are in greatest concentration in shallow, warmer water (where the snails are), swimmers should seek to avoid these areas.

Sea Bather's Eruption

Sea bather's eruption is similar to swimmer's itch, but occurs only in seawater and tends to involve areas of the skin covered by the bathing suit, rather than exposed areas. The skin involved is similar in distribution and appearance to that affected by seaweed dermatitis, but no seaweed is found on the skin. Sea bather's eruption is managed in a fashion identical to that used for swimmer's itch.

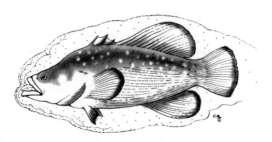

FIGURE 70. *Soapfish, enveloped by a cloud of irritant mucus secreted by the fish.*

Soapfish Dermatitis

The tropical soapfish, *Rypticus saponaceus*, is covered with a soapy mucus (Fig. 70). When exposed to this slime, the victim's skin develops redness, itching, and slight swelling. Treatment involves a good wash with soap and water, followed by cool compresses, application of calamine lotion, and treatment for a mild allergic reaction similar to that for hives (below).

Fish Handler's Disease

When cleaning marine fish or shellfish, the handler frequently creates small nicks and scrapes in his skin, usually on the hands. If these become infected with the bacteria *Erysipelothrix insidiosa*, a typical skin rash may develop within 2–7 days. It appears as a red to violet-colored area of raised skin surrounding the small cut or scrape, with warmth, slight tenderness, and a well-defined border (Fig. 71). The sufferer should be treated with penicillin, cephalexin, or erythromycin for one week.

HIVES

Hives are one skin manifestation of an allergic reaction. They appear as raised, red, irregularly bordered welts or thickened

186 · MINOR MEDICAL PROBLEMS

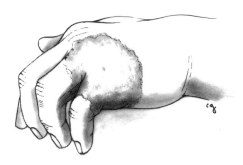

FIGURE 71. *Typical rash of fish handler's infection.*

patches of skin (Fig. 72). Often, the patient will also complain of itching and/or fever. The treatment is to administer an antihistamine (such as Benadryl) at 6-hour intervals until the rash has disappeared, and to observe the victim closely for progression to a serious allergic reaction. If the patient complains of shortness of breath or wheezing, or has a swollen tongue (muffled voice), immediately proceed to the section on allergic reactions (see page 58) and prepare to administer epinephrine.

HEAT RASH

Heat rash is a skin irritation that is composed of small raised spots that coalesce to form large areas of redness, particularly in the

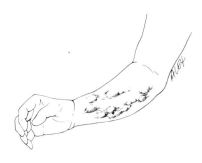

FIGURE 72. *Hives.*

groin, under the arms, in the creases of the elbows, over the chest, under the neck, and under the breasts. It rarely itches, but more often becomes irritated, particularly with rubbing. It should be treated with cool compresses, light cotton clothing that will absorb sweat, and if painful, with thin applications of 0.5–1.0% hydrocortisone lotion twice a day.

IMPETIGO

Impetigo is a skin infection caused by the bacteria *Streptococcus* and/or *Staphylococcus*. It is seen as discrete weeping sores, with crusted scabs (with or without yellow pus), of the sort often associated with infected insect bites, small scrapes, or areas frequently scratched. Once a few sores have become infected, they crop up all over the body (particularly in children), and can cause fevers, fatigue, and swollen regional lymph glands.

Treatment involves the administration of oral penicillin, cephalexin, or erythromycin for one week, and improved skin hygiene. The skin should be washed twice a day with pHisoHex scrub or plain soap and water, and the sores covered thinly with bacitracin ointment.

ABSCESS

An abscess (boil) is a collection of pus. Although these can occur anywhere in the body, they are most frequently found in the skin, particularly in areas of high perspiration, friction, and bacteria (*Staphylococcus*) population, such as near the hair follicles under the arms (Fig. 73). The early abscess first appears as a firm tender red lump, which develops over the course of a few days into a reddish-purple soft tender raised area, occasionally with a white or yellowish cap ("comes to a head"). The surrounding skin is reddened and thickened, and regional lymph glands may be swollen and tender. Fever, swollen lymph glands, and red streaking that travels in a linear fashion from the infected site toward the

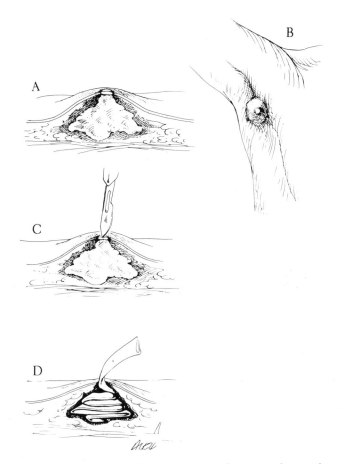

FIGURE 73. *Abscess cavity. (A) Cross-section of a pus pocket, with a soft cap. (B) External appearance of an abscess in the armpit. (C) To drain an abscess, a stab wound is made in the center of the softest area. (D) After the pus is removed and the cavity is rinsed, a gauze wick is layered into the cavity.*

trunk indicate the spread of infection into the lymphatic system (Fig. 78).

Treatment involves drainage of the pus and dead tissue from within the core of the soft abscess. This is performed by taking a sharp blade and cutting a line into the roof of the abscess at the softest point (Fig. 73C). The incision must be large enough (generally, half the size of the soft area) to allow all of the pus to run out. Unless no help can be obtained for 4–5 days, this procedure should be performed only by a qualified medical technician. After the pus is allowed to drain, the cavity should be rinsed well and then packed snugly with a small piece of gauze to prevent the skin from sealing closed over a large empty space (Fig. 73D). Each day, the packing is removed (quickly, to minimize pain) and the wound irrigated and then repacked until the cavity shrinks to a small size. If the abscess is adequately drained, there is no need to begin antibiotic administration.

DO NOT SQUEEZE AN ABSCESS TO CAUSE RUPTURE, particularly on the face. This may force bacteria into the bloodstream and create a much more serious infection elsewhere (such as behind the eye or in the brain).

If the infection has not yet softened, but is still red, painful, and hard, begin the patient on warm soaks and administer dicloxacillin, erythromycin, or cephalexin. Continue soaks until the abscess softens and a white or yellow cap becomes apparent. If the abscess is soft, but there is evidence of lymphatic infection (described above), begin antibiotics.

BLISTERS

Blisters are the bane of all hikers. These clear-fluid or blood-filled vesicles have probably ended more outings than all major illnesses combined. They can be prevented by keeping feet dry, wearing adequate and properly fitted socks, and padding all rough edges within hiking boots.

If a blister is caused by pressure (ill-fitting boots), you have a couple of choices. If the blister site can be padded with moleskin or other adhesive foam, so that rubbing no longer occurs, the blister should be ringed with a doughnut of padding and left intact (Fig. 74). For a better cushion, a piece of Spenco 2nd Skin can be laid into the doughnut hole and the entire area covered with a second layer of moleskin. If no such padding is available, if continued rubbing will rupture the blister, or if it interferes with walking, then the blister may be drained of fluid by using a "sterile needle" (heat a sewing needle to red hot and allow it to cool) to punch a small hole at the edge. If the blister appears infected, it should be unroofed in its entirety, an appropriate dressing applied, and the patient treated with dicloxacillin, erythromycin, or cephalexin for 5 days or until the skin appears normal.

Blisters or reddened skin may also be caused by an allergic ("contact") reaction to chemicals, such as formaldehyde or rubber. If a rash is confined to the soles of the feet (shoe inserts) or tops of the feet (shoe tongue dye), suspect this problem. If this is the case, the footgear must be changed.

If a blister is caused by a thermal burn, it should be immediately immersed in cold water (DO NOT apply ice directly to the burn) for a period of 10–15 minutes, in order to relieve pain and lessen the ultimate injury. The wound is then dried and a soft sterile dressing applied. Unless there is a reason to suspect infection (cloudy fluid or pus, fever, surrounding redness and swell-

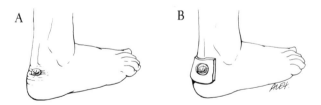

FIGURE 74. (A) *Blister on the heel.* (B) *A cushion of moleskin protects the area from further irritation.*

ing, swollen lymph glands), burn blisters should be left intact. Opening an uninfected blister or sticking a needle into it risks introducing bacteria that can cause an infection. Topical antibacterial creams such as silver sulfadiazene should be applied if the blister is broken, or to prevent the dressing from sticking to the wound.

ATHLETE'S FOOT AND JOCK ITCH

Athlete's foot and jock itch are both caused by fungal infections that develop in warm, moist areas, such as between the toes or in the groin. Athlete's foot can be recognized as a red rash, moist or scaling, with small blisters and frequent weeping. Itching is the major symptom. Jock itch is a red rash with a well-demarcated border that causes itching and irritation in the groin and occasionally over the genitals. Both rashes are more common in summer, particularly in those who do a lot of sweating and bathe infrequently. Either rash is managed with antifungal cream (ketoconazole 2%: Nizoral), lotion, and powder, such as tolnaftate (Tinactin) or clotrimazole (Lotrimin), applied 2 or 3 times a day. Because the rash is contagious, socks and underwear should not be shared. Cotton underclothing that absorbs sweat should be worn.

LICE AND MITES

In a situation of poor hygiene and shared living quarters, particularly overseas, a person may acquire head and/or body mites or lice, which make their homes predominantly in hair-covered areas of the body. The overwhelming symptom is itching. Upon close inspection, you may discover nits (eggs) or tiny crawling forms, particularly in the scalp or pubic hair. Fortunately, mites and lice cannot leap or fly.

The treatment is to lather the body and scalp vigorously with lindane 1% shampoo (Kwell) or crotamiton 10% lotion (Eurax).

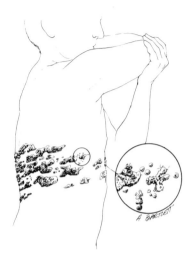

FIGURE 75. *Shingles (herpes zoster) eruption.*

Children may be treated with 5% permethrin (Elimite cream) in a single application; this is safe for infants over 2 months of age. The cream should be rubbed into the skin and scalp, and washed off after 8–12 hours. The hair should be combed thoroughly to remove all nits. To be most effective, the process should be repeated in one week. All clothing and bedding (including sleeping bag) should be washed thoroughly with laundry soap in hot water or dry cleaned.

SHINGLES

Shingles is the common name for herpes zoster, a skin eruption that is frequently activated during times of stress. The varicella virus (the same agent that causes chicken pox in children) is carried silently in nerve roots by individuals, and upon appropriate stimulation, causes the outcropping of a series of blisters in patterns that correspond with skin areas served by particular nerve roots that originate from the spinal cord (Fig. 75). Classically, the patient will have a day or two of unexplained itching or burning pain in the area to be involved, and will then notice the outbreak of the rash. The discomfort can be tremendous and will frequently require the liberal use of pain medication. The rash itself should be kept clean and dry, and covered with a light dry dressing to prevent further irritation from rubbing or the sun. The disorder is self-limited, and will resolve spontaneously over the course of approximately 10 days to 3 weeks. If the victim appears to be moderately ill (fever, chills, severe headache), or if the rash involves the eyes, mouth, or genitals, a physician should be seen immediately.

FEVER BLISTERS

See page 157.

Minor Bruises and Wounds

THIS section deals with all of the assorted bumps and bruises that occur in the out-of-doors. One should be conservative and evacuate anyone whose injury is not easily managed by the therapies suggested in this section.

BRUISES

Bruises are collections of blood that develop in soft tissue (muscles, skin, and fat), caused by a direct blow to the body part or by a tearing motion (such as a twisted ankle). Small blood vessels are torn or crushed, and leak blood into the tissue, so that it rapidly becomes discolored. Pain and swelling are proportional to the degree of injury.

The immediate (within the first 48 hours) treatment of a bruise is to apply cold compresses or to immerse the injured part in cold water (such as a mountain stream). This decreases the leakage of blood, minimizes swelling, and helps to reduce pain. This should be done for intermittent 10-minute periods until a minimum total application time of 1 hour is attained. Do not apply ice directly to the skin (to avoid frostbite); rather, wrap the ice in a cloth before application.

If the swelling is rapidly progressive (such as bleeding into a thigh), an elastic wrap may be applied snugly to try to contain the swelling (cold applications should continue over the wrap). It is important to keep the wrap loose enough to allow free circulation (fingertips and toes should remain pink and warm; wrist and foot pulses should remain brisk), and to elevate the injured body part as much as possible. Elastic wraps are indicated only if pain and swelling will not allow the victim to extricate himself in order to seek medical attention.

One should never attempt to puncture or cut into a bruise in order to drain it. This is fraught with the risk of uncontrolled bleeding and the introduction of bacteria that cause infection. The only exception to this rule is a tense and painful collection of blood under the fingernail (see below).

Elevation of the bruised and swollen part above the level of the heart is essential, in order to allow gravity to keep further swelling to a minimum.

After 48–72 hours, the application of moist or dry heat will help promote local circulation and resolution of the swelling and discoloration. Heat ointments or liniments are ineffective, as they only irritate nerve endings in the outermost layers of the skin and give a false impression of warmth. If you stick a thermometer into a tube of heat ointment, the temperature recorded is not elevated.

Persons who have slow blood-clotting times and/or who have large bruises should avoid aspirin-containing products, which might cause increased bleeding.

BLACK EYE

A black eye is a darkened blue or purple discoloration in the region around the eye. It can be caused by a direct blow (bruise) or by blood that has settled into the area from a broken nose, skull fracture, or laceration of the eyebrow or forehead. If it is due to a direct injury (with swelling and pain), first examine the eyeball for injury (see page 145). The skin discoloration may be treated with intermittent cold compresses for 24 hours.

BLOOD UNDER THE FINGERNAIL

When a fingertip is smashed between two objects, there is frequently a rapid blue discoloration of the fingernail, which is caused by a collection of blood underneath the nail. Pain from the pressure may be quite severe. To relieve the pain, it is necessary to create a small hole in the nail directly over the collection of blood, to allow the blood to drain and thus relieve the pressure. This can be done during the first 24 hours following the injury by heating in a flame a paperclip or similar-sized metal wire to red-hot temperature (taking care not to burn your fingers holding the other end of the wire; use a needle-nose pliers if available) and quickly pressing it through the nail (Fig. 76). If you are successful, as soon as the nail is penetrated, the victim will yank his finger away, blood will spurt out, and the pain will be considerably lessened. Another method is to twirl the tip of a knife blade gently to create a small hole in the nail. Before and after the procedure, the finger should be washed carefully. If the procedure was not performed under sterile conditions, and antibiotics are available, the patient should be administered dicloxacillin, erythromycin, or cephalexin for 4 days.

PUNCTURE WOUNDS

Puncture wounds are most frequently caused by nails, tree branches, fishhooks, and the like. Because they do not drain

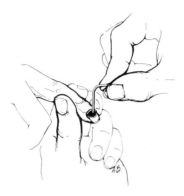

FIGURE 76. *Hot paperclip technique to drain blood from under the fingernail.*

freely, these wounds carry a high risk for retained bacteria and subsequent infections. All puncture wounds should be irrigated copiously (use at least 1–2 liters) with the cleanest solution that is at hand, and left open to heal. Bleeding washes bacteria from the wound, so a small amount of bleeding should be encouraged. If this does not occur spontaneously, it can be promoted by applying the Extractor suction device (see page 256) for 10–15 minutes. NEVER suture or tape a puncture wound closed; if you do, you are asking for a serious infection. Similarly, do not occlude the opening of a puncture wound with a "grease seal" of medicinal ointment. If the wound is more than ¼ inch at the opening, a piece of sterile gauze can be left in the wound as a wick for a day or two, to allow drainage and prevent the formation of an abscess cavity (see pages 189, 190). If antibiotics are available, treat the victim with dicloxacillin, erythromycin, or cephalexin 250 mg 4 times a day for 5 days. If the wound develops the appearance of infection (see page 203), apply warm soaks 4 or more times a day.

SCRAPES

Scrapes (abrasions) are injuries that occur to the top layers of the skin when it is abraded by a rough surface (rocks, asphalt, sharkskin). They are generally very painful, because large surface areas with numerous nerve endings are involved. Bleeding is of an oozing, rather than free-flowing, nature.

Abrasions should be scrubbed until every last speck of dirt is removed. Although it hurts just to think about this, it is necessary for two reasons. The first is the obvious infection potential, when such a large area of injured skin is exposed to dirt and debris. The second is that if small stones or pieces of dirt are left in the wound, it in essence becomes a tattoo, and the victim can be left with permanent markings that require surgical removal. Soap and water scrubbing with a good final rinse should be followed with a bland antiseptic ointment (such as bacitracin or Silvadene) and a sterile dressing. Alternately, if the surface area is not particularly large and on an easily exposed area, it may be left open to the air. The pain of cleansing may be relieved by applying pads soaked with lidocaine ointment (2.5%) to the abrasion for 10–15 minutes prior to scrubbing. To avoid lidocaine toxicity, this should not be done if the surface area of the abrasion exceeds 5% of the total body surface area (an area approximately 4–5 times the size of the victim's fingers and palm).

CUTS (LACERATIONS)

Cuts are easily managed according to the following principles:
1. Control bleeding. This may be done in almost every instance by direct pressure (see page 48). If the wound is not gushing forth blood (in other words, if there is no danger of shock from blood loss), carefully irrigate it with the cleanest water available to remove dirt and blood clots. Examine the wound and remove all obvious foreign debris. After cleansing (use nothing stronger than soap and water), apply firm pressure to the wound,

using a wadded sterile compress, cloth, or direct hand contact. Hold the wound for a full 10–15 minutes without releasing pressure. If this does not stop the bleeding, reapply pressure for 20–25 minutes. If this does not stop the bleeding, apply a sterile compress and wrap with an elastic wrap, taking care not to wrap so tightly as to occlude the circulation (remember, always check for warm and pink fingers and toes). During all of these maneuvers, keep the patient calm and elevate the injured part as much as possible.

2. Do not pour tincture of iodine, rubbing alcohol, merthiolate, mercurochrome, or any other over-the-counter antiseptic (except for potentially rabid animal bites — see page 302) into the wound. These inhibit wound healing and are extremely painful. Although recommended by healers in ancient civilizations, herbal doctors, and professional woodsmen, the use of butter, pine sap, ground charcoal, hard liquor, or wine as an antiseptic is not recommended.

3. Reapproximate the anatomy as best possible. Most cuts do not involve tissue loss, so that the edges fit together like a jigsaw puzzle. Because of the infection risk away from the hospital or doctor's office (a relatively germ-free environment), one should not close a wound tightly with stitches of thread (sutures). Instead, bring the wound edges loosely together with Steri-Strips (paper tape with adhesive specifically made for wound closure) or butterfly bandages. The latter may be fashioned from regular surgical adhesive tape (Fig. 77). A small scar is preferable to a wound infection caused by tight closure that requires hospitalization for surgical management of a wound infection. If nothing else is available to hold together the edges of a widely gaping wound that prevents the victim from seeking help, a safety pin may be used.

Another method of wound closure using tape, one which may be more appropriate for a longer wound, is to cut two strips of adhesive tape 1 inch longer than the wound. Fold one-quarter of each strip of tape over lengthwise (sticky to sticky) to create a long

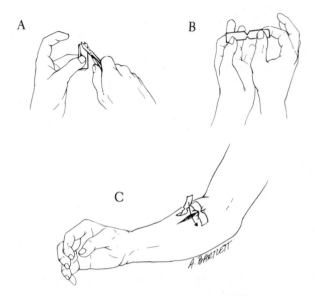

FIGURE 77. *Fashioning a butterfly bandage. (A) Fold a piece of tape and cut off both corners at the crease. (B) The straightened tape reveals the "butterfly." (C) The bandage is used to hold the wound edges close together.*

nonsticky edge on each piece. Lay one strip of the tape on each side of the wound, ¼ to ½ inch from the wound, with the folded (nonsticky) edge toward the wound. Using a needle and thread, sew the folded edges together, cinching them tight enough to bring the wound edges together properly. The tape will stick much better if you first apply a thin layer of benzoin to the skin (see item 4 below).

4. If the skin is moist and tape will not stick well, first apply a thin layer of tincture of benzoin. Take care not to get any benzoin in the wound, because it stings terribly.

5. Dress the wound. Antiseptic cream or ointment may be sparingly applied to the surface of the wound, provided there is good drainage and there are no large open pockets in the wound.

If the wound is deep, a thick antiseptic grease seal that prevents drainage may actually promote the development of a deep space infection.

Bandages should be fashioned of the most sterile material available (usually prepackaged squares or rolls of gauze). If sterile dressings are not available, use clean white cloth (the more absorbent, the better). Apply the dressing snugly enough to control bleeding, but not to impede circulation (as judged by warm and pink fingers and toes). All dressings should be changed as frequently as they become soaked; if there is no significant drainage, they should be changed daily. You should use an antiseptic cream or ointment to prevent the dressing from sticking to the wound, but again, take care to use it sparingly, to avoid applying a grease seal to any deep cuts or puncture wounds. Alternately, a nonstick bandage (Metalline or Telfa) may be applied to the wound. If tape is used to secure the dressing, tincture of benzoin may be used to increase the stickiness of the skin. Do not get any benzoin into the wound. When dressings are applied, keep the body part in the "position of function" (normal resting position) (Fig. 28). Check all dressings daily for soaking, a snug fit, and underlying infection. If you have enough supplies, change dressings daily. Bandaging techniques are addressed in the next section.

6. There is always the risk of infection in an open wound. If the wound is an animal bite, if it is in the hand or foot, if it is a puncture wound, if it has inadequate drainage, has resulted from a crush injury, is very dirty, or if you are more than 24 hours from medical care, this is a high-risk situation and the patient should be treated with oral antibiotics (penicillin, erythromycin, or cephalexin) until the wound is healed or help is reached. This is also true for any large wound. For a cat bite, use penicillin or tetracycline.

7. Splint the wound (see page 64). For instance, if the injury involves the hand, place the arm in a sling to minimize motion of the injured part. Movement delays healing and promotes the spread of infection.

8. Seek appropriate medical attention. Field cleansing and dressing are no substitute for proper irrigation, trimming, and wound management undertaken in a medical facility. Small nicks do not require fancy intervention, but if you are in doubt as to the seriousness of the injury, get good advice.

BANDAGING TECHNIQUES

Bandage application is an art form. The only way to become proficient is to practice. There is no inviolable rule other than to avoid excessive tightness. The following tips should prove useful.

Finger bandage: Fold a 1-inch rolled gauze back and forth over the tip of the finger to cover and cushion the wound. Wrap the gauze around the finger until the bandage is snug and not overly bulky. On the last turn around the finger, pull the gauze over the top of the hand, so that it extends beyond the wrist. Split this tail lengthwise. Tie a knot at the wrist, and wrap the two ends around the wrist; tie again to secure the bandage.

Hand bandage: The hand should be bandaged as it is for a fracture, in the position of function (see page 71). Take care to place gauze or cotton padding between the fingers to separate and cushion them.

Arm or leg bandage: Cover the wound(s) with a gauze pad(s). Overwrap the wound using simple turns of rolled gauze or a figure-of-eight pattern. Secure the bandage with adhesive tape in a spiral pattern to avoid a tourniquet effect. Whenever possible, don't apply tape directly to the skin.

Foot bandage: The foot should be bandaged as it is wrapped for an ankle sprain, using gauze instead of elastic wraps (see page 208).

Chest bandage: To wrap the chest with gauze, circle the chest and upper abdomen for a few turns. To keep the bandage from slipping toward the hips, bring the bandage up over the shoulder every third or fourth turn. Secure the bandage with adhesive tape.

WOUND INFECTIONS

Despite your best efforts, a wound may become infected. The most common bacteria that cause these infections are *Staphylococcus aureus* and *Streptococcus pyogenes*. The common signs of an infection include redness and swelling surrounding the wound, pus or cloudy discharge (pink, green, or cream-colored), a foul odor (this is variable), fever, increased wound tenderness, red streaking that travels to the trunk from the wound, fever, and swollen tender regional lymph nodes (Fig. 78).

If a wound is infected, the edges should be spread apart to allow the drainage of any pus. To do this, you need to remove all

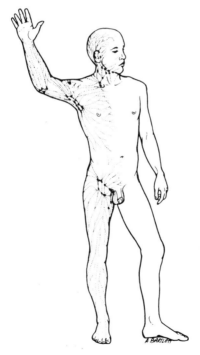

FIGURE 78. *Location of the lymph glands (nodes).*

fastening bandages. The wound should then be irrigated copiously, and dressed with a dry sterile bandage *without bringing the wound edges tightly together.* Begin to apply warm moist compresses, using disinfected water, to the wound at least four times a day and place the patient on antibiotics (penicillin, cephalexin, or erythromycin). For a cat bite, use penicillin or tetracycline.

If a wound infection is present the victim should be brought rapidly to a physician. If you see gas bubbles in a wound, if it is draining foul reddish-gray fluid, and/or if there is a feeling of "Rice Krispies" (crepitus) in the skin surrounding a wound, it may be the onset of gangrene. This is a life-threatening infection and requires immediate advanced surgical attention.

ABSCESS (BOIL)

See page 188.

SCALP LACERATION (CUT ON THE HEAD)

See page 57.

FISHHOOK REMOVAL

See page 355.

SPLINTER REMOVAL

See page 356.

BLISTERS

See page 190.

Musculoskeletal Injuries

OVERUSE SYNDROMES

Whenever a muscle is overused — that is, exercised past its state of conditioning — there is actual destruction of the muscle tissue and generation of lactic acid in the region. Given a reasonable rest period, the products of metabolism are carried away in the circulation and the muscle tissue regenerates to a healthy, sometimes even stronger, condition. However, if the exercise has been vigorous and unrelenting, the participant may suffer from a variety of aches and pains that are generally categorized as overuse syndromes.

Muscle Fatigue

Simple fatigue, with depletion of energy sources within the muscle, is manifested as weakness, pain on exertion, soreness to the touch, and cramping. In many cases, this is compounded by dehydration, deficiencies in electrolytes (usually sodium and/or potassium), lack of sufficient caloric intake, or a specific injury. The sufferer has been informed by his body that it is time to rest. Sufficient time should be allowed to remove waste products, restore energy sources, correct dehydration, and regenerate muscle tissue. The victim should avoid vigorous physical activity for 12–24 hours, and should eat and drink amply. Pharmaceutical muscle relaxants are of little value, and pain medication is generally not necessary. Massage of the involved muscle groups is relaxing, although it probably does not hasten recovery.

Shin Splints

Shin splints is a term used to describe a painful disorder generated by excessive walking, running, or hiking. In this case, the sufferer has irritated the thin membrane that connects the two lower leg bones where it attaches to the bones. With every footstep, there is further irritation of the membrane, so that it can become impossible to walk rapidly. The victim should attempt to curtail running or vigorous walking activity and may benefit from the administration of aspirin or a nonsteroidal anti-inflammatory agent (ibuprofen or naproxen). A shoe that is well cushioned (particularly the ball and heel) is very important for prevention and recovery.

Torn Muscle

A torn muscle (pulled muscle) is recognized as sudden excruciating pain in a muscle group, associated with a particular vigorous exertion, such as sprinting or lifting a heavy object. Depending on the severity of the injury, there may be associated bruising, swelling, loss of mobility, and/or weakness. For instance, a small tear in the deltoid muscle of the shoulder may cause minor discomfort upon lifting the arm over the head, while a complete separation of the quadriceps group in the anterior thigh will cause inability to straighten the leg at the knee, extreme local pain, blue discoloration of the knee, and a defect in the shape of the muscles above the knee that is readily felt and seen.

In general, a minor muscle injury can be distinguished from a bone injury by evaluating active and passive range of motion. Active range of motion is the range of normal activity the victim can manage without rescuer assistance; this will be painful with both muscle and bone injuries. Passive motion is movement of a body part performed only with the aid of the rescuer; no effort is provided by the victim, who should attempt to relax the muscle completely. If there is no pain on passive (assisted) motion, but there is pain present on active motion, then the injury is most likely muscular, because an injured bone will hurt no matter how it is moved.

Minor muscle injuries should be treated in the first 24 hours with immobilization, the application of cold (remember, never apply ice directly to the skin) for 30–45 minutes every 2–3 hours, and elevation. After 48–72 hours, the application of heat (warm water or a heating pad, *not* ointments) and gentle movement should be started. If a significant injury is suspected (for example, complete tear of the biceps muscle or quadriceps group), the injury should be immobilized as for a fracture (see page 64) and the victim transported to a hospital.

Sprains and Strains

Sprains and strains are injuries to ligaments (which attach one bone to another) or tendons (which attach muscle to bone) that are incurred by twisting, direct blunt trauma, or overexertion. Symptoms include pain, swelling and/or deformity, decreased range of motion secondary to pain, and bruising. The treatment is the same as for a suspected fracture: that is, the injured part should be elevated, immobilized (see page 64), and treated with cold applications for the first 24–48 hours. After 72 hours, heat may be applied. It is important to avoid reinjury to the affected joint (ankles are notorious for reinjury) by proper wrapping or the application of a splint. Because the involved joint is immediately weakened, it should not be relied upon for great exertion. Evaluation by a physician is advised upon return to civilization.

The most common sprain is the ankle sprain. If the injury is minor (no chance of a fracture) and/or if the victim needs to put weight on the ankle in order to seek help, the ankle may be wrapped snugly with an elastic wrap in a figure-of-eight method (Fig. 79) or taped in a crisscross weave (Fig. 80). If the sprain is severe, splint the ankle as for a fracture (Figs. 49 and 50).

ARTHRITIS

Arthritis is irritation and inflammation of a joint that can be caused by overuse, infection, or different diseases (such as gout or rheumatoid arthritis). Symptoms include pain in the joint with motion, swelling (fluid collections), redness, and warmth. If the

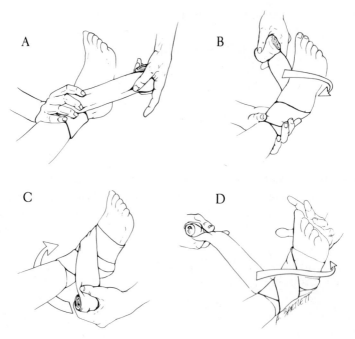

FIGURE 79. *Wrapping the ankle with a figure-of-eight bandage. (A) Start above the ankle and (B) wrap down under the foot. (C) Cross back and forth over the top of the foot and (D) continue in a figure-of-eight pattern to secure the ankle.*

joint is infected (contains pus), then the condition is very serious and must be evaluated by a physician as soon as possible. Generally, persons with such infections have high fevers, shaking chills, weakness, and a recent infection elsewhere on the body or recent direct injury to the joint. The differentiation between an arthritic and an infected joint is often quite impossible to make until the physician sticks a needle into the joint to see if bacteria or pus is present and to obtain fluid for a culture. If infection is a possibility, the person should be started on penicillin, erythromycin, or cephalexin immediately.

If there is little chance of infection, and the joint problem is

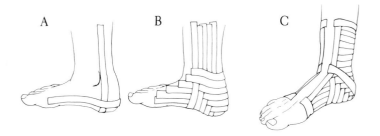

FIGURE 80. *Taping a sprained ankle. (A) Strips of adhesive tape are placed perpendicular to each other to (B) lock the ankle with a tight weave. (C) The tape edges are covered to prevent peeling.*

known to be due to overuse, the patient should take aspirin or another anti-inflammatory drug, such as ibuprofen or naproxen. Rest the affected joint, keep it elevated if it is swollen, and adjust goals for the trip accordingly.

BURSITIS

Bursitis is irritation and inflammation of the lubricating sac (bursa) that allows muscles to move freely around the joints. Common areas of irritation include the sacs in front of the knee-cap (irritated by prolonged kneeling), behind the elbow (irritated by a fall), in the shoulder (irritated by arm swinging), and on the outside of the hip (irritated by walking, hiking, or falling) (Fig. 81). Evaluation and treatment are the same as for arthritis.

THROMBOPHLEBITIS

Thrombophlebitis is inflammation in a vein associated with the development of a blood clot. This occurs in conditions of injury to the veins (cuts, bruises), after periods of prolonged rest in a single position (sitting on a plane, cramped in a cave), or associated with other risk factors (pregnancy, cigarette smoking, cancer, varicose veins). A blood clot irritates the lining of the vein

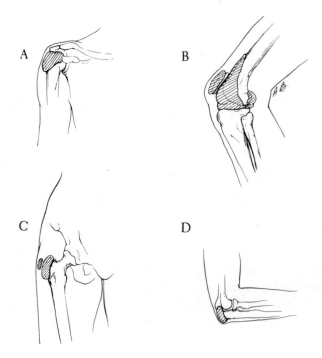

FIGURE 81. *Bursitis affects the lubricating sacs (bursae) near the (A) shoulder, (B) knee, (C) hip, and (D) elbow.*

(most often in the leg) and causes local redness, swelling, warmth, and pain. If the clot enlarges, an entire limb can become affected. If the clot is in a deep vein, it may break off and travel to the lungs, where it causes a serious condition known as pulmonary embolism (see page 41).

It is easy to confuse the presentation of thrombophlebitis with that of an infection. If the former is suspected, the victim should elevate the limb, and apply hot packs or soaks for 60 minutes every 3 hours. Seek immediate medical attention. If you are more than 24 hours from help and not absolutely sure what you are treating, there is no harm in also starting antibiotics (penicillin, erythromycin, or cephalexin).

BACK PAIN

The most common back injury is muscle strain. Symptoms include muscle pain and spasm in the lower back, adjacent to the lumbar vertebrae. Treatment consists of maximal rest while lying

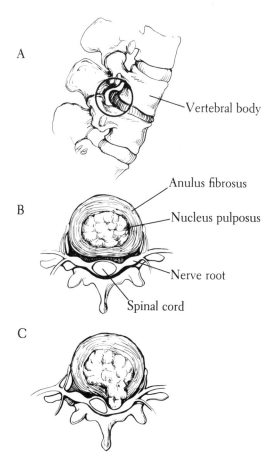

FIGURE 82. *Herniated (slipped) disc. (A) Posterior protrusion of the disc into the spinal cord canal. (B) Cross-section of the normal disc. (C) Protruding disc impinges on the spinal cord nerve root.*

supine on a firm supporting surface. The knees may be drawn up on a pillow or rolled blanket. All possible lifting and forward bending should be discontinued. The victim should take aspirin, ibuprofen, or naproxen to control inflammation, and pain medicine as necessary. Gentle massage and the application of moist heat or a heating pad are often soothing.

If one of the cushioning discs that lie between the vertebrae has been injured, additional symptoms may be noted, which include numbness and/or tingling of parts of the leg (indicates impingement of the disc upon a nerve root arising from the spinal cord), shooting pains through the buttocks and posterior leg (indicates irritation [sciatica] of the sciatic nerve), weakness of the legs, constipation, or difficulty with urination (Fig. 82). The immediate treatment is the same as for muscular back strain. A physician should be seen as soon as possible.

Disorders of the Kidneys and Bladder

THE urinary tract is commonly subject to infections, kidney stones, or injury. By far the most common problem is bladder infection, followed by kidney infections and stones.

BLADDER INFECTION

Bladder infections occur frequently in females, particularly children, because the shorter female urethra does not protect the bladder from bacteria as efficiently as does the male organ. A person with a bladder infection complains of discomfort (sharp pain, cramping, or burning) upon urination, frequent urination, difficulty initiating urination, lower abdominal cramping, and occasional blood in the urine, which may be as severe as small clots. Similar symptoms may be suffered by males who harbor infections in the prostate gland. Treatment involves the administration of antibiotics, and increased fluid intake. Because many antibiotics are well concentrated in the urine, there are a number of acceptable treatment regimens. For the sake of simplicity, the female patient may be treated with ampicillin 500 mg 4 times a day or trimethoprim with sulfamethoxazole (Septra or Bactrim) 1 double-strength tablet twice a day for 10 days. An alternative drug is norfloxacin (Noroxin) 400 mg twice a day. Chlamydia are bacteria-like "germs" that are increasingly the cause of reproductive-tract infections in women and, very frequently, genitourinary-tract infections in men. Because the penicillins (such as ampicillin) are not effective against Chlamydia, any male with a bladder or prostate infection should be treated with tetracycline (500 mg 4 times a day) or trimethoprim with sulfamethoxazole (1 double-strength tablet twice a day) for 2 weeks. Any male who develops a bladder or prostate infection should be seen by a physician when he returns from his journey.

KIDNEY INFECTION

Kidney infection is considerably more serious than bladder infection. Symptoms may include all of those for bladder infection, as well as flank or lower back pain, severe abdominal pain, fever, chills, nausea and vomiting, weakness, and cloudy urine with a foul odor. The back pain is characterized as aching, and may be exquisite when one punches gently just under the ribs adjacent to the spine.

The field treatment is just the same as for bladder infection. However, the patient is more ill and may require hospitalization for intravenous antibiotics. Therefore, anyone who is suspected to have a kidney infection should be evacuated immediately.

KIDNEY STONES

See page 116.

BLOOD IN THE URINE

Blood in the urine is caused by bladder and kidney infections, the passage of stones, blunt or penetrating injuries to the flank (kidney) region, or by tumors of the urinary tract. After heavy exertion or high fever, a person may break down small amounts of muscle tissue, and release myoglobin (an oxygen-carrying protein found in muscle) into the bloodstream. In cases of burns, severe injuries, or certain infections, red blood cells can be destroyed and will release their oxygen-containing protein (hemoglobin) into the bloodstream. Hemoglobin and myoglobin are filtered through the kidneys and may be concentrated in the urine, giving it a pink to reddish-brown hue. If the urine is not made dilute (by drinking large amounts of fluid to increase the urine volume), the concentration of these pigments in the kidney can clog the filtration system and cause sudden kidney failure. Although after vigorous exercise some individuals may normally pass a small amount of reddish urine, any person who develops darkened urine after fever or exertion should be placed at maximal rest, cooled to a normal body temperature (see page 235), encouraged to drink as much fluid as possible, and rapidly transported to a medical facility. If you are more than 24 hours away from a doctor, the urine rapidly clears with rest and increased fluids, and the patient appears in good health, the journey may continue.

Urine can be discolored by the ingestion of chemical agents, such as urinary tract anesthetics (blue-green or orange), beets (pink-red), or bile pigments (brown, seen with hepatitis).

Psychiatric Emergencies

THE wilderness experience can be quite stressful, and occasionally a member of the party may behave in an unusual fashion. This may be directly related to the events at hand or reflect an underlying psychiatric disorder. It is imperative that someone recognize warning signs early and evacuate anyone who cannot retain mental stability, to avoid placing the impaired individual and his traveling companions at risk for injury.

ANXIETY

Anxiety is the most common psychiatric symptom, and may range from appropriate and adaptive minor doubts about success to a full-blown panic reaction. Minor anxiety is expressed as general discomfort about a situation; the excessive worrier may become timid and withdrawn, and may lose his enthusiasm for participation. His anxiety may be clothed in criticism of plans or refusal to cooperate. It is important that every member of the expedition voice fears and objections at the outset, so as not to be caught in a panic when performing hazardous crossings or rescues. The treatment is reassurance and support. Frequently, practice sessions that build up to a completed effort will relieve anxiety and improve the performance of the group. In no case should anyone be made to feel ashamed of his fears. Rather, the leader should seek to help the victim conquer them.

Approach all problems directly; do not beat around the bush. Most persons do much better if fear is identified and managed than if it is never confronted.

PANIC

Panic is anxiety taken to the extreme. The victim loses all judgment and becomes consumed with efforts at escape and self-preservation. Panic renders the victim unable to make reasonable decisions and immediately places him and all around him at risk for injury. The rescuer must assume a strong authoritative posture with the panic victim, and assure him in no uncertain terms that the situation is under control and that the panic behavior is intolerable. Depending on the nature of the situation, this can be done with verbal explanations, convincing arguments, or demonstrations of safety. If the victim places any other individuals at immediate risk for injury, he should be subdued with force if necessary.

Persons who use cocaine or who smoke marijuana or phencyclidine (angel dust, PCP) cigarettes occasionally suffer from panic reactions. The management of these reactions is no different from that previously outlined, with the exception being the risk of true violent behavior from a person under the influence of PCP. If a person appears to be under the influence of psychotropic drugs, do your best to keep him from hurting anyone, but be careful not to become injured in the process.

HYPERVENTILATION

One manifestation of anxiety that verges on panic is the hyperventilation syndrome, in which the victim, overcome with his fears, begins to breathe at an inappropriately rapid rate (40–100 times per minute). This causes the level of carbon dioxide in the blood to fall precipitously and induces dizziness, fainting spells, numbness and tingling in the hands, feet, and around the mouth, muscle spasm in the hands and wrists, and, occasionally, seizures. If the rescuer is certain that the victim is hyperventilating because of anxiety (that is, there is no reason to suspect a collapsed lung, pneumonia, etc.), he should place a paper bag or similar object over the victim's mouth and nose for about 5 minutes. The victim breathes in and out of this bag, and rebreathes expired carbon dioxide, allowing normalization of the level in the bloodstream and correction of the symptoms. At the same time, the victim should be reassured that he will be all right, and an attempt should be made to identify the cause of the anxiety.

DEPRESSION

Depression occurs in the outdoor setting in response to situations that are perceived as hopeless. Some victims who are injured, lose their way, or who are weakened by starvation and exposure may lose the will to continue. They become listless, fatigued out of proportion to their physical condition, uninterested, inattentive, without appetite, sleepy, and tearful. Clearly, the rescuer must encourage all party members to maintain their survival instincts, to continue to help others and to help themselves. In a cold environment, it is important to remember that hypothermia (see page 221) is a significant cause of apathy and should be corrected if possible. An individual with chronic depression may go on a vacation trip with the enthusiastic expectation that his psychiatric disease may be alleviated or that his most recent depression has lifted. The sudden realization that such expectations are not fulfilled may put that person at risk for severe mood depression. Do not be afraid to inquire about a past history of psychiatric illness.

REACTION TO AN INJURY OR ILLNESS

Persons react differently to stress, and may become irrational, angry, apathetic, confused, or withdrawn following an accident or harsh environmental exposure. The most common reaction, given the presence of a strong leader, is to become dependent. It is crucial for the rescuer to bolster the victim's self-confidence and self-esteem at every opportunity, for it may take extraordinary physical and mental effort to survive a catastrophe in the wilderness.

Different individuals react differently to the same situation, so try to individualize your approach to each person. To best understand the changing needs of victims and families, try to maintain regular dialogue intended solely for the purpose of psychological support. Stay with the victim as much as possible. Use frequent touch and reassurances to relay your sense of concern and to comfort him. As best possible, involve the victim in his treatment and rescue, so that his thoughts are attuned to survival rather than to fear or grief.

When you are under stress, do your best to be supportive to others with less emotional control. Anger is rarely successful and commonly worsens an already difficult situation.

Equally important, the rescuer must constantly be alert for true medical problems that masquerade as psychological disorders. The uninterested victim may be hypothermic, the belligerent climber hyperthermic, the intoxicated hiker hypoglycemic, or the irritable child stricken with acute mountain sickness.

PART ✿ FOUR

DISORDERS RELATED TO
SPECIFIC ENVIRONMENTS

Injuries and Illnesses Due to Cold

COLD injuries include hypothermia, frostbite, frostnip, immersion foot (chilblains), and trench foot. The appropriate first aid can save a life or limb; mismanagement can be catastrophic.

HYPOTHERMIA (LOWERED BODY TEMPERATURE)

Mild hypothermia is defined as a core (rectally measured) body temperature less than 98.6°F (37°C) and greater than 95°F (35°C); moderate hypothermia is defined as a core body temperature less than 95°F (35°C) and greater than 90°F (32.2°C); severe hypothermia is defined as core body temperature less than 90°F (32.2°C). The body generates heat through metabolic processes that can be maximized with involuntary shivering to roughly 5 times the basal level (up to 10 times with maximal exercise). However, shivering is abolished after a few hours of exposure, because of exhaustion and depletion of muscle energy supplies. At the time when a victim loses the ability to shiver, the cooling process becomes quite rapid. Skin, surface fat, and superficial muscle layers then act as an insulating "shell" for the "core" of vital organs (heart, lungs, liver, kidneys, etc.). Normal skin temperature in cool weather is 90–93°F (32.2–33.9°C), which can drop to 70–73°F (21.1–22.8°C) before core cooling begins.

Heat is lost from the body to the environment by direct contact (conduction), air movement (convection), infrared energy emission (radiation), the conversion of liquid (sweat) to a gas (evaporation), and the exhalation of heated air from the lungs (respiration). It is important to note that heat loss via conduction is increased fivefold in wet clothes and twenty-fivefold in cold-water immersion. Windchill refers to the increase in the rate of heat loss (convection) that would occur when a victim is exposed to moving air (Fig. 83). This chill can be compounded further if the victim is wet (conduction, convection, and evaporation).

Immersion hypothermia refers to the particular case in which a victim has become hypothermic because of sudden immersion into cold water. A person immersed in cold water loses heat approximately 25 times as fast as does someone exposed to cold air. A sudden plunge into cold water causes the victim to hyperventilate (see page 216), which may lead to confusion, muscle spasm, and loss of consciousness. The cold water rapidly cools the muscles and the victim loses the ability to swim or tread water. Any person pulled from cold water should be presumed to be hypothermic.

The progression of hypothermia leads to predictable physiologic responses, which roughly correspond to different body temperatures. Although not invariable, the signs and symptoms are as follows:

95–98.6°F (35–37°C): Sensation of cold; shivering; increased heart rate; urge to urinate; slight incoordination in hand movements.

90–95°F (32.2–35°C): Increasing muscular incoordination; stumbling gait; decreased or absent shivering; weakness; apathy/drowsiness/confusion; slurred speech.

85–90°F (29.4–32.2°C): Loss of shivering; confusion progressing to coma; inability to walk or follow commands; paradoxical undressing (inappropriate behavior); complaints of loss of vision.

Below 85°F (29.4°C): Rigid muscles, decreased blood pressure, heart rate, and respirations; dilated pupils; appearance of death.

THE FIRST PRINCIPLE OF THERAPY IS TO SUSPECT THE DISORDER. *Any person who is found in a cold environment should be suspected of suffering from hypothermia.* The definition of cold environment is variable. A person who is wet,

WIND SPEED (MPH)	OUTSIDE AIR TEMPERATURE (°F)																
	35	30	25	20	15	10	5	0	−5	−10	−15	−20	−25	−30	−35	−40	−45
	EQUIVALENT TEMPERATURE (°F)																
5	32	27	22	16	11	6	0	−5	−10	−15	−21	−26	−31	−36	−42	−47	−52
10	22	16	10	3	−3	−9	−15	−22	−27	−34	−40	−46	−52	−58	−64	−71	−77
15	16	9	2	−5	−11	−18	−25	−31	−38	−45	−51	−58	−65	−72	−78	−85	−92
20	12	4	−3	−10	−17	−24	−31	−39	−46	−53	−60	−67	−74	−81	−88	−95	−103
25	8	1	−7	−15	−22	−29	−36	−44	−51	−59	−66	−74	−81	−88	−96	−103	−110
30	6	−2	−10	−18	−25	−33	−41	−49	−56	−64	−71	−79	−86	−93	−101	−109	−116
35	4	−4	−12	−20	−27	−35	−43	−52	−58	−67	−74	−82	−89	−97	−105	−113	−120
40	3	−5	−13	−21	−29	−37	−45	−53	−60	−69	−76	−84	−92	−100	−107	−115	−123
45	2	−6	−14	−22	−30	−38	−46	−54	−62	−70	−78	−85	−93	−102	−109	−117	−125

FIGURE 83. Windchill determination. To determine windchill, find the ambient air temperature on the top line, then read down the column to the line that corresponds with the current wind speed. Example: When the air temperature is 10°F and the wind speed is 20 miles per hour, the rate of heat loss is equivalent to minus 24°F under calm conditions.

improperly dressed, and intoxicated with alcohol can become hypothermic in 70°F weather. Do not use yourself as an indicator of warmth — you may be perfectly comfortable when your companion is lapsing into hypothermia.

Unless the victim is found frozen in a block of ice or has been recently pulled from frigid waters, the most likely clue to a hypothermic state is altered mental status. The winter hiker who gradually loses interest and lags behind the group ("Just leave me behind, I'll catch up"), who dresses inappropriately for the weather or begins to undress, or who begins to stumble and make slightly inappropriate remarks, should be immediately evaluated for low body temperature. *Never leave a victim of even mild hypothermia to fend for himself.*

THE SECOND PRINCIPLE OF THERAPY IS TO MEASURE THE VICTIM'S TEMPERATURE, IF POSSIBLE. This must be done with a thermometer calibrated to read below 94°F (34.4°C), which is the cutoff for most standard oral thermometers. Hypothermia thermometers with a range of 75–105°F (23.9–40.5°C) are available from Dyna-Med, Carolina Biological Products, and Zeal G. H., Ltd. (see pages 331–332). Temperature should be measured rectally. Oral and axillary (armpit) temperatures are unreliable in this situation, and should be used only to screen for low body temperature. That is, if they are normal, the victim will have a normal core temperature; however, if they are low, they may grossly understate how cold the victim really is, and should be followed by a rectal measurement.

Before proceeding further, it is important to mention that unless the victim has suffered a full cardiopulmonary arrest, the hypothermia itself may not be harmful. That is, unless tissue is actually frozen, cold is in many ways protective to the brain and heart. However, if a hypothermic victim is improperly transported or rewarmed, the process may precipitate ventricular fibrillation, in which the heart does not contract, but quivers in such a fashion as to be unable to pump blood. THE BURDEN OF RESCUE IS TO TRANSPORT AND REWARM THE VIC-

TIM IN SUCH A WAY SO AS NOT TO PRECIPITATE VEN-
TRICULAR FIBRILLATION.

The following general rules of therapy apply to all cases:

1. Handle all patients gently. Rough handling can cause the heart to fibrillate (cause a cardiac arrest).

2. If necessary, protect the airway (see page 18) and cervical spine (see page 31).

3. Prevent the victim from becoming any colder. Provide a shelter. Remove all his wet clothing and replace it with dry clothing. Don't give away all of your own clothing, however, or *you* may become hypothermic. Be sure to cover the victim's head and neck. Insulate the victim from above *and below* with blankets. If possible, put him in a sleeping bag sandwiched between two rescuers. Do not count on a sleeping bag to be adequately pre-warmed by a normothermic rescuer's body heat. In this situation, no heat is really contributed by the bag itself. Hot water in bottles, *well insulated with clothing to prevent skin burns*, may be placed next to the victim in areas of high heat transfer, such as the neck, chest wall, and groin.

4. Do not attempt to warm the patient by vigorous exercise, rubbing the arms and legs, or immersing in warm water. This is "rough handling," and can cause the heart to fibrillate if the victim is severely hypothermic.

5. Seek assistance as soon as possible.

Mild Hypothermia
(core temperature above 95°F/35°C)

The mild hypothermic is awake, can answer questions intelligently, and complains of being cold. He may or may not be shivering. PREVENT THE PATIENT FROM BECOMING ANY COLDER. GENTLY remove wet items of clothing and replace them with dry garments. If no dry replacements are available, the clothed victim should be covered with a waterproof tarp or poncho to prevent evaporative heat loss. Cover the head, neck, hands, and feet. Insulate the patient both above and below with blankets. If the patient is coherent and can swallow without difficulty, encourage the ingestion of warm sweetened fluids. If a dry sleeping bag is available, one or more rescuers should climb in with the victim and share body heat. Do not apply commercial heat packs directly to the skin; they must be wrapped in blankets or towels to avoid serious burns.

Moderate Hypothermia
(core temperature 90–95°F/32.2–35°C)

The moderate hypothermic has become apathetic and mildly confused, wishes to be left behind, and is uncooperative. Speech is often slurred and logic is on the wane. The victim rapidly becomes uncoordinated and clumsy, often stumbling. He has ceased to shiver, and shows signs of muscle stiffness. Unless you have a thermometer to measure this victim's temperature, you must assume that he is severely hypothermic, or will soon become so. Follow the directions for the mild hypothermic, with the added caution that it is best not to allow this victim to walk about until he is fully alert. Do not give the victim fluids to drink until he becomes wide awake and understands what is going on.

Severe Hypothermia
(core temperature less than 90°F/32.2°C)

Depending on the body temperature, a victim who appears to be asleep may be in a complete coma. Below 65°F (18.3°C), man becomes like a snake, and takes on the temperature of the environment. Examine the patient carefully and gently for signs of life. Listen closely to the nose and mouth and examine chest movement for spontaneous breathing. Feel gently at the groin (femoral artery) and neck (carotid artery) for a weak and/or slow pulse (see page 25).

If the patient shows any signs of life (movement, pulse, respirations), do not initiate the chest compressions of CPR. If the victim is breathing regularly, even at a subnormal rate, then his heart is beating. Because hypothermia is protective, the victim does not require a "normal" heart rate, respiratory rate, and blood pressure. Pumping on the chest unnecessarily is "rough handling," and may induce ventricular fibrillation.

If the victim is breathing at a rate of less than 6–7 breaths per minute, you should begin mouth-to-mouth breathing (see page 24).

If help is on the way (within 1–2 hours) and there are no signs of life whatsoever, or if you are in doubt, you should begin standard CPR (see page 26). If possible, continue CPR until the victim reaches the hospital. There have been documented cases of hypothermic victims' "miraculous" recoveries from complete cardiopulmonary arrest after prolonged resuscitation, presumably because of the protective effect of the cold. However, all of these victims were ultimately resurrected in the hospital, after they had been rewarmed.

THE SEVERE HYPOTHERMIC CANNOT BE REWARMED IN THE FIELD. IF A HYPOTHERMIC VICTIM SUFFERS WHAT YOU DETERMINE TO BE A CARDIAC ARREST IN THE WILDERNESS, transport should be the first priority. If enough rescuers are present to allow CPR and simultaneous transport, then do both. If you are the only person present, do not bother with CPR, because you will not be able to resuscitate the victim until he is rewarmed. Your only hope is that the victim is in a cold-protected state ("metabolic icebox"), and that you can extricate him (as gently as possible!) to sophisticated medical attention. Remember, no one is dead until he is warm and dead.

In any case of severe hypothermia, transport should be undertaken as soon as possible. Take care to cover the patient with dry blankets, and to handle him as gently as possible. Rapid rewarming or restoration of circulation will release cold acidotic blood from the limbs back to the core organs, which may cause a profound deterioration of the victim.

A *Special Note About the Victim of Cold-Water Drowning*

If a victim is pulled from icy waters, and appears to be clinically dead (fixed dilated pupils, no respirations, no detectable pulse), perform CPR until a qualified medical person is available to intervene. Because of the physiology of cold-water immersion, the victim may be sufficiently protected to survive the event. DO NOT GIVE UP until you are exhausted, or the situation becomes hopeless.

Prevention of Hypothermia

1. Carry adequate food and thermal wear, such as Thermax, Capilene, and/or polypropylene or wool undergarments. Anticipate the worst possible weather conditions. Dress in layers, so that clothing may be adjusted for overcooling, overheating, perspiration, and external moisture. Use a foundation layer to wick moisture from the body to outer layers. Add an insulation layer to provide incremental warmth. Carry windproof and waterproof outer garments, mittens or gloves, socks, and a hat (in very cold weather, over 60% of generated heat may be lost by radiation from the uncovered head). Stay dry. Carry properly rated (for the cold) sleeping bags with Hollofil II, Quallofil, or down stuffing.

2. Do not exhaust yourself in cold weather. Avoid becoming overheated and perspiring in cold weather. Do not sit down in the snow without insulation under you.

3. Seek shelter in times of extreme cold and high winds. Don't sit on cold rocks or metal. Insulate yourself from the ground with a pad, backpack, log, or tree limb.

4. Do not become dehydrated. In the cold, dehydration is caused by evaporation from the respiratory tree, increased urination, and inadequate fluid intake. Drink at least 3–4 liters of fluid

daily. Ingesting snow is an inefficient way to replace water, as it worsens hypothermia. Do not skip meals. Do not consume alcoholic beverages in cold weather. They cause an initial sensation of warmth because of dilatation of superficial skin blood vessels, but this same effect markedly contributes to heat loss.

FROSTBITE

Frostbite is an injury that is caused by the actual freezing of tissues. Factors that predispose a person to frostbite include poor circulation (caused by previous cold injuries, cigarette smoking, alcohol ingestion, diseases of the blood vessels, constricting garments, poorly fitted boots, old age) and extremes of cold exposure. Windchill contributes markedly to frostbite risk. For instance, at an air temperature of 20°F (minus 6°C), a 45 mph wind causes the same rate of heat loss as a 2 mph breeze at minus 22°F (about minus 30°C). During exposure, once the temperature of the skin drops below 50°F (10°C), the skin becomes numb, and injury may go unnoticed until it is too late. Tissue freezes at or below a temperature of 28°F (minus 2°C).

The injury of frostbite may be present in a number of stages, much like a burn injury. These are recognized as:

First degree — numbness, redness, swelling
Second degree — superficial blistering
Third degree — deep blistering
Fourth degree — extremely deep involvement (including bone)

The major immediate symptom of a frostbite injury is numbness, occasionally preceded by itching or prickling. The frostbitten area will appear to be white, with a yellow or bluish waxy tint. If the injury is superficial, as commonly occurs on the face, the skin is firm and may indent with a touch, as the underlying tissue is still soft and pliable. If the injury is deep, the skin may feel hard and actually be frozen solid. The most common areas to be affected are the fingertips and toes (particularly in cramped footwear), followed by earlobes, nose tips, and other exposed skin. These parts have little heat-generating capability and no significant insulation.

Rapid rewarming is the standard of therapy. However, *do not thaw out a frostbitten body part if it cannot be kept thawed.* In other words, if you come upon a lost hiker 10 miles back in the woods who has frostbitten toes, do not use your stove to heat water to thaw his feet, if he will then have to put his wet boots back on and hike out, in the process refreezing his toes. Frostbitten tissue is damaged and is prone to reinjury; refreezing causes damage that will far exceed the initial frostbite injury. It is much better to walk out on frostbitten toes until safety is reached than to thaw and allow refreezing.

Once you have reached a location where you can be sure that refreezing will not occur, immerse the frostbitten part in water heated to 108°F (42.2°C). Do not induce a burn injury by using hotter water; 108°F water can be estimated by considering it to be water in which normal skin can be submersed for a prolonged period with minimal discomfort. Never use a numb frostbitten finger to test water temperature. Circulate the water to allow thawing to proceed as rapidly as possible. If the skin is frozen to mittens or metal, use heated water to remove them. NEVER REWARM THE SKIN BY VIGOROUS RUBBING, OR BY USING THE HEAT OF A CAMPFIRE, CAMP STOVE, OR CAR EXHAUST, as you will most certainly damage the tissues.

Thawing of the skin usually requires 30–45 minutes; it is complete when the skin is soft and pliable and color and sensation have returned. Moderate burning pain may occur during the last 5–10 minutes of rewarming. If the victim is hypothermic, thawing should not be undertaken until the core body temperature has reached 95°F (35°C) (see page 225). If blisters are present, leave them intact. After thawing the skin, protect it with fluffy sterile bandages (aloe vera lotion, gel, or cream may be applied if available) and transport the victim to an appropriate facility. Administer ibuprofen 400–600 mg or 1 aspirin 3 times a day. If the frostbite involves the feet, try to minimize walking. Do not allow tobacco smoking or the drinking of alcohol.

Prevention of Frostbite

1. Wear adequate properly fitted clothing. Take care to cover the hands, feet, and face (particularly the nose and ears). Wear mittens in preference to gloves, to decrease the surface area available for heat loss from the fingers. Carry pocket, hand, and/or foot warmers and use them properly. Choices include fuel-burning warmers or chemical packs, such as Heat Wave, reusable sodium acetate thermal packs (Eptek, Inc.; see page 332), or air-activated, single-use Mycoal Grabber hand and pocket warmer (John Wagner Associates, Inc.; see page 333).
2. Keep clothing dry.
3. Do not touch bare metal with bare skin. Remember that certain liquids (such as gasoline) become colder than frozen water before they freeze, and can cause frostbite. Cover all metal handles with cloth, tape, or leather.
4. Do not maintain one position in the cold for a prolonged period of time. Avoid cramped quarters.
5. Wear sunscreens with a cream or grease base to prevent windburn.

FROSTNIP

Frostnip is reversible ice-crystal formation that occurs on the surface of the skin. It is distinct from frostbite in that actual freezing of the tissues does not occur. However, because the symptoms (numbness, frosted appearance) may resemble those of frostbite, it should be taken as a serious warning that the skin is not adequately protected.

IMMERSION FOOT (CHILBLAINS)

Immersion foot (affecting lower extremities) and chilblains (affecting hands and feet) are similar disorders caused by prolonged exposure to cold water. Symptoms include numbness, tingling, and burning pain. These progress to skin numbness and muscle cramps. The skin looks red at first, and then becomes mottled or pale with a gray-blue tint. Eventually, the skin becomes infected, with oozing, blisters, and occasional gangrene. Trench foot is a milder version that is due to having the foot confined and damp for prolonged periods.

If immersion foot (chilblains) is suspected, the limb should be carefully cleansed and dried, and rewarmed in an environment where it can be kept warm. If left unattended, immersion foot, trench foot, or chilblains can lead to prolonged disability. Seek immediate medical attention.

SNOW BLINDNESS

See page 149.

Illnesses and Injuries Due to Heat

THIS section will consider the various ways in which high environmental temperatures may affect the otherwise healthy individual. Burn injuries are discussed on page 90.

Human core temperature is maintained at 98.6°F (37°C), with little variation from individual to individual. Heat is generated by all of the metabolic processes that contribute to life, from the blink of an eyelid to the completion of a marathon, and must be shed constantly to avoid a condition of overheating. The resting person generates enough heat (60 kilocalories) to raise body temperature 1.8°F (1°C) per hour; vigorous exercise can increase heat production tenfold. As outlined in the section on hypothermia (see page 221), heat is lost to the environment through conduction, convection, radiation, and evaporation. In the normal situation, the skin is the largest heat-wasting organ, and radiates approximately 65% of the daily heat loss. The skin is also largely responsible for evaporation (of sweat); extreme humidity impedes this process and greatly diminishes human temperature control. (The National Weather Service heat index, Figure 84, roughly correlates air temperature, relative humidity, and "apparent temperature.") When maximally effective, the complete evaporation of 1 liter of sweat from the skin removes 600 kilocalories of heat (equivalent to the total heat produced with strenuous exercise in 1 hour).

When heat control mechanisms are overloaded, the body responds unfavorably. As opposed to hypothermia, in which moderate cooling may offer a protective effect, the syndromes of true hyperthermia (in which core body temperature is measurably elevated) can rapidly become life threatening, as the heat destroys the vital organs, and dismembers chemical systems essential to life. Therefore, it is crucial to be familiar with heat illness, and to be prepared to respond promptly and decisively.

HEAT EXHAUSTION AND HEATSTROKE

Heat exhaustion and heatstroke are part of the same process, but of differing severity. Heat exhaustion is illness caused by an elevation of body temperature that does not result in permanent damage; heatstroke is life threatening and can permanently disable the victim. I will define each by symptoms and then discuss the therapy for management of the overheated individual.

The signs and symptoms of heat exhaustion are minor confu-

	AIR TEMPERATURE (°F)										
	70	75	80	85	90	95	100	105	110	115	120
RELATIVE HUMIDITY (%)	APPARENT TEMPERATURE (°F)										
0	64	69	73	78	83	87	91	95	99	103	107
10	65	70	75	80	85	90	95	100	105	111	116
20	66	72	77	82	87	93	99	105	112	120	130
30	67	73	78	84	90	96	104	113	123	135	148
40	68	74	79	86	93	101	110	122	137	151	
50	69	75	81	88	96	107	120	135	150		
60	70	76	82	90	100	114	132	149			
70	70	77	85	93	106	124	144				
80	71	78	86	97	113	136	157				
90	71	79	88	102	122	150	170				
100	72	80	91	108	133	166					

FIGURE 84. *Heat index. Humidity contributes greatly to the accumulation of heat; when both are excessive, human temperature control is diminished.*

sion, irrational behavior, a rapid weak pulse, dizziness, nausea, diarrhea, headache, and mild temperature elevation (up to 105°F or 40.5°C). It is important to note that SWEATING MAY BE PRESENT OR ABSENT and that THE SKIN OF THE VICTIM MAY FEEL COOL TO THE TOUCH. It is the core temperature that is elevated and that must be measured (rectally).

The signs and symptoms of heatstroke are extreme confusion (in many cases, unconsciousness), low blood pressure or shock, seizures, increased bleeding (bruising, vomiting blood, bloody urine), diarrhea, vomiting, shortness of breath, darkened ("machine oil") urine, and major core body temperature elevation (up to 115°F/46.1°C has been reported in the medical literature). Again, it is important to note that *sweating may be present or absent*. It is rare for someone to feel cool externally when his temperature exceeds 105°F (45°C), but it is not impossible. *You must take a rectal temperature.*

The skin will usually be warm or hot to the touch when a victim suffers heat exhaustion or heatstroke, but, again, this is not absolutely reliable. *Carry a thermometer, so you can take a temperature.*

The most important aspect of therapy is to GET THE TEMPERATURE DOWN AS QUICKLY AS POSSIBLE. The body may lose its ability to control its own temperature at 106°F (41.1°C), so from there temperature can skyrocket.

IF YOU SUSPECT HEAT ILLNESS, MEASURE THE TEMPERATURE. Use a rectal thermometer. If a thermometer is not available, and you are fairly certain that the victim is suffering from heat exhaustion or heatstroke, proceed with therapy.

Manage the airway (see page 18) and administer oxygen, 10 liters per minute, by face mask if available. Do not give liquids by mouth unless the victim is awake and coherent. Cooled liquids do not assist the cooling process enough to risk choking the uncooperative victim.

Cooling the Victim

1. Remove the victim from obvious sources of heat. Shield the victim from direct sunlight and remove his clothing.

2. Wet the victim down and begin to fan him vigorously. Evaporation is a very efficient method of heat removal. Use cool or tepid water. If electric fans are available, use them. Do not be concerned with shivering, so long as you continue aggressively to cool the victim. *Do not sponge the victim with alcohol.*

3. If ice is available, place ice packs in the armpits, behind the neck, and in the groin. There is some controversy surrounding total body immersion in ice water for hyperthermia, one argument being that such action causes constriction of superficial blood vessels and redirection of hot blood to the core circulation, temporarily increasing core temperature. This is of no concern in a life-threatening field situation. If the only method available for cooling is immersion in a cold mountain stream, do it.

4. Recheck the temperature every 5–10 minutes, to avoid cooling much below 98.6°F (37°C). When you have cooled the victim to 99.5–100°F (37.5–37.8°C), taper the cooling effort. After the victim is cooled, recheck the temperature every 30 minutes for 3–4 hours, as there will often be a rebound temperature rise.

5. *Do not use aspirin or acetaminophen unless the victim has an infection.* These drugs are used to combat fever caused by the release of chemical substances from infectious agents (bacteria, viruses, etc.) into the bloodstream. These chemicals affect the portion of the brain (hypothalamus) that serves as the body's thermostat, causing it to raise the body temperature. Aspirin or acetaminophen acts to block this chemical interaction in the brain, and thus eliminate the fever. If elevated body temperature is not caused by an infection (fever), then aspirin will not work and may in fact be harmful, as it increases the incidence of bleeding disorders.

6. If the victim is alert, begin to correct dehydration.

MUSCLE CRAMPS

Muscle cramps in a warm environment are an accompaniment of overuse (see page 205) or of water and salt losses in the individual who exerts strenuously. A well-trained athlete can lose 2–3 liters of sweat per hour (a potential 20-gram sodium loss each day). In most cases, cramps are caused by replacement of water without adequate salt intake. Treatment for muscle cramps consists of gentle motion and stretching of the affected muscles, accompanied by adequate fluid and salt replacement. This may be done by drinking water and balanced salt solutions such as Gatorade, ERG, Exceed, or Pripps Plus prior to and during heavy exertion. With proper fluid and electrolyte replacement, salt tablets (which irritate the stomach lining) are usually unnecessary.

HEAT SWELLING

In warmer climates, normal persons, particularly the elderly, may suffer from swelling of the feet and ankles. This effect is noted after prolonged periods of walking or sitting, and usually occurs in individuals who have no underlying heart disease. Often the swelling will disappear as the person becomes adjusted to the warm environment (several days). The swelling is painless, and there is no sign of infection (redness). Body temperature is not elevated.

Treatment for heat swelling is to minimize periods of walking, and to use support stockings (with a minimum length to mid-thigh). The legs should be kept elevated whenever possible. There is no reason to use fluid pills (diuretics). If the sufferer is short of breath or otherwise ill in association with the leg swelling, he should seek the advice of a physician.

FAINTING

Fainting has many causes (see page 134). Fainting due to heat exposure occurs when a person (particularly an elder) adapts by dilating blood vessels in the skin and superficial muscles in order to deliver warm blood to the surface of the body, where the excess energy can be delivered back to the environment. The expansion of the superficial blood vessels allows a greater-than-normal proportion of the circulating blood volume to be away from the central circulation (which supplies, among other organs, the brain). This lack of sufficient central pressure is worsened when a person is on his feet for a prolonged period of time, as gravity allows a significant blood volume to collect in the lower extremities. Combined with fatigue and mild dehydration, the diversion of blood leads to a fainting episode, as not enough blood (with oxygen and glucose) is pumped to the brain.

A victim who has suffered a fainting episode in the heat should be examined for any head or neck injuries, as well as other possible breaks or cuts. Other causes of fainting must be considered (low blood sugar, abnormal heart rhythm, etc.). If the faint is due to the heat, the victim will reawaken shortly, as the horizontal position returns blood to the brain and solves the major problem. In general, body temperature is not elevated.

The victim of a fainting spell due to heat should be rested in a horizontal position for 15–30 minutes, and should not immediately assume a standing posture without first sitting for 5 minutes. He should be encouraged to consume a pint or two of cool sweetened liquid (such as Gatorade). To avoid further episodes, efforts should be made to avoid dehydration, missing meals, or standing in one position for a prolonged period. Support hose may be of benefit, as is regular leg muscle exercise. The victim should learn to recognize the warning signs of a fainting spell, which include dizziness, light-headedness, nausea, weakness, sweating, blurred vision, or seeing flashing lights. When these warning signs occur, the victim should immediately assume a horizontal position or should sit and lower his head to between his knees.

AVOIDING HEAT ILLNESS

To avoid serious heat illness, the traveler is advised to:

1. Avoid dehydration. Drink at least 1 pint to 1 quart of liquid with adequate electrolyte supplementation (see below) each hour during heavy exercise with sweating in a hot environment. ADEQUATE WATER INGESTED DURING EXERCISE IS NOT HARMFUL, DOES NOT CAUSE CRAMPS, AND WILL

PREVENT A LARGE PERCENTAGE OF CASES OF HEAT ILLNESS. If the urine becomes darkened or scant, then fluid requirements are not being met. As a general rule, persons outdoors should consume at least 3 quarts of fluid each day; with moderate activity, this should be increased to at least 4–5 quarts. Do not rely upon thirst as an absolute guide to fluid requirements. In general, merely quenching thirst does not adequately replace fluid losses in heat stress (or high altitude) conditions.

With a normal diet, there is no need to take salt tablets; electrolyte requirements can be met with food salted to taste. Electrolyte- and sugar-enriched drinks such as Gatorade, Squincher, or Bodyfuel should be used when normal meals cannot be eaten or when sweating is excessive (during athletic training or military forced marching). The normal daily diet may be safely supplemented during times of extreme sweating (greater than ½–1 quart per hour) with 5–10 grams of sodium (the normal daily dietary intake is 4–6 grams; most adults would be fine with 1–3 grams) and 2–4 grams of potassium. Supplemental salt is advised when weight loss from sweating exceeds 5 pounds in a single session, particularly early in the acclimatization period, when salt losses in sweat are great. Consume ½ gram (¹⁄₁₀ teaspoon) of sodium chloride (table salt) with a pint of water for each pound of weight loss over 5 pounds. A home brew (see page 164) may be used if Gatorade is not available. If large quantities of electrolytes are lost and not replaced (for instance, if large quantities of water are consumed without salt), a person can become quite ill. Similarly, salt without water can be harmful. Salt tablets can be very irritating to the stomach, and should not be used unless salt-containing solutions are not available. Coffee, tea, and alcohol-containing beverages cause increased fluid loss through excessive urination and should be avoided.

2. Be watchful of the very young and very old. Their bodies do not regulate body temperature efficiently and can rapidly become too hot or too cold. Do not bundle up infants in warm weather.

3. Stay in shape. Obesity, lack of conditioning, insufficient

rest, ingestion of alcohol, and illicit drugs all contribute to an increased risk for heat illness.

4. Condition yourself for the environment. Gradual increased exposure to work in a hot environment for a period of 10 days will allow an individual to acclimatize. Acclimatization is manifested as increased sweat volume with a decreased electrolyte concentration (more "efficient" sweating), greater peripheral blood vessel dilatation (more efficient heat loss), lowered heart rate, increased water and salt conservation by the kidneys, and enhanced metabolism of energy supplies. Eat potassium-rich vegetables and fruits, such as broccoli and bananas.

5. Wear clothing appropriate for the environment. Dress in layers, so that clothing can be added or shed as necessary. Keep out of the sun on a hot day, and wear a loosely fitted broad-brimmed hat. Do not wear plastic or rubber "sweat" suits in the heat.

Wildland Fires

THE wilderness adventurer or casual day hiker in a forest or timbered park may find himself face-to-face with a wildland fire. Dry timber, drought conditions, lightning storms, careless placement of campfires, and reckless behavior with flames lead to a large number of destructive blazes each year. The outdoor enthusiast should be prepared to protect himself and others in a confrontation with fire.

This section will discuss high-risk situations, survival techniques, and medical considerations. The sections on burns (see page 90), lightning injuries (see page 290), heat illness (see page 232), and inhalation injuries (see page 95) should be reviewed.

HIGH-RISK SITUATIONS

The risk for a wildland fire is increased under certain environmental conditions. Pay heed to posted warnings of fire hazard, and do not venture into the woods unprepared to escape. Be particularly cautious when:

1. There are drought conditions. Low humidity, higher air temperatures, and gusty winds create dry fuel for a fire.

2. You are in an area rich with abundant fuel, such as dead grass, pine needles, shrubs, fallen trees, etc.

3. You travel through gullies, canyons, along steep slopes, or other regions where wind and fuel are ideal for rapid advance of an established fire.

4. Fires have occurred recently in the vicinity.

STANDARD FIRE ENCOUNTER PRINCIPLES

The following basic principles are recommended for all people who deal with a wildland fire:

1. Have advance knowledge of weather conditions prior to undertaking an expedition. Do not travel in hazardous regions in times of high fire risk. Local ranger stations are the best source of information. NEVER PLAN AN EXTENDED JOURNEY WITHOUT LEAVING AN ITINERARY WITH THE PROPER AUTHORITIES.

2. At every campsite, take a few moments to prepare mentally for an evacuation, and plan at least two escape routes.

3. If a fire is in the area, pay attention to it. If there is any chance that it can involve your party, GET OUT EARLY.

4. If smoke or fire is seen at a distance, post a lookout to watch for any changes that might indicate increased danger.

5. In all situations, stay calm and act with authority. Give orders concisely and be sure that they are understood.

6. Do not attempt to fight the fire. Your first responsibility is

to evacuate all potential victims and provide necessary first aid. Leave fire fighting to professionals.

7. Do not sleep near a wildland fire. If the wind and fire direction change, you may be overcome with smoke and not be able to escape.

WHAT TO DO WHEN CAUGHT IN A WILDLAND FIRE

If you are caught in a fire, the following information may help you and others to survive:

1. Try not to panic. This is your most difficult task, but if anything will save your life, it will be a clear head.

2. If possible, don't move downhill toward a fire, as fires have a tendency to run uphill.

3. Unless the path of escape is clear, don't start running. Conserve your strength, and seek the flank of the fire. Continually observe changes in speed and direction of fire and smoke to choose travel away from fire hazards. Be alert, keep calm, and avoid injury from rolling or falling debris.

4. Enter a burned area, particularly an area with little fuel (grass or low shrubs). Although there is a chance that the area might burn again, you are better off here than in an area of fresh fuel. If you have to cross the fire line, cover your skin as well as possible, take a couple of deep breaths, and dash through the lowest flames (less than 3 feet deep, and where you can see through them). If smoke is dense, crawl along the ground for better air and visibility.

5. Try to avoid breathing smoke. Hold a moistened cloth over your mouth. If the air is very hot, use a dry cloth (dry heat is less damaging to the lungs than is steam).

6. Seek refuge from the radiant heat. Take shelter in a trench, pond, behind rocks, in a stream, vehicle, or building. Do not climb into elevated water tanks, wells, caves, or any other place where you may be trapped or quickly use up the available oxygen.

7. If all else fails and you cannot escape the advancing flames, lie facedown on the ground and cover your exposed skin as well as possible. This is better than standing upright or kneeling.

8. If you are near a vehicle, and there is no route for escape, it is better to stay in the vehicle than to run from the fire. Try to position the auto in an area of little natural vegetation. Avoid driving through dense smoke. Turn off the headlights and ignition. Roll up the windows, close the air vents, and shield yourself from the radiant heat by covering up with floor mats or hiding under the dash. Stay in the vehicle as long as possible (it is rare for gas tanks to explode, and it takes a minute or two for the car to catch on fire). Do not be overly alarmed if the vehicle rocks, or if smoke and sparks enter the vehicle. When the fire passes, cover your nose and mouth with a moistened cloth, to avoid inhaling fumes from burning plastics and paint. Use urine if no other liquid is available.

HOW TO REPORT A FIRE

If you suspect a wildland fire, IMMEDIATELY report it to local fire protection authorities. You should be prepared to give the following information:

Your name and location

Location of the fire

Description of the fire (flames, color, smoke)

Any persons in the area, with their most exact location

MEDICAL CONSIDERATIONS

The three most common medical problems in a wildland fire situation are burns, smoke inhalation, and dehydration. Burns and smoke inhalation are discussed on pages 90 and 95. All persons exposed to the constant and intense heat of a forest fire should consume at least a pint to a quart of fluid per hour (see page 238).

CARBON MONOXIDE POISONING

In general, there is no shortage of oxygen in the region of an outdoor fire, so long as there is adequate ventilation. However, in enclosed spaces, oxygen may be rapidly depleted as toxic gases and smoke accumulate. The most common inhaled toxin is carbon monoxide, which is the odorless and colorless product of incomplete combustion. Symptoms of carbon monoxide intoxication include:

Mild — decreased exercise tolerance, decreased ability to concentrate, headache, nausea
Moderate — severe headache, vomiting, poor coordination, decreased vision, decreased hearing, shortness of breath
Major — fainting, unconsciousness, gasping respirations, seizures, shock, death

If a person is suspected to have inhaled any toxic gas, he should be moved to fresh air as soon as possible, and have oxygen, 5–10 liters per minute, administered by mask. Anyone overcome with smoke inhalation should be rapidly transported to a hospital. Be prepared to manage the airway (see page 18).

Altitude-Related Problems

GREAT numbers of travelers seek their recreation in environments at high altitude, which is considered to begin at 8,000 feet above sea level. This section describes the different problems encountered at altitude, and their treatment.

GENERAL INFORMATION

Altitudes of 8,000 to 14,000 feet are attained regularly by skiers, hikers, and climbers in the continental United States. Outside this country, mountain climbers may reach altitudes of up to 29,000 feet (Mount Everest).

Most difficulties at high altitude are a direct result of the lowered concentration of oxygen in the atmosphere. Although the percentage of oxygen in the air is relatively constant at about 20%, the absolute amount of oxygen decreases with the declining barometric pressure. Thus, at 18,000 feet there is half the oxygen that is available at sea level. This condition causes a generalized decreased tolerance for exercise and physical stress. To a certain extent, man can adapt to high altitude and become more efficient in the oxygen-poor environment. Adaptation requires gradual exposure to altitude, with a rate of ascent not to exceed 1,500 feet per day above 8,000 feet. Rest days at a constant altitude are essential at heights above 10,000 feet. A discussion of prevention of high-altitude illnesses is found at the end of this section.

HIGH-ALTITUDE PULMONARY EDEMA

Pulmonary edema is excessive fluid in the lungs, either in the lung tissue itself or in the space normally used for gas exchange (oxygen for carbon dioxide). Fluid in the lungs renders them unable to perform their normal task, and thus the victim cannot get enough oxygen.

High-altitude pulmonary edema (HAPE) usually occurs in the unacclimatized individual who rapidly ascends to an altitude that exceeds 8,000 feet, particularly if heavy exertion is involved. Prior traditional physical conditioning is not a factor, as many cases involve young, previously healthy individuals. If the victim exercises above 8,000 feet, but sleeps at a lower (6,000 feet) altitude, the chance for developing HAPE is much less.

Symptoms begin 1–3 days after arrival at high altitude; they include shortness of breath, cough, weakness, easy fatigue, and difficulty sleeping. As greater amounts of fluid accumulate in the lungs, the victim develops drowsiness, severe shortness of breath, and rapid heart rate; his coughing produces white phlegm and then blood; he exhibits confusion and cyanosis (bluish discoloration of the skin). If the examiner places an ear to the victim's chest, he may hear gurgling noises. Rapidly, the patient becomes extremely agitated, disoriented, sweaty, and in obvious extreme respiratory distress. Coma and collapse follow.

As soon as the earliest signs of HAPE are present, the victim should be evacuated (carried if necessary) to a lower altitude at which there were previously no symptoms. Such warning signs include rapid heart rate (greater than 90–100 beats per minute at rest), weakness, shortness of breath, cough, difficulty walking, inability to keep up, and poor judgment. Maximal rest is advised. The definitive treatments are *descent* and the administration of oxygen; if it is available, oxygen should be administered by mask at 10 liters per minute. Improvement is rarely noted until oxygen is administered or descent of at least 1,000 feet is accomplished. IN NO CASE SHOULD A VICTIM BE LEFT TO DESCEND BY HIMSELF; ALWAYS HAVE A HEALTHY PERSON ACCOMPANY THE VICTIM. If the victim must be carried down, he should be kept in a sitting position if possible. The administration of fluid pills (diuretics) is controversial and should be done only under strict medical supervision. Some aid stations in high-altitude regions are equipped with inflatable pressure bags (Gamow bags) large enough to enclose a human. These are used to simulate conditions at lower altitude and may be used by experienced rescuers to treat moderate or severe high-altitude illness.

Once a victim has been judged to suffer from any degree of HAPE, he should no longer be a candidate for high-altitude travel until cleared by a physician. Such a precaution does not include routine jet airplane transportation.

HIGH-ALTITUDE CEREBRAL EDEMA

High-altitude cerebral edema (HACE) is the medical term for a disorder (tentatively linked to brain swelling) that involves an alteration of mental status seen at high altitude, related to diminished atmospheric oxygen. Symptoms include difficulty walking (inability to walk a straight line, staggering, or frank inability to walk), headache, confusion, difficulty in speaking, drowsiness, vomiting, and in severe cases, unconsciousness or coma. Patients may suffer from HACE and HAPE at the same time.

The treatment for HACE is the same as for HAPE; that is, immediate descent to an altitude below where there were previously no symptoms and the administration of high-flow oxygen. In addition, administration of the steroid drugs prednisone (80 mg) or dexamethasone (Decadron 4 mg) each day until descent is accomplished may be helpful. Again, rescuers are admonished never to leave a potentially seriously ill victim to fend for himself. A person who suffers from HACE or HAPE may deteriorate rapidly, and most such patients will need to be carried down the mountain. Because the early symptoms of mountain sickness and HACE are similar, pay close attention to the condition of ill members of your climbing party.

MOUNTAIN SICKNESS

Acute mountain sickness (AMS) is the most common altitude-related disorder; it affects many persons who ascend to altitudes above 8,000 feet without proper acclimatization. Symptoms, which may be quite subtle in the beginning, include headache (mild to severe), insomnia, fatigue, loss of appetite, drowsiness, weakness, and apathy. Children are prone to nausea and vomiting. The lips and fingernails may have a blue discoloration (cyanosis) if HAPE is present.

The most common and disabling symptom of AMS is headache, which typically occurs on the second or third day at high altitude, and may be complicated by difficulty in walking (if HAPE is present) and impaired memory. Mild symptoms of HACE accompany AMS; they include decreased appetite, mood swings, and lack of interest in activity. The illness may be compared in symptoms to a hangover.

One hallmark of AMS is an alteration of the normal sleeping pattern, known as periodic breathing. Sleep is fitful, with periods of wakefulness and disturbing dreams. The pattern of breathing in sleep is irregular, such that the sleeper has periods of rapid breathing (very deep breaths) alternated with periods of no breathing. The latter can be quite startling to the casual observer, for intervals of 10 seconds may pass without a breath.

Treatment of AMS includes rest, adequate fluid intake to avoid dehydration, and mild pain medicine for the headache. Sleeping medicines are not advised, because they might mask the symptoms of HACE. If the victim is severely ill, he should be brought (carried if necessary, preferably in the sitting position) to a lower altitude (below 5,000 feet), and administered oxygen by mask. Because the victim of AMS will adjust to the altitude in 3–4 days, he may remain at altitude if symptoms are mild. IN NO CASE SHOULD ONE ATTEMPT TO CLIMB TO A HIGHER ALTITUDE UNTIL THE SYMPTOMS OF AMS HAVE COMPLETELY SUBSIDED. With mild AMS, if acetazolamide (Diamox) is available, it can be administered in a dose of 250 mg by mouth every 8–12 hours until symptoms diminish. If AMS is severe and HACE is felt to be present, administer prednisone or dexamethasone, as previously recommended for HACE.

PREVENTION OF SERIOUS ALTITUDE-RELATED DISORDERS

The prevention of altitude-related disorders is most intelligently accomplished by gradual acclimatization to the lowered oxygen content of atmospheric air. This is achieved by adhering to a schedule of ascent:

For any climb above 8,000 feet, all members of the party should spend an initial 2–4 days at 5,000–7,000 feet. The first day should be a rest day. If any member of the party shows signs of altitude-related illness, additional time should be spent at that altitude.

For any climb above 13,000 feet, all members of the party should add 2–4 days for acclimatization at 10,000–12,000 feet. Subsequent climbing should not exceed 1,500 feet per day. Scattered rest days are advised. The party should sleep at the lowest altitude that does not interfere with the purpose of the expedition.

In addition, the drug acetazolamide (Diamox) has proven to be useful in stimulating breathing, diminishing the sleep disorder associated with AMS, facilitating the body's normal adjustment to high altitude, and thus improving nocturnal oxygenation. It is administered in a dose of 250 mg twice a day beginning the day before the ascent, and continued for a period of 2–3 days. Diamox has a diuretic (increased urination) effect, so that it is important to drink sufficient fluids to prevent dehydration. Fluid losses are generally greater at high altitude, so do not rely upon thirst as a gauge to adequate fluid intake. Drink enough to keep the urine clear and light-colored. DIAMOX IS NO SUBSTITUTE FOR PROPER ACCLIMATIZATION!

MINOR DISORDERS OF HIGH ALTITUDE

Fluid Retention

Swelling of the face, hands, and feet may occur after 4–10 days at increased altitude. Women are more commonly affected than men, and they note puffiness of the hands, feet, eyelids, and face, particularly in the morning after a night's sleep or just prior to a menstrual period. Ten or more pounds may be gained in fluid retention. The swelling persists for 1–3 days after return to lower altitude, and then spontaneously disappears (increased urination is noted at this time). The disorder is a nuisance, but of no real hazard. Salt intake should be controlled so as not to be excessive. Fluid pills (diuretics) should be avoided, as they promote dehydration and rarely reduce the swelling to any significant degree.

High-Altitude Flatus Expulsion (HAFE)

HAFE is the spontaneous and unwelcome passage of increased quantities of rectal gas noted at high altitude. It may become an embarrassment but is of no true medical concern. Trekkers should avoid those foods, such as chili and beans, that are known to induce flatulence at low altitudes, and should show consideration for other members of the party in sleeping arrangements. If stricken, a traveler may benefit from chewable tablets of simethicone (Mylicon 80 mg).

Altitude Throat

Altitude throat is a sore throat caused by nasal congestion and mouth breathing during exertion at high altitudes. Because the air is dry and cold, the protective mucous coating of the throat is dried out, and the throat becomes extremely irritated, with redness and pain. In general, this can be distinguished from a bacterial or viral infection (see page 155) by the absence of fever, swollen lymph glands in the neck, or systemic symptoms (fatigue, muscle aches, sweats, etc.). Prevention is difficult and treatment is only mildly satisfying. The victim should keep the throat moist by sipping liquids and sucking on throat lozenges or Life Savers. As soon as convenient, nighttime breathing of warm humidified air should be instituted. Anesthetic gargles should be avoided, since they will mask the signs of a true infection.

SNOW BLINDNESS

See page 149.

Snakebite

No animal invokes so much fear in man as does the snake. In reality, the medical management of a snakebite outside the hospital is simple and should be well understood by all members of an expedition.

POISONOUS SNAKES

General Information

There are two types of poisonous snakes indigenous to the United States. These are pit vipers (rattlesnake, cottonmouth [water moccasin], copperhead) and the coral snakes. Their distributions are as follows:

Northeast — cottonmouth, copperhead, timber rattlesnake

Southeast — cottonmouth, copperhead, eastern diamondback rattlesnake, pygmy rattlesnake, eastern coral snake

Central — cottonmouth, copperhead, massasauga rattlesnake, timber rattlesnake, prairie rattlesnake

Southwest — cottonmouth, copperhead, pygmy rattlesnake, massasauga rattlesnake, northern black-tailed rattlesnake, prairie rattlesnake, sidewinder, Mojave rattlesnake, western diamondback rattlesnake, red diamondback rattlesnake, Texas coral snake, Sonoran coral snake

Pacific coast — northern Pacific rattlesnake, southern Pacific rattlesnake, Great Basin rattlesnake, western diamondback rattlesnake, red diamondback rattlesnake, sidewinder, Mojave rattlesnake

In addition, many "nonvenomous" species, such as colubrid (rear-fanged) snakes (e.g., the red-neck keelback), are capable of producing venomous bites.

Pit vipers are typified by rattlesnakes, which have a character-istic triangular head, vertical elliptical pupils ("cat's eyes"), two hinged fangs in the front part of the jaw, heat-sensing facial pits on the sides of the head, a single row of scales on the underbelly leading to the tail (not seen in nonpoisonous snakes), and rattles on the tail (Fig. 85). Because fangs are replaced every 6–10 weeks

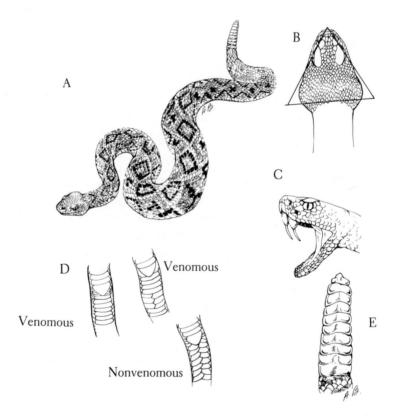

FIGURE 85. *Rattlesnake. (A) Typical rattlesnake appearance with fea-tures of identification that include (B) triangular head, (C) hinged fangs, (D) single row of underbelly scales leading up to the anal plate, and (E) a rattle on the tail.*

in the adult rattlesnake, bites may demonstrate from 1 to 4 large puncture marks.

Coral snakes are characterized by their color pattern, with red, black, and yellow or white bands encircling the body (Fig. 86). A general rule is "red on yellow — kill a fellow [venomous]; red on black — venom lack [nonvenomous]." The fangs are very short, the snakes have round pupils, and the snakes bite with a chewing, rather than striking, action.

Signs of Envenomation

Most snakebites do not result in envenomation, either because the snake does not release venom, because the skin is not penetrated, or because the venom is not potent. Therefore, it is important to recognize the signs of envenomation, in order to avoid needless worry, evacuation, and improper therapy.

The most common signs of envenomation are:

PIT VIPERS

1. One or more fang marks. Most snakebites (venomous and nonvenomous) will demonstrate rows of markings from the teeth.

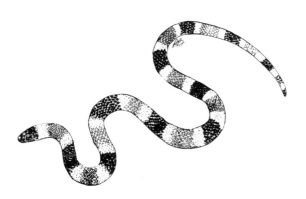

FIGURE 86. *Coral snake.*

In the case of venomous snakes, there will be 1–4 larger distinct markings from the elongated fangs which introduce the venom (Fig. 87).

2. Burning pain at the site of the bite. THIS MAY NOT BE PRESENT WITH THE BITE OF THE MOJAVE RATTLE-SNAKE.

3. Swelling at the site of the bite. This usually begins within 5–10 minutes of envenomation, and may become quite severe. THIS MAY NOT BE PRESENT WITH THE BITE OF THE MOJAVE RATTLESNAKE.

4. Numbness and tingling of the lips, face, and scalp 30–60 minutes after the bite. (This can also be present if the victim hyperventilates with fear and excitement. If a victim of a snake-

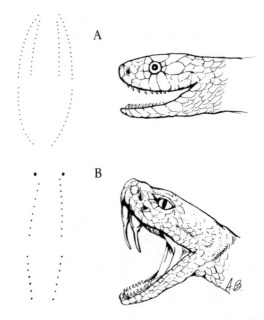

FIGURE 87. *Snakebite patterns. (A) Nonvenomous snake. (B) Venomous snake.*

bite has *immediate* symptoms, they are likely to be due to hyperventilation.)

5. Twitching of the mouth and eye muscles 30–90 minutes after the bite.

6. Rubbery or metallic taste in the mouth 30–90 minutes after the bite.

7. Sweating, weakness, nausea, vomiting, and fainting 1–2 hours after the bite.

8. Bruising at the site of the bite. This usually begins within 2–3 hours. Large blood blisters may develop within 6–10 hours.

9. Difficulty breathing, increased bleeding (bruising, bloody urine, vomiting blood), and collapse 6–12 hours after the bite.

CORAL SNAKES

1. Burning pain at the site of the bite may be present or absent. There is generally very little local swelling or bruising.

2. Numbness and/or weakness of a bitten arm or leg within 90 minutes.

3. Twitching, nervousness, drowsiness, giddiness, increased salivation and drooling in 1–3 hours.

4. Slurred speech, double vision, difficulty talking and swallowing, and impaired breathing within 5–10 hours.

5. Death from heart and lung failure.

Treatment of Snake Venom Poisoning

If a victim is bitten by a snake that could be poisonous, the rescuer should be prepared to act swiftly, according to a pre-arranged plan. THE DEFINITIVE TREATMENT FOR SNAKE VENOM POISONING IS THE ADMINISTRATION OF ANTIVENIN. THE MOST IMPORTANT ASPECT OF THERAPY IS TO GET THE VICTIM TO AN APPROPRIATE MEDICAL FACILITY AS QUICKLY AS POSSIBLE.

1. Avoid panic. Most bites, even by poisonous snakes, do not result in medically significant envenomations. Reassure the vic-

tim and keep him from acting in an energy-consuming, purpose-less fashion. If the victim has been envenomed, increased activity may increase his illness by spreading the venom. If the victim is hyperventilating, manage according to the instructions on page 216.

2. Retreat out of the striking range of the snake.

3. Locate the snake. If possible, identify the species. If you cannot do this with confidence, kill the animal with a blow on the neck from a long heavy stick. Collect the snake and bring it along for proper identification. Doing this may be extremely important in estimating the amount of antivenin necessary. Take care to carry the dead animal in a container that will not allow the head of the snake to bite another victim (the jaws can bite in a reflex action 20–60 minutes after death). If you are not sure how to collect the snake, it is best just to get away from it, to avoid another bite.

4. Apply the Extractor suction device according to the man-ufacturer's instructions (Fig. 88). This removes venom without the need for a skin incision.

5. If possible, splint the bitten body part, to avoid unnecessary

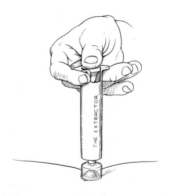

FIGURE 88. *Application of the Extractor to a snakebite wound.*

motion. Maintain the bitten arm or leg at a level below the heart.

6. Transport the victim to the nearest hospital.

7. DO NOT APPLY ICE DIRECTLY TO THE WOUND OR IMMERSE THE PART IN ICE WATER. An ice pack placed over the wound is of no proven value. Application of extreme cold can cause an injury similar to frostbite.

8. If the victim is more than 2 hours from medical attention, and the bite is on the arm or leg, place a 2″ x 2″ cloth pad (¼″ thick) over the bite and apply an elastic wrap firmly around the involved extremity directly over the padded bite site with a margin of 4–6 inches on either side of the wound, taking care to check for adequate circulation in the fingers and toes (normal feeling and color). Such a wrap may impede absorption of venom into the general circulation.

9. The only indications for incision and suction are if all four of the following conditions are present: the bite is from a rattlesnake (incision and suction are valueless for the bite of coral snakes), the victim is more than 1 hour from medical care, the Extractor cannot be applied, and the procedure can be performed within 5 minutes of the bite. The incisions should be made *only by a person experienced in the procedure* with a sterile razor blade or sharp knife directly over the fang marks, in a parallel fashion (not crisscross) ⅛″–¼″ long and ⅛″–¼″ deep. Apply suction for 30 minutes with the rubber device from a snakebite kit; the mouth should be used only as a last resort. *The impression of most snake experts is that incision and suction as traditionally taught are of little value and should probably be abandoned.* It appears that little venom can actually be removed from the bite site unless a perfectly placed incision is made immediately after the bite and followed by superb suction. Furthermore, mouth contact with a crisscross incision invariably creates a nasty infection that leaves a noticeable scar.

10. "Snakebite medicine" (whiskey) is of no value and may actually be harmful if it increases circulation to the skin.

11. There is not yet scientific evidence that electrical shocks applied to snakebites are of any value. To the contrary, animal experiments thus far refute this concept.

12. The bite wound should be washed vigorously with soap and water, and the victim treated with penicillin, erythromycin, or cephalexin.

Once the victim is in the hospital, the severity of envenomation will be ascertained, and the patient treated with antivenin if necessary. Such therapy must be carried out under the supervision of a physician, as serious allergic reactions to presently available antivenins are common. New purification techniques may soon allow the preparation of a less hazardous antivenin product.

Avoidance of Poisonous Snakes

The best way not to get bitten is to avoid poisonous snakes. The following rules should be observed:

1. Avoid the known habitats of poisonous snakes.

2. Do not reach into areas that you cannot see first. Walk on clearly marked trails, and use a walking stick to move suspicious objects.

3. Wear adequate protective clothing, particularly boots to cover the feet and lower legs.

4. Never hike alone in snake territory. Carry the Extractor and an elastic wrap.

5. Avoid hiking at night in snake territory. Carry a flashlight and walking stick.

6. Do not handle snakes unless you know what you are doing. Remember that you can be bitten and envenomed by seemingly dead or nonvenomous snakes.

NONPOISONOUS SNAKEBITES

Many snakes (for example, the gopher snake or king snake) are nonvenomous and do not create serious medical problems with a bite. However, identifying a snake from the bite puncture wounds is often extremely difficult for the amateur. Unless the snake can be positively identified as a nonvenomous species, the victim should be considered to have been bitten by a poisonous snake and managed appropriately. The snake should be captured for identification. If the snake is known to be nonvenomous, the wound should be washed vigorously with soap and water, and the victim treated with penicillin, erythromycin, or cephalexin.

GILA MONSTER

The Gila monster and beaded lizard, which can be up to 35 cm (14 inches) long, are found in the Great Sonoran Desert area in southern Arizona and in northwestern Mexico (Fig. 89). They possess grooved teeth and venom glands that may be used to envenom victims. Most envenomations occur when an animal bites and holds on, or when a tooth is shed into the bite wound.

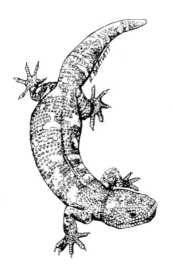

FIGURE 89. *Gila monster.*

If the Gila monster holds on, the grip may need to be loosened with mechanical means or with incision of the jaw muscles.

Symptoms of an envenomation include burning pain at the site of the bite, swelling of the bite wound, bluish discoloration, weakness, and sweating. Low blood pressure is the most serious complication.

The wound should be washed vigorously and all pieces of teeth removed. The victim should have the arm or leg splinted and should be transported to a hospital. Severe reactions are unusual, as most victims recover uneventfully. Be prepared to treat the victim for shock (see page 53). Do not administer alcohol, stimulants, or narcotic pain medicines. Do not apply ice directly to the wound.

Hazardous Marine Life

THERE are a great number of marine animals that can sting, bite, or poison unwary victims. This section will describe these animals and suggest first aid measures. In general, a person who acquires an infection following a marine wound should be treated with trimethoprim-sulfamethoxazole, ciprofloxacin, tetracycline, or cephalexin (the latter two only if one of the first two drugs is not available).

SHARKS

Sharks injure their victims by biting them. The jaws of the shark contain rows of razor-sharp teeth, which can bite down with a force that is measured in tons per square inch (Fig. 90). The result is a wound with loss of tissue which bleeds freely and can lead rapidly to shock.

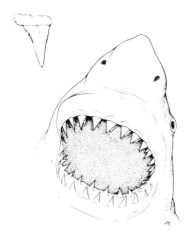

FIGURE 90. *Jaws of the great white shark, with advancing rows of razor-sharp ripsaw teeth.*

The basic management of a major bleeding wound is outlined beginning on page 48. Even if the shark bite appears minor, the wound should be washed out and bandaged, and the victim taken to an appropriate emergency facility. Often the wound will contain pieces of shark teeth, seaweed, or sand debris, which must be removed in order to avoid a bad infection. This can be properly done only in the hospital. Like other animal bites, shark bites should not be sewn or taped tightly shut, in order to allow drainage. This helps to prevent serious infection. The patient should be placed on trimethoprim with sulfamethoxazole (ciprofloxacin may be used as an alternative).

The skin of many sharks is rough like sandpaper, and can cause a bad scrape. If this occurs, it should be managed like a second-degree burn (see page 93).

Shark Avoidance

The best way to manage a shark bite is to not get bitten! The following safety rules must be obeyed:

1. Avoid shark-infested waters, particularly at dusk and after dark. Do not dive in known shark feeding grounds.

2. Swim in groups. Sharks tend to attack single swimmers.

3. When diving, avoid deep dropoffs, murky water, or areas near sewage outlets.

4. Do not tether captured (e.g., speared) fish to your body.

5. Do not corner or provoke sharks.

6. If a shark appears, leave the water with slow, purposeful movements. DO NOT PANIC OR SPLASH. If the shark approaches a diver in deep water, he should attempt to position himself so that he is protected from the rear. If a shark moves in, attempt to strike a firm blow to the snout.

BARRACUDA

Barracuda may bite victims and create nasty wounds with their long caninelike teeth (Fig. 91). These wounds are managed like shark bites. Because barracuda seem to be attracted to shiny objects, the swimmer or diver is well advised to not wear bright metallic objects, such as anklets, bracelets, or flashy belts.

MORAY EELS

Although they appear quite ferocious, moray eels seldom attack humans, unless unduly provoked. They have muscular jaws

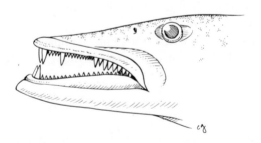

FIGURE 91. *Barracuda, with large caninelike teeth.*

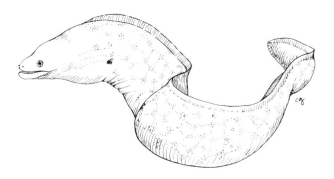

FIGURE 92. *Moray eel.*

equipped with sharp fanglike teeth, which can inflict a vicious bite (Fig. 92). Morays tend to bite and hold on; in some instances, it is necessary to break the eel's jaws to get it to release.

A moray bite should be managed like a shark bite. Even if the bite is very small, it should be examined by a physician, to be sure that all tooth fragments have been removed. If the bite is on the hand, foot, or near a joint, the patient should be placed on trimethoprim with sulfamethoxazole, ciprofloxacin, or tetracycline.

SPONGES

Sponges handled directly from the ocean can cause two types of skin reaction. The first is an allergic type similar to that caused by poison ivy (see page 181), with the exception that the reaction generally occurs immediately after the sponge is handled. The skin becomes red, with burning and itching. The second type of reaction is caused by small spicules of silica from the sponges which are broken off and embedded in the outermost layers of the skin. The results are irritation, redness, and swelling.

Because it is difficult to tell which type of reaction has occurred, if a person develops a skin reaction after carrying a sponge, the following therapy should be undertaken:

1. Soak the affected skin with vinegar (5% acetic acid) for 10–15 minutes. This may be done by wetting a gauze pad or cloth with vinegar and applying it to the skin. Dry the skin.

2. Apply the sticky side of adhesive tape to the skin and peel it off. This will remove most sponge spicules that are present.

3. Repeat the vinegar soak for 5 minutes or apply rubbing (isopropyl 40%) alcohol for 1 minute.

4. Apply hydrocortisone lotion (0.5–1.0%) thinly twice a day until the irritation is gone.

5. If the rash worsens (blistering, increasing redness or pain, swollen lymph glands), this may indicate an infection, and the patient should be treated with trimethoprim-sulfamethoxazole, ciprofloxacin, or cephalexin.

JELLYFISH

Jellyfish is the name commonly used to describe an enormous number of marine animals (coelenterates) that are capable of inflicting a painful, and occasionally life-threatening, sting. This occurs when the skin comes into contact with the creature's tentacles, which carry millions of small stinging cells, each equipped with venom and a microscopic stinger. Depending on the species, size, geographic location, time of year, and other natural factors, stings can range in severity from mild burning and skin redness to excruciating pain and severe blistering with generalized illness (nausea, vomiting, shortness of breath, low blood pressure, etc.). Broken-off tentacles that are fragmented in the surf or washed up on the beach can retain their toxicity for months and should not be handled.

The dreaded box jellyfish of northern Australia contains one of the most potent animal venoms known to man (Fig. 94). A sting from one of these creatures can induce death in minutes, generally from immediate cessation of breathing, abnormal heart rhythms, and profound low blood pressure (shock).

The following therapy is recommended for all unidentified

jellyfish and other creatures with stinging cells, including Portuguese man-of-war (bluebottle) (Fig. 93), box jellyfish (sea wasp) (Fig. 94), Irukandji, fire coral (Fig. 95), stinging hydroid, sea nettle, and sea anemone (Fig. 96):

1. Immediately rinse the skin with seawater. *Do not rinse with fresh water or apply ice directly to the skin.* A dry cold pack or ice bag may relieve pain following a man-of-war sting, but care must be taken to avoid skin contact with melted fresh water or condensation from the bag.

2. Apply soaks of vinegar (5% acetic acid) or rubbing (isopropyl 40–70%) alcohol for 30 minutes or until the pain is relieved. *In the case of the Australian box jellyfish (sea wasp), use vinegar in preference to alcohol.* If these are not available, apply soaks of dilute (¼ strength) household ammonia or urine. A paste made from unseasoned meat tenderizer (do not exceed 15 minutes application time, particularly upon the sensitive skin of small

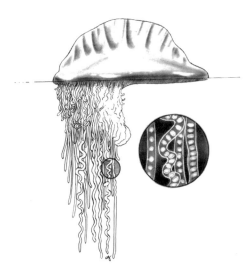

FIGURE 93. *Portuguese man-of-war (bluebottle), with a close-up of stinging cells located on the tentacles.*

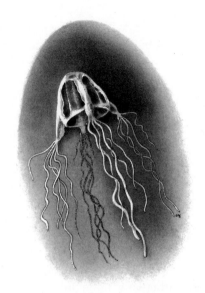

FIGURE 94. *Indo-Pacific box jellyfish (sea wasp).*

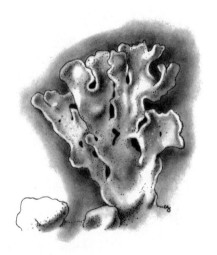

FIGURE 95. *Fire coral.*

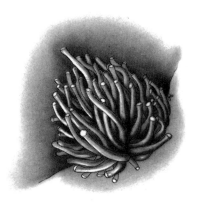

FIGURE 96. *Sea anemone.*

children) or papaya fruit may be helpful. Do not apply any organic solvents, such as kerosene, turpentine, or gasoline.

3. Remove large tentacle fragments, using forceps. Take care not to handle the tentacles with bare hands.

4. Apply a lather of shaving cream or a paste of baking soda (in an isolated area, you can use a paste of sand or mud in seawater), and shave the affected area with a razor. If a razor is not available, use a sharp-edged object, such as a clamshell.

5. Reapply the vinegar or rubbing alcohol soak for 15 minutes.

6. Apply a thin coating of hydrocortisone lotion 0.5–1.0% twice a day.

7. If the victim has a large area involved (entire arm or leg, face, or genitals), is very young or very old, or shows signs of generalized illness (nausea, vomiting, weakness, shortness of breath, chest pain, etc.), seek help from a doctor. If tentacle fragments are placed in the mouth (only small children or intoxicated adults will do this!), immediately have the victim swish and spit a mouthful of whatever potable liquid is available. If there is already swelling in the mouth (muffled voice, difficulty in swallowing, enlarged tongue and lips), do not give anything by

mouth, protect the airway (see page 18), and rapidly transport the victim to a hospital.

8. If a person is stung by an Australian box jellyfish, in addition to the maneuvers listed above, pay immediate attention to the airway (see page 18) and seek assistance. In Australia, an antivenin has been prepared against the effects of the venom.

CORAL AND BARNACLE CUTS

Cuts and scrapes from sharp-edged coral and barnacles tend to fester and become infected wounds if not managed properly. Treatment for these cuts is as follows:

1. Scrub the cut vigorously with soap and water, then flush the wound with large amounts of water.

2. Flush the wound with a ½-strength solution of hydrogen peroxide in water. Rinse again with water.

3. Apply a thin layer of bacitracin ointment, and cover with a dry sterile dressing. If no ointment or dressing is available, the wound can be left open. Thereafter, it should be cleaned twice a day.

4. If the wound shows signs of infection (extreme redness, pus, swollen regional lymph glands), the patient should be given trimethoprim with sulfamethoxazole, ciprofloxacin, or tetracycline.

SEA URCHINS

Sea urchins are covered with sharp venom-filled spines that can easily penetrate and break off into the skin (Fig. 97). These create painful wounds, most often of the hands or feet. If a person receives many puncture wounds, the reaction may be so severe as to cause difficulty in breathing, weakness, and collapse. The treatment for a sea urchin sting is as follows:

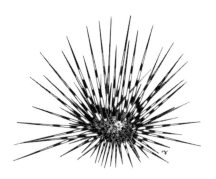

FIGURE 97. *Sea urchin.*

1. Immerse the area in hot water to tolerance (110–113°F/ 43.3–45°C). This frequently provides pain relief. Administer appropriate pain medicine.

2. CAREFULLY REMOVE ANY READILY VISIBLE SPINES. Do not dig around in the skin to try to fish them out; you will only crush the spines and make them more difficult to remove. Do not intentionally crush the spines.

3. Seek the care of a physician. If the spines have entered the skin in the hand or foot, or near a joint, they may need to be removed surgically, to minimize infection and damage to nerves or important blood vessels.

4. If the wound shows signs of infection (extreme redness, pus, swollen regional lymph glands), the victim should be given trimethoprim-sulfamethoxazole, ciprofloxacin, or tetracycline.

SEA CUCUMBERS

Sea cucumbers are sausage-shaped creatures that produce a liquid called holothurin, which is a contact irritant to the skin and eyes (Fig. 98). Because some sea cucumbers dine on jellyfish, they may excrete jellyfish venom as well. Therefore, anyone who sustains a skin irritation from a sea cucumber may benefit from

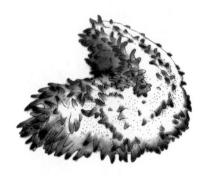

FIGURE 98. *Sea cucumber.*

the treatment for jellyfish stings described above. If the eyes are involved, they should be irrigated vigorously with at least a quart of water, and immediate medical attention should be sought. If the victim is out at sea, treat the eye injury as a corneal abrasion (see page 144).

STINGRAYS

A stingray does its damage by lashing upward in defense with a muscular tail, which carries up to 4 sharp, swordlike stings (Fig. 99). The stings are supplied with venom, so that the injury created is both a deep puncture or laceration and an envenomation. The pain from a stingray wound can be excruciating, and accompanied by bleeding, weakness, vomiting, headache, fainting, shortness of breath, paralysis, collapse, and, occasionally, death. Most wounds involve the legs and feet, as unwary waders and swimmers tread upon the creatures hidden in the sand. (Tide poolers, beware! Always wear adequate footgear and shuffle your feet in stingray territory.) If a person is struck by a stingray, immediately do the following:

1. Rinse the wound vigorously with whatever water is available (seawater is acceptable). Immediately immerse the wound in

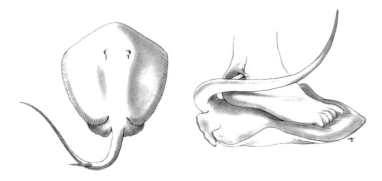

FIGURE 99. *Stingray. The ray thrusts upward in self-defense with venom-laden spine(s) into the foot of an unwary victim.*

hot water to tolerance (110–113°F/43.3–45°C) for pain relief. Generally, it is necessary to soak the wound for 30–90 minutes.

2. If medical attention is not available, scrub the wound vigorously with soap and water. Remove any visible fragments of the sting(s). Do not try to sew or tape it closed, as doing so could create a serious infection.

3. Apply a dry dressing and seek medical help. If more than 12 hours will pass before a doctor can be reached, administer trimethoprim with sulfamethoxazole, ciprofloxacin, or tetracycline.

4. If the patient is fully awake, administer pain medication.

CATFISH

Catfish sting their victims with dorsal and pectoral fin spines, which are charged with venom. When the fish is handled, the spines are extended and "locked" into position. The wound can be exceedingly painful; it resembles the sting of a stingray. The treatment is the same as that for a stingray wound. Soaking in hot water to tolerance (110–113°F/43.3–45°C) may provide dramatic relief of pain.

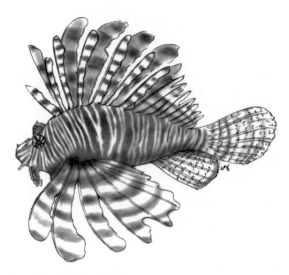

FIGURE 100. *Zebrafish (lionfish)*.

SCORPIONFISH

Scorpionfish include zebrafish (lionfish), scorpionfish, and stone-fish (Fig. 100). Like catfish, they possess spines that are venom-charged and can create extremely painful, and occasionally life-threatening, wounds. The treatment is the same as that for a stingray wound. Soaking in hot water to tolerance (110–113°F/43.3–45°C) produces dramatic relief of pain. If the victim appears intoxicated (weak, vomiting, short of breath, unconscious), seek immediate advanced medical aid. Scorpionfish stings frequently require weeks to months to heal, and therefore need the attention of a physician. In Australia, an antivenin is available to physicians to help manage the sting of the dreaded stonefish.

SEA SNAKES

Sea snakes are the most abundant reptiles in the world, though they are found only in the Pacific and Indian oceans. They may attain a length of nine feet and are equipped with a paddlelike tail that allows them to swim forward and backward with considerable speed (Fig. 101).

A sea snake can bite a victim with two to four fangs. The venom is extremely toxic, and causes paralysis, destruction of red blood cells, and widespread muscle damage.

The diagnosis of a sea snake envenomation is determined as follows:

1. One must be in the water to be bitten by a sea snake. The animals cannot move easily on land and do not survive very long there. However, one must be cautious when exploring regions of tidal variation, particularly in mangrove vegetation or near inlets where snakes breed.

2. Sea snake bites rarely cause much pain at the bite site.

3. Fang marks. These are like pinholes, and may number from 1 to 4 (rarely, up to 20).

4. Development of symptoms. If these do not occur within 6–8 hours of the bite, then significant poisoning has not occurred. They include weakness, paralysis, lockjaw, drooping eyelids, difficulty speaking, and vomiting. Later, the victim will develop darkened urine and difficulty in breathing.

If a person is bitten by a sea snake, seek IMMEDIATE medical attention. The proper therapy is similar to that for a land snake

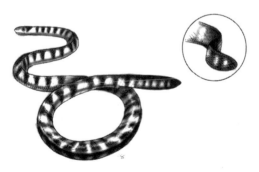

FIGURE 101. *Sea snake, with paddle-shaped tail.*

bite: namely, the administration in a hospital of the proper anti-venin (see page 255). A sea snake envenomation is a true medical emergency.

SKIN RASHES CAUSED BY AQUATIC PLANTS (SWIMMER'S ITCH)

See page 184.

TOXIC (POISONOUS) MARINE LIFE

There are a large number of illnesses that can occur from eating toxic (absolute or seasonal) or contaminated seafood. The following are the most commonly encountered, frequently by travelers to new and exotic locations.

Scombroid Poisoning

Scombroid poisoning is caused by improper preservation (inadequate refrigeration or drying) of fish in the family Scombridae, which includes tuna, mackerel, bonito, skipjack, and wahoo. Nonscombroid fish that can also cause this syndrome include mahi-mahi (dolphin), anchovies, sardines, and Australian ocean salmon. Most of these fish are dark-fleshed. When fish are not preserved properly, bacteria in the fish break down chemicals in the flesh to produce the chemical histamine, which causes an allergic reaction in the victim. Although the fish may have a peppery or metallic taste, they may also have normal color and flavor.

Minutes after eating the fish, the victim becomes flushed, with itching, nausea, diarrhea, low-grade fever, abdominal pain, and the development of hives (see page 186). Occasionally, victims become weak and short of breath with wheezing. The reaction is similar to that seen with monosodium glutamate (MSG) sensitivity ("Chinese food syndrome"). Treatment is the same as for an allergic reaction (see page 58). If the victim does not improve with diphenhydramine (Benadryl), he may benefit from administration of cimetidine (Tagamet) 300 mg by mouth. Administer either drug every 6–8 hours until symptoms resolve (generally, for 12–24 hours).

Puffer Poisoning

Certain puffers (blowfish, globefish, porcupine fish, etc.) contain tetrodotoxin, one of the most potent poisons in nature (Fig. 102). These fish are prepared as a delicacy (*fugu*) in Japan by specially trained and licensed chefs; amateur preparation results in occasional mishaps. The toxin is found in the entire fish, with greatest concentration in the liver, intestines, reproductive organs, and skin. After the victim has eaten the fish, symptoms can occur as quickly as 10 minutes later or be delayed by a few hours. They

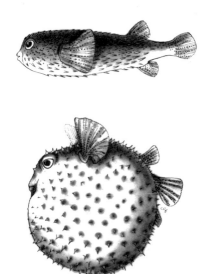

FIGURE 102. *Porcupine fish (puffer).*

include numbness and tingling about the mouth, light-headedness, drooling, sweating, vomiting, diarrhea, abdominal pain, weakness, difficulty in walking, paralysis, difficulty in breathing, and collapse. Many victims die.

If a person is suffering from puffer poisoning, immediately transport him to a hospital. Pay attention to his ability to breathe, and help him if necessary (see page 24). Unfortunately there is no antidote, and the victim will need sophisticated medical management until he metabolizes the toxin. Eating puffers, unless they are prepared by the most skilled chefs, is dietary Russian roulette.

Ciguatera Fish Poisoning

Ciguatera fish poisoning involves a large number of tropical and semitropical bottom-feeding fish that dine on plants or smaller fish which have accumulated toxins from the microscopic di-noflagellate *Gambierdiscus toxicus*. Therefore, the larger the fish, the greater the toxicity. The ciguatoxin-carrying fish most commonly ingested include the barracuda, jack, grouper, and snapper. Symptoms, which usually begin 15–30 minutes after the victim eats the contaminated fish, include abdominal pain, nausea, vomiting, diarrhea, tongue and throat numbness, tooth pain, difficulty in walking, blurred vision, skin rash, tearing of the eyes, weakness, and occasional difficulty in breathing. A classic sign of ciguatera intoxication is the reversal of hot and cold sensations (hot liquids seem cold, and vice versa). Unfortunately, the symptoms may persist in varying severity for weeks to months.

Treatment is purely supportive; there is no specific antidote. Although there is a test that can be used to identify ciguatoxin in fish flesh, there is no blood test to identify ciguatera poisoning in man. If, after eating fish, someone becomes ill as described above, he should be seen by a physician immediately.

Paralytic Shellfish Poisoning

Paralytic shellfish poisoning is caused by eating shellfish that contain concentrated toxins produced originally by certain planktons and protozoans in the ocean. These same microorganisms are responsible for so-called red (blue, brown, white, black, etc.) tides, which occur in warm summer months. The shellfish (such as California mussels, which are quarantined each year from May through October, and New England clams) dine upon the microorganisms and concentrate the poison in their digestive organs and muscle tissues. Generally, crabs, shrimp, and abalone are safe to eat.

Minutes after eating contaminated shellfish, the victim complains of numbness and tingling inside and around the mouth, and of the tongue and gums. He soon becomes light-headed, weak, and incoherent, and begins to suffer from drooling, difficulty in swallowing, incoordination, headache, thirst, diarrhea, abdominal pain, blurred vision, sweating, and rapid heartbeat. Curiously enough, even if a victim becomes paralyzed, he may continue to be aware of what is happening, unless he does not receive enough oxygen to the brain (because he stops breathing).

The victim of paralytic shellfish poisoning should be brought immediately to a hospital. If he is having difficulty breathing, be prepared to help him (see page 24).

Insect and Arthropod Bites

BEES, SPIDERS, SCORPIONS, AND OTHER SMALL BITERS

Problems with insects range from the nuisance of mosquito bites to life-threatening allergic reactions caused by bees and wasps.

This section will enable the reader to treat insect and arthropod bites and stings and will suggest ways to avoid unnecessary contact with the most dangerous species.

Bees, Wasps, and Ants

This group of insects includes honeybees, bumblebees, wasps, hornets, and yellow jackets. Each of these insects possesses a stinger, which is used to introduce venom into the victim. Most stings occur on the head and neck, next most commonly on the arms and legs. A honeybee leaves its stinger and venom sac in the victim after a sting (this kills the bee). Hornets, yellow jackets, bumblebees, and wasps do not lose their weapons and may sting a victim repeatedly. Pain is immediate, usually with rapid swelling, redness, warmth, and itching at the site of the sting. If the person is allergic to the insect, a dangerous reaction may follow rapidly (within minutes, but occasionally delayed by up to 2 hours). This consists of hives, shortness of breath, difficulty in breathing, swelling of the tongue, weakness, vomiting, and collapse. Persons have swallowed bees (undetected in beverage bottles) and sustained stings of the esophagus, which are enormously painful. A severe allergic reaction may also follow the sting(s) of a fire ant, as it marches along the victim and leaves a trail of small painful blisters.

TREATMENT FOR BEE STINGS

1. If a person is stung by a bee, wasp, or fire ant, be prepared to deal with a severe allergic reaction (see page 58). If the victim develops hives, shortness of breath, profound weakness, and appears to be deteriorating, IMMEDIATELY administer epinephrine. This is injected subcutaneously (see page 352) in a dose of 0.3–0.5 ml for adults and 0.01 ml per 2.2 lb (1 kg) for children (not to exceed 0.3 ml). Epinephrine is available in allergy kits (Ana-Kit, Hollister-Stier; EpiPen and EpiPen Jr., Center Laboratories) with instructions for use. ANYONE KNOWN TO

HAVE INSECT ALLERGIES WHO TRAVELS IN THE WIL-
DERNESS AWAY FROM MEDICAL CARE SHOULD
CARRY EPINEPHRINE. Take particular care to handle preloaded syringes properly, to avoid inadvertent injection into a
finger.

2. Administer diphenhydramine (Benadryl) by mouth, 50–
100 mg for adults and 1 mg per 2.2 lbs of weight (1 kg) for
children. This antihistamine drug may be used by itself for milder
allergic reactions.

3. Stingers or pieces of stingers left in the skin should be
scraped off with a knife or razor edge (Fig. 103). Do not attempt
to remove a honeybee stinger with tweezers or the fingers (pinching action), because often the venom sac is still attached to the
stinger. If it is grasped, more venom may be squeezed into the
wound, worsening the reaction. An alternative is to use the Extractor device immediately after the sting (Fig. 88).

4. Apply ice packs to the site of the sting.

5. Apply directly to the wound a paste made from an *unsea-*

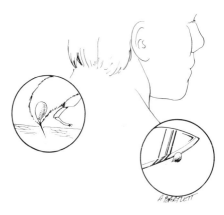

FIGURE 103. *Honeybee sting. Because the venom sac is still attached to the
stinger, it must be scraped free from the skin without squeezing more
venom into the victim.*

soned papain-containing meat tenderizer (for example, Adolph's unseasoned meat tenderizer) and water for no more than 15–20 minutes. A paste of baking soda is of no value. Do not apply mud. If a person is allergic to meat tenderizer, a 20% aluminum salt–containing preparation (e.g., many household antiperspirants) may be effective. The commercial product After Bite (Tender Corporation, Littleton, New Hampshire), a mixture of ammonium hydroxide and mink oil, is moderately effective for relief of pain and itching following insect bites, but will not abort an allergic reaction. Stingeze liquid (Wisconsin Pharmacal, Jackson, Wisconsin) is a mixture of camphor, phenol, benzocaine, and diphenhydramine; this is a good agent to control itching and mild pain following any insect bite: Itch Balm Plus (Sawyer Products; see page 334) is a similar mixture of hydrocortisone, diphenhydramine, and tetracaine.

6. If a person stung by an insect develops more than a mild local reaction, transport the victim to a hospital.

AVOIDING STINGING INSECTS

1. Store garbage, particularly fruit, at a distance from the campsite.

2. Remove (CAREFULLY) beehives and wasp nests from children's play areas.

3. Avoid wearing sweet fragrances that make you smell like a flower.

4. Do not anger bees or wasps. If confronted by a swarm, cover your face and move rapidly from the area. Do not poke sticks or throw rocks into bee holes.

SPIDERS

Although over 20,000 different types of spiders live in the United States, only a few pose any real hazard to man. Troublemakers are those that bite and introduce toxic venom from venom glands into the wound. The nature of the reaction relates to the type and quantity of venom.

Black Widow Spider

In the United States, the female black widow spider (*Latrodectus mactans*) is 15 mm (about ⅝ inch) in body length, black or brown, with a characteristic red hourglass marking on the underside of the abdomen (Fig. 104). It is found scattered about the United States in rural regions, in barns, harvested crops, and around outdoor stone walls.

The bite of the black widow spider is rarely very painful (no more than a pinprick) and causes little swelling or redness. However, if much venom has been deposited, the victim develops a typical reaction within an hour. This consists of muscle cramps, particularly of the abdomen and back; muscle pain; numbness and tingling of the palms of the hands and bottoms of the feet; headache; vomiting; fever; and high blood pressure. Untreated, most people recover without help over the course of 8 hours to 2 days. However, very small children and elderly victims may suffer greatly, with possible death.

TREATMENT FOR A BLACK WIDOW SPIDER BITE
1. Apply ice packs to the bite.
2. IMMEDIATELY transport the victim to a medical facility.

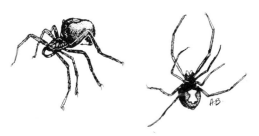

FIGURE 104. *Female black widow spider with typical hourglass marking on the underside of the abdomen.*

3. Once the victim is in the hospital, the doctor will have a number of therapies he can use, which include muscle relaxant medicines for muscle spasm; antihypertensive drugs for elevated blood pressure; pain medicine; and in very severe cases, antivenin to the venom of the black widow spider.

Brown Recluse Spider

The brown recluse spider (*Loxosceles reclusa*) is found most commonly in the South and southern Midwest; however, interstate commerce has created new habitats in many other parts of the country for the brown recluse and related species. The spider is brown, with a body length of 10 mm (just under ½ inch). A characteristic dark violin-shaped marking is found on the top of the upper section of the body (Fig. 105). The brown recluse spider is found in dark sheltered areas, such as under porches, in woodpiles, and in crates of fruit.

The bite of the brown recluse spider may cause very little pain at first. Within 1–5 hours, a painful red blister appears, surrounded by a bull's-eye of whitish-blue discoloration. In some cases, the victim develops chills, fever, weakness, and a gener-

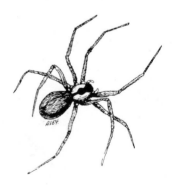

FIGURE 105. *Brown recluse spider with typical violin-shaped marking on the top side of the cephalothorax.*

alized red skin rash. Severe allergic reactions within 30 minutes of the bite occur infrequently.

TREATMENT FOR A BROWN RECLUSE SPIDER BITE: Because the bite of the brown recluse spider typically causes severe tissue destruction over the course of 1–2 weeks, the victim should see a physician as soon as possible. In the meantime, apply cold packs to the wound for as long as possible and administer erythromycin or cephalexin. Depending upon the severity of the reaction, the doctor will either administer additional drugs or suggest surgical excision of the bite. An antivenin has been developed and is currently being tested.

SCORPIONS

Scorpions are generally found in deserts and warm tropical climates, hidden under stones, fences, and garbage. In the United States, the most dangerous species is the nocturnal *Centruroides exilicauda* (*sculpturatus*), which is found almost exclusively in

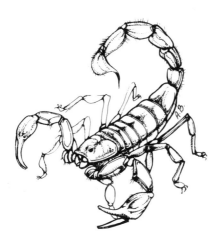

FIGURE 106. *Scorpion.*

the southwestern states and can be up to 5 cm (2 inches) long. This yellowish-brown (straw-colored) solid or striped species is distinguished from other scorpions by its slender body and a small tubercle (telson) at the base of the stinger (Fig. 106). The sting is inflicted with the last segment of the tail. The sting is immediately exquisitely painful; the pain is made much worse by tapping on the site of the injury. Other symptoms include excitement, increased salivation, sweating, numbness and tingling around the mouth, nausea, double vision, nervousness, muscle twitching and spasm, rapid breathing, shortness of breath, high blood pressure, seizures, paralysis, and collapse. Children under the age of 2 are at particular risk for severe reactions. Stings by nonlethal scorpion species are similar to bee stings.

If someone is stung by a scorpion, immediately apply ice packs to the wound, and immobilize the affected body part. Seek immediate care, particularly for stings of *C. exilicauda*. In Arizona and New Mexico, antivenin is available to physicians for treatment.

MOSQUITOES

Female mosquitoes bite humans in quest of a blood meal, in order to lay eggs. Because they breed in water, they are most frequently found in marsh and wetland or wooded areas. Although many tend to swarm at dusk, different species feed at different times. The insects are attracted to host odors (long-range), exhaled carbon dioxide (mid-range), and heat and moisture (short-range). During a bite, mosquito saliva is injected into the victim. This liquid contains the substances that cause the classic reaction of a small white or red bump that itches, then disappears. Persons who have been sensitized because of previous bites can have delayed (12–48 hours) reactions, which include intense local swelling and itching. In addition, mosquitoes transmit diseases such as malaria (see page 121) and various types of encephalitis. There is not yet evidence that mosquitoes transmit human immunodeficiency virus (HIV), the cause of AIDS.

Therapy for mosquito bites is limited to cool compresses and skin hygiene to prevent infections. If a person is bitten intensely and suffers a bad delayed allergic reaction, he may benefit from a course of prednisone similar to that for poison ivy (see page 183).

Insect repellents are discussed on page 288.

TICKS

Ticks are ubiquitous in wooded regions and fields, and readily attach to the skin of victims, most commonly in the scalp, armpits, groin, and other cozy (for a tick) areas (Fig. 107). They like shade and moist skin, and may wander for a while in search of a comfortable spot. Once in place, they hang on with the mouth parts and feed on the victim's blood. The tick is the intermediate host for many diseases, such as Rocky Mountain spotted fever (see page 126), Colorado tick fever, and Lyme disease (see page 127).

The proper way to remove a tick is to grasp it close to the mouth parts with tweezers or with the fingernails and pull it straight out with a slow and steady motion (Fig. 108). Do not

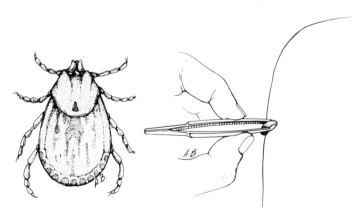

FIGURE 107. *Tick.*   FIGURE 108. *Removing a tick with tweezers.*

twist the tick. If you must remove it with your fingers, use tissue paper or cloth to prevent skin contact with infectious tick fluids. THE TICK SOLUTION is a precision instrument (Instruments of Sweden, Inc., Waterbury, Connecticut) designed to allow spring-loaded pincers to grasp a tick in such a fashion that it can be properly removed. Do not touch the tick with a hot object (such as an extinguished match head) or cover it with mineral oil, alcohol, kerosene, camp stove fuel, or Vaseline; these remedies might cause the tick to struggle and regurgitate infectious fluid into the bite site. If a tick head is buried in the skin, you can apply permethrin (Permanone insect repellent), using a cotton swab, to the upper and lower body surfaces of the tick. After 10–15 minutes, the tick will relax and you will be able to pull it free. After the tick is removed, carefully inspect the skin area for remaining head parts, and gently scrape them away.

If a person (particularly a young girl with long hair) is traveling in tick country and begins to complain of fatigue and weakness, you may have discovered a case of "tick paralysis." Certain ticks attach to the skin and slowly release a toxin that causes profound lethargy and muscle weakness in the victim. Search the skin (particularly the hair-covered areas) thoroughly for ticks and remove them. Recovery occurs in 24–48 hours after removal of the tick. When traveling in forests and fields, it is a good idea to inspect the body thoroughly (particularly the hairline, groin, underarms, navel, scalp, and other hair-covered areas) for ticks each day. Don't forget to brush ticks out of the fur of all dogs and pack animals.

Wear proper clothing to prevent tick attachment. Keep shirts tucked into pants and trouser cuffs tucked into socks. Light-colored clothing displays ticks. The deer tick, which transmits the infectious agent of Lyme disease, is extremely small, particularly in juvenile stages. The best repellent is permethrin (Permanone) applied to clothing, not to skin (see page 290), but DEET is also effective.

CATERPILLARS

The puss caterpillar, *Megalopyge opercularis*, is found in the southern United States (Fig. 109). The gypsy moth caterpillar, *Lymantria dispar*, is found in the northeastern United States (Fig. 110). The numerous bristles that cover the bodies of both species cause skin irritation. Shortly after exposure, the victim suffers a dermatitis with redness, itching, burning discomfort, and hives. If a large area of skin is involved, the victim can become nauseated and weak and can suffer from high fever. If the small bristle hairs are inhaled, shortness of breath may follow. If

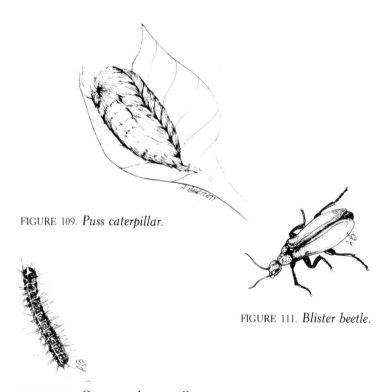

FIGURE 109. *Puss caterpillar.*

FIGURE 111. *Blister beetle.*

FIGURE 110. *Gypsy moth caterpillar.*

the eyes come in contact, symptoms include redness, itching, tearing, and swollen eyelids.

Treatment of the skin consists of the application of adhesive tape to attempt to remove the bristles, followed by an application of calamine lotion. Management of an allergic reaction similar to that from poison ivy is described on page 183. If the redness and swelling are persistent, the patient should be treated with ibuprofen for five days.

BEETLES

Blister beetles, *Epicauta* species, are found throughout the eastern and southern United States (Fig. 111). These insects are usually about ½ inch long and extremely agile. When they make contact with the skin, they release a chemical substance (cantharidin) that is very irritating. Within a few hours, blisters appear, which are not particularly painful unless they are large. If a blister beetle is squashed on the skin, an enormous blister follows.

The treatment is the same as for a second-degree burn (see page 93). If "beetle juice" enters the eye, it should be irrigated with water copiously, and the injury managed as one would snow blindness (see page 149).

INSECT REPELLENTS

In insect-laden areas, where contact is inevitable, the traveler must wear proper clothing. Cover the head and neck with a hat (with or without netting) and scarf (temperature permitting), and shield the ankles and wrists. Nylon (particularly double-layered) and sailcloth are more difficult for insects to hang onto or penetrate and are generally preferred over cotton or cloth with a loose weave. Insect repellents applied to clothing are extremely effective and avoid skin irritation. It is a good idea to test the repellent on a small area of clothing before general application, to be certain that it will not blemish the fabric.

Chemical insect repellents are mandatory whenever one travels through mosquito, sand fly, or tick territory. Different repellents work by different mechanisms and therefore their effectiveness varies for different types of insects, but I will make some general recommendations that will be applicable in most situations.

The best repellents contain the chemicals DEET (N,N-diethyl-meta-toluamide), Indalone (butyl 3,4-dihydro-2,2-dimethyl-4-oxo-2H-pyran-6-carboxylate), Rutgers 612 (2-ethyl-1,3-hexanediol), and DMP (dimethyl phthalate). Brand names include Muskol, 6–12, Cutter, OFF, and Repel (see Appendix One). Citronella and Skin-So-Soft bath oil are far less effective (1 hour protection versus 7 hours with 25% DEET). To be effective, the repellents should be applied liberally to the skin (liquid) and clothing (spray). After a person swims, bathes, or perspires excessively, the repellent should be reapplied. In windy conditions, repellents evaporate quickly and may need to be reapplied (judiciously). Children under 2 years of age should not have insect repellent applied to the skin more than once in 24 hours (it is more effective to apply it to the clothing, anyhow). With regard to DEET-containing products, do not use repeated applications or concentrations greater than 15% in children under the age of 6. In adults, skin irritation and/or rare severe side effects may be seen following use of concentrated (75–100%) products. Most authorities recommend avoidance of concentrated products, noting good effectiveness of a 50% concentration in jungle settings. A concentration not to exceed 30–50% for routine adult use seems reasonable. It has been stated that a 20–30% concentration applied to clothing is 90% effective in preventing tick attachment.

The following recommendations are offered to avoid toxicity:

1. Apply repellent sparingly only to exposed skin or clothing. Keep it out of the eyes.

2. Avoid high-concentration products on the skin, particularly with children.

3. Do not inhale or ingest repellents.

4. Use long-sleeved clothing and apply repellent to fabric rather than to skin.

5. Don't use repellent on children's hands that may be rubbed in the eyes or placed in the mouth.

6. Do not reapply repellent in normal weather conditions.

7. Wash repellent off the skin after the insect bite risk has ended.

Permethrin (Permanone Tick Repellent) is a synthetic form of pyrethrin (insecticide) that may be applied to clothing and footwear. As the name implies, it is most effective against ticks. N-octyl bicycloheptene dicarboximide synergist combined with DEET (Sawyer Products DEET Plus; S. C. Johnson Ticks OFF or Deep Woods OFF) is a tick repellent, also effective against biting flies and gnats, that can be applied directly to the skin.

Fleas, horseflies, blackflies, sand flies, deerflies, chiggers, gnats, and other assorted nuisances may not be scared off by insect repellents. Protective netting and a lot of swatting may be your only defenses. After the insect has bitten you, nothing is better than cold applications and perseverance.

Lightning Strike

LIGHTNING strikes the earth at least 100 times per second during an estimated 3,000 thunderstorms per day. Fortunately, the odds of being struck by lightning are not very high; however, 200–400 persons per year are victims of fatal strikes in the United States. The wise traveler respects the incredible forces generated by thunderheads and seeks shelter at all times during a lightning storm.

Lightning is the electrical discharge associated with thunderstorms; it releases a charge of up to 100 million volts. However, when this charge strikes a person directly (or splashes at him from a tree or building), it may largely flow around the outside of the body, which causes a unique constellation of signs and symptoms. The victim is frequently thrown, clothes may be burned or torn, metallic objects (such as belt buckles) may be heated, and shoes removed. The victim often undergoes severe muscle contractions and may travel a great distance. In most cases, the person struck is confused and rendered temporarily blind and/or deaf. In more severe cases, there are feathered (fernlike) or sunburst patterns of burns over the skin (Fig. 112), loss of consciousness, ruptured eardrums, and inability to breathe. Occasionally, victims cease breathing and suffer a cardiac arrest.

If a victim is found confused, burned, or collapsed in the vicinity of a thunderstorm, consider the possibility that he was struck by lightning.

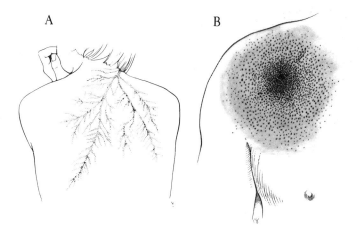

FIGURE 112. *(A) Ferning lightning burn. (B) Punctate (starburst) lightning burn.*

1. Maintain the airway and assist breathing (see pages 18–25). Continue to perform artificial respiration and CPR (see page 26) until sophisticated help can be obtained. Victims of lightning strike may have paralysis of the breathing mechanism for a period of 15–30 minutes, and then make a remarkable recovery. A seemingly lifeless individual may be saved if you breathe for him promptly after the injury.

2. Assume that the victim has been thrown a considerable distance. Protect the cervical spine (see page 31).

3. Examine the victim for any other injuries and treat accordingly.

4. Transport the victim to a hospital.

LIGHTNING AVOIDANCE

1. Know the weather patterns for your area. Don't travel in times of high thunderstorm risk. Avoid being outdoors during a thunderstorm.

2. If a storm enters your area, immediately seek shelter. Enter a hard-roofed auto or large building if possible. Tents and convertible autos offer no protection from lightning. Indoors, stay away from windows, open doors, fireplaces, and large metal fixtures.

3. Do not carry a lightning rod, such as a fishing pole or golf club. Avoid tall objects, such as ski lifts and power lines.

4. In the woods, avoid the tallest trees or hilltops. Shelter yourself in a stand of smaller trees. Avoid clearings (you become the tallest tree). In the open, crouch down or roll into a ball. *If you are in the water, get out.* Avoid being near boat masts or flagpoles. Do not seek refuge near power lines or tall metal structures.

5. Stay in your car, unless it is a convertible. If it is a convertible, huddle on the ground at least 50 yards from the vehicle.

6. If you are part of a group of people, spread the group out, so that everyone isn't struck by a single discharge.

TORNADO AVOIDANCE

1. Watch the cloud formations in a stormy sky. If you see revolving, funnel-shaped clouds, you are in danger.

2. Take shelter immediately. The best location is an underground cave or concrete structure. Do not remain in a tent or camper.

3. If you are caught outside in open country, hunker down or lie flat in a depression, ditch, culvert, or ravine. Cover your head with your arms.

4. Do not try to outrun a tornado. There is no way to predict when it will change direction.

Underwater Diving Accidents and Near-Drowning

As greater numbers of travelers become certified scuba (self-contained underwater breathing apparatus) divers and travel to the tropical waters off domestic and exotic foreign shores (where medical care is frequently difficult to obtain), there will be an increasing incidence of afflictions that require prompt recognition and specific management. Every diver should be familiar with all of the material in this chapter.

AIR EMBOLISM

An air embolism occurs where there is a rupture in the barrier between the air space of the lungs and the blood vessels in the lung that carry oxygenated blood back to the heart (where it can be distributed to the body). In effect, bubbles of air are released into the arterial bloodstream, where they act as barriers to circulation, and can cause a stroke (see page 120), heart attack (see page 46), headache, and/or confusion. Typically, the victim is a diver who ascends too rapidly without exhaling, thus allowing overexpansion of the lungs — and rupture of the tissue — as the external water pressure decreases with ascent. In other words, as a diver ascends from the depths, the air in the lungs (which was delivered from the scuba tank at a pressure regulated to be equal to the surrounding water pressure on the lungs, thereby allowing normal lung expansion) expands. If the rate of exhalation does not keep pace with the lung expansion, the increased pressure within the lungs causes air to be forced through the lung tissue in bubble form, where it appears in the bloodstream and travels directly to the heart. From the heart, the air circulates to and may occlude critical small blood vessels that supply the heart, brain, and spinal cord. The most common symptoms are unconsciousness, confusion, seizures, and/or chest pain immediately upon surfacing. Any disorder that appears in a previously normal diver more than 10 minutes after surfacing is probably not due to air embolism. If the expanding air ruptures through the lung into the pleural space between the lung and the inside of the chest wall, a pneumothorax may be created. (The hazards of a pneumothorax are discussed on page 36.)

Anyone suspected of having suffered an air embolism should be placed in a head-down position (with the body at a 15–30 degree tilt), turned on the left side, be assisted in breathing if necessary (see page 24), and IMMEDIATELY TRANSPORTED TO AN EMERGENCY FACILITY. The treatment for arterial gas embolism is recompression in a hyperbaric chamber, which pressurizes the victim's environment and shrinks the bubbles. This must be accomplished as rapidly as possible to save the victim's life, or to avoid serious disability. If oxygen is available, it should be administered by face mask at a flow rate of 10 liters per minute.

DECOMPRESSION SICKNESS (BENDS)

When a diver descends in the water, nitrogen present in the compressed air he breathes is absorbed into the tissues of the body. This process is analogous to the introduction of carbon dioxide into carbonated beverages. In the human case, there is a limit to the time and depth that a diver can tolerate before exceeding the amount of nitrogen that can be absorbed safely. If this limit is exceeded, and/or if the diver ascends too rapidly, this nitrogen leaves the tissues and enters the bloodstream in the form of microscopic bubbles (like opening a bottle of soda pop). The signs and symptoms caused by these bubbles in the body represent decompression sickness, also known as the bends. Symptoms may begin immediately after ascent from a dive or may be delayed by a number of hours. These include joint pain, numbness and tingling of the arms and legs, back pain, fatigue, weakness, inability to control the bladder or bowels, paralysis, headache, confusion, dizziness, nausea, vomiting, difficulty in speaking, itching, skin mottling, shortness of breath, cough, and collapse.

If someone is suspected of having suffered the bends, immediately have him begin to breathe oxygen (10 liters per minute by face mask) and begin rapid transport to a hospital. The definitive treatment is recompression in a hyperbaric chamber. DO NOT PUT THE DIVER BACK INTO THE WATER TO ATTEMPT IN-WATER RECOMPRESSION; this is very hazardous.

Because the pressure inside a commercial jet aircraft at 30,000 feet is equivalent to an unpressurized environmental altitude of 8,000 feet, a diver should not fly for 12 hours following a no-decompression dive and for 24 hours following a decompression dive.

NITROGEN NARCOSIS

When absorbed into the bloodstream in sufficient concentration, nitrogen acts as an anesthetic agent. Thus, at depths that exceed

90 feet, divers are at risk for euphoria, confusion, inappropriate judgment, and unconsciousness induced by nitrogen absorbed into the bloodstream from air breathed under pressure. The treatment is prompt (but cautious) ascent, to allow the absorbed levels of nitrogen to decrease. NO ONE SHOULD EVER DIVE ALONE. ALWAYS PAY ATTENTION TO YOUR DIVE BUDDY'S BEHAVIOR. IF HE ACTS IN A STRANGE MANNER, ASSIST HIM TO THE SURFACE.

EAR SQUEEZE

As a diver descends in the water, the external water pressure on the eardrum increases rapidly. If the diver cannot equalize this pressure from within by forcing air into the eustachian tube (a small passageway that connects the middle ear and the throat) and into the middle ear, the eardrum stretches inward (extremely painful) and then ruptures (Fig. 113). This break allows water to

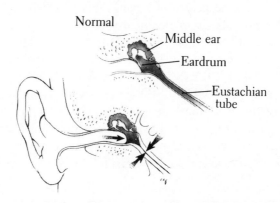

Normal

Middle ear

Eardrum

Eustachian tube

FIGURE 113. *Middle ear squeeze. When a diver descends, air in the middle ear contracts, the eustachian tube collapses, and the eardrum bulges inward, causing pain. If the external water pressure is sufficient, the eardrum may rupture.*

rush into the middle ear, with resultant severe pain, vertigo (see page 137), nausea, vomiting, and disorientation. If the diver cannot make his way to the surface, he may drown. If the eardrum is injured but not ruptured, the pain is similar to that of an ear infection.

Inability to "clear" the ears (equalize pressure from within) in order to prevent inward bulging and rupture of the eardrum should keep the diver out of the water. A person with an upper respiratory tract infection (and narrowed eustachian tube) should not dive and should avoid travel in unpressurized aircraft.

If a diver suddenly feels pain in his ear and is stricken with dizziness, nausea, or visual difficulty, he should remain calm and slowly ascend to the surface. The ear should be allowed to dry on its own. Do not insert cotton swabs into the ear, as you may increase damage to the eardrum. Do not instill any medicines into the ear. Immediately transport the victim to an ear specialist. Suspend all diving activities until the eardrum is healed or repaired. If dizziness is profound, administer drugs for motion sickness (see page 326). Begin antibiotic administration with trimethoprim-sulfamethoxazole or ciprofloxacin. Because sudden dizziness may also be due to air embolism or the bends, the victim should be observed closely for worsening of this condition.

SINUS SQUEEZE

Sinus squeeze occurs if pressurized air cannot be forced into the sinuses during descent. In such a case, the air within the sinus contracts, causing the walls of the sinus to bleed, accompanied by intense sharp pain. Symptoms include pain over the affected sinus and nosebleed. A "reverse squeeze" occurs during ascent, when air expands in the sinus without being able to escape. This is also very painful, but fortunately self-limited, as the air is absorbed slowly into the tissues that line the sinuses.

If a sinus squeeze occurs, slowly ascend to the surface. This generally alleviates most of the pain, but it may take a while for the bleeding to stop. Because the sinus is now blood-filled, the victim is at great risk for developing sinusitis (see page 154) and should be placed on ampicillin, erythromycin, or penicillin for 4 days, along with oral and nasal decongestants to promote drainage. If the pain is severe and persists for more than 12 hours after the initial incident, the patient may benefit from a short course of prednisone (60 mg the first day, 40 mg the second, 20 mg the third). This combats the inflammation of the "squeeze" and should not be given if the patient has symptoms of a sinus infection (foul nasal discharge, fever, facial tenderness).

NEAR-DROWNING

One of the most common tragic accidents, particularly of children, is near-drowning. Near-drowning can occur in a variety of settings, but the problems encountered seldom vary:

1. Lack of oxygen. This occurs because the lung tissue is injured by water, and oxygen transfer into the bloodstream is inhibited. Another factor is occasional spasm of the vocal cords, which blocks the passage of air through the windpipe (most commonly seen in cold-water drownings).

2. Body chemistry abnormalities. Because of the lack of oxygen delivery to the organs and tissues of the body, there is the rapid accumulation of waste products that cannot be effectively removed. This results in an accumulation of acid and other chemicals that alter the function of the heart, brain, kidneys, liver, etc. (Victims who drown in the Red Sea often have abnormally high sodium concentrations in the blood because of the high salt content of the water.)

3. Accompanying problems, such as hypothermia (see page 221), injuries, and serious illnesses (for example, heart attack, stroke). Sadly, alcohol figures prominently in adult boating and near-drowning accidents.

If a near-drowning incident occurs, the rescuer should do the following:
1. SEND SOMEONE FOR HELP.
2. Suspect a broken neck in the appropriate circumstances. For instance, someone who has been seen to collapse in a swimming pool probably hasn't broken his neck. (If he *dove* into the pool, that is another story!) However, someone who tumbles into the waves off a surfboard and washes up onto the beach unconscious may well have a neck injury. Do what is necessary to aid the victim, but remember to protect the neck (page 31).
3. Check for breathing by feeling over the mouth and nose while watching the chest rise. Open the mouth and sweep it clean with two fingers. Align the victim on the ground with the head at a level below the feet. Begin mouth-to-mouth or (for a child) mouth-to-mouth and nose breathing if necessary (pages 24, 30).
4. Check for pulses and begin chest compressions if necessary (page 26).
5. If it is impossible to perform mouth-to-mouth breathing because the stomach is full (most victims swallow a fair amount of water in the drowning process), turn the victim on his side (with his head at a level below the feet) and perform the Heimlich maneuver (see page 22). Sweep the mouth clear and resume mouth-to-mouth breathing.
6. Hypothermia (see page 221) is commonly associated with near-drowning. Cover the victim above and below with blankets. Gently remove all wet clothing. Because hypothermia may be protective for the heart and brain (with regard to lack of oxygen) to a considerable degree, if the victim is cold, continue the resuscitation until trained rescuers arrive or until you are fatigued (see page 227). Remember, no one is dead until he is warm and dead.
7. If the victim responds to your measures, he should be transported to an emergency facility. Even if he feels 100% normal,

he should still be evaluated by a physician, because delayed worsening of lung function is common. A person who is already short of breath and coughing is headed for big trouble soon.

8. Administer oxygen, 10 liters per minute, by face mask.

PREVENTION OF NEAR-DROWNING

1. Watch your children. Toddlers are at greatest risk for drowning.

2. Fence in all pools and swimming areas. Maintain the water level in a pool as high as possible to allow a person who reaches the edge to pull himself out.

3. Teach all children to swim.

4. Never place nonswimmers in high-risk situations; small sailboats, whitewater rafts, inflatable kayaks, etc.

5. When boating or rafting, always wear a good life vest with a snug fit and a head flotation collar. In a kayak, wear a proper helmet.

6. Do not mix alcohol and water sports.

7. Know your limits. Feats of endurance and demonstrations of bravado in dangerous rapids or surf are for idiots.

8. Be prepared for a flash flood. In times of unusually heavy rainfall, stay away from natural streambeds, arroyos, and other drainage channels. Use your map to determine your elevation and stay off low ground or the very bottom of a hill. Know where the high ground is and how to get there in a hurry. Absolutely avoid flooded areas and unnecessary stream and river crossings. Do not attempt to cross a flowing stream where the water is above your knees. Abandon a stalled vehicle in a flood area.

Animal Attacks

MOST animal attacks are from man's best friend, the pet dog. Other animals that will attack man, given the provocation, include the cat, rat, tiger, lion, skunk, squirrel, camel, elephant, bear, alligator, bat, wolf, and rhinoceros. Although there are unique variations to the nature of the wounds created by different animals (in most part related to size of the animal, types of teeth and claws, and risk of infection), the basic out-of-hospital management of an animal bite or mauling is the same for all creatures.

GENERAL TREATMENT

1. If a person is bitten or mauled by an animal, apply pressure to stop any brisk bleeding, and follow the instructions for management of bleeding and cuts (see pages 48, 198).

2. In particular, it is very important to clean the wounds vigorously. Flush any injury that has broken the skin with at least 2 quarts of water, scrub with mild soap, and flush again. If you are carrying povidone-iodine (Betadine) solution (not soap or scrub), benzalkonium (Zephiran) liquid, or Bactine antiseptic, you should rinse the wound with one of these for 1 minute (to help kill rabies virus), and then rinse away the solution until there is no discoloration of the wound.

3. Do not suture (sew) or tape closed any animal bite, unless it is absolutely essential to allow rescue. If a large tear is present, the wound edges can be held together with dry wraps. Tight closure of a contaminated wound (all animal bites and scratches introduce bacteria into the wound) can lead to a horrible infection.

4. If the victim is more than 5 hours from a doctor, administer dicloxacillin, penicillin, cephalexin, or ciprofloxacin. If the bite is from a cat, administer antibiotics as soon as possible.

5. Any wound larger than a scratch requires a doctor's attention.

SPECIAL CONSIDERATIONS

High-Risk Wounds

Wounds at high risk for infection include bites to the hands and feet, and all puncture wounds (see page 196). These should be rinsed copiously and *never* taped closed. All persons who sustain such wounds should be given antibiotics (as suggested above). Cat, human, and monkey bites are enormously prone to infection, and require prompt attention by a physician.

Rabies

Rabies virus infection occurs more frequently in wild than in domestic animals. In some foreign countries where immunization of animals is infrequently practiced, the risk is greater than in the United States for domestic transmission of the disease. The virus is carried in saliva and is transmitted by bite or lick (if the skin is broken). Dogs, foxes, coyotes, skunks, wolves, bats, and raccoons are the most common carriers. Although rabbits, rats, guinea pigs, and ferrets may be rabid, they are rarely involved in transmission of rabies to humans. Because of rabies risk, all wild animal bites and bites of unregistered or strangely behaving cats and dogs should be reported to the appropriate public health authority. If the animal is a pet with otherwise normal behavior, it should be observed for 10 days. If the animal is rabid, it will become very ill or die during that time, and its brain tissue can be analyzed for the presence of rabies. If the animal is a pet with unusual behavior, or a captured high-risk wild animal, it should be killed and examined. *If it is a high-risk wild animal, and cannot be captured, it must be presumed to be rabid.*
Immediately scrub the wound vigorously with soap and water.

If benzalkonium chloride (Zephiran), Bactine antiseptic, or 10% povidone-iodine (Betadine) solution is available, one of them should be used to swab the wound, since they may kill rabies virus.

If rabies is a consideration, the victim should seek the assistance of a physician, who will determine the need for postexposure rabies vaccination (a series of 5 injections) and the administration of antirabies serum. Preexposure vaccination against rabies is now available, and should be administered to persons at high risk of exposure (animal handlers, cavers, hunters and trappers in rabies-endemic areas, and travelers to certain foreign countries). This is given as a series of 3 injections over 30 days.

Bubonic Plague

Cases of bubonic plague are still reported in the United States. The disease is transmitted by the bites of fleas that have acquired the plague bacillus from infected squirrels, rats, and mice. Rarely, the disease can be contracted from direct contact with infected pets. Pay attention to local public health warnings, and do not travel with pets in areas of plague infestation. Take care to spray or dust your canine companions with flea repellent regularly (after each time they get wet) when traveling in wooded areas. Do not allow children to handle small dead animals.

AVOIDING HAZARDOUS ANIMALS

Most wild animal encounters can be avoided with caution and a little common sense. Follow these rules:

1. Do not provoke animals. Unless starving, senile, or ill, most animals will not attack humans without provocation. Do not corner or provoke carnivores, and do not tease animals by handling them or approaching their young.

2. Do not disturb feeding animals. Do not explore into their feeding territory or disrupt mating patterns.

3. Do not separate fighting animals using your bare hands. If possible, drive animals apart using a long stick or club.

4. In bear country, hang all food off the ground in trees away from the campsite. Never keep food or captured game inside a tent. Make noise when hiking, particularly on narrow paths or through tall grass. If attacked by a bear, do not try to outrun it (you can't). Cover your head and neck with your arms and curl into a fetal position.

5. Never leave a small child alone with an animal, regardless of how friendly you think the animal is.

Wild Plant and Mushroom Poisoning

Toxic plants and mushrooms may be eaten by curious children or by hikers and amateur herbalists who mistake their selections for edible species. The poisoning of at least 15,000 Americans by plants each year results in about 100 deaths.

Because it takes an experienced botanist or mycologist to identify species, I will discuss the general evaluation and treatment of a person who has ingested a potentially toxic plant or mushroom. Although you have read and heard this a thousand times, it bears repeating: *never eat wild plants, mushrooms, or berries unless you know what you are doing.*

MEDICAL HISTORY

Although the narrative description of the ingestion will have little bearing on the immediate patient management, it is important to gather as much information as possible, for the benefit of the physician who will ultimately care for the victim.

1. When was the plant eaten?

2. What parts of the plant were eaten? How many different plants were eaten?

3. What symptoms does the victim have? What were the initial symptoms (e.g., sweating, hallucinations, nausea, vomiting, abdominal pain)? What was the time interval between the ingestion and the onset of symptoms? Did anyone who did not eat the plant(s) develop similar symptoms? Did everyone who ate the plant(s) become ill?

4. Was the plant eaten raw, or was it cooked? How was it cooked? Was alcohol consumed within 72 hours of the plant ingestion?

It is important to obtain as much of the original plant as possible for identification. If the patient regurgitates, save his vomitus, because it may contain part of the plant or spores that can be identified by an expert.

There are few specific antidotes for toxic plant ingestions, so that most victims are managed according to their symptoms, which may include sweating, nausea, vomiting, diarrhea, shortness of breath, slow or rapid heartbeat, pinpoint or dilated pupils, salivation, increased frequency of urination, weakness, difficulty in breathing, hallucinations, and many others.

If it is known that someone has ingested a toxic plant or mushroom within the last 2 hours, he should immediately be forced to vomit (if he has not done so already). This may be done by administering syrup of ipecac (adult dose 2 tablespoons; pediatric dose, age greater than 12 months, 1 tablespoon) followed by at least a pint of warm water (½ pint for a small child). *If the victim is drowsy, do not induce vomiting.* After vomiting is induced, immediately seek the attention of a physician.

COMMONLY INGESTED TOXIC PLANTS AND MUSHROOMS

The following are toxic plants that are most commonly ingested:

1. Oleander is a shrub, up to 20 feet tall, commonly found along highways and in gardens (Fig. 114). It is an extremely hardy plant, requiring minimal soil and care. Its attractive red, pink, or white clusters of flowers make oleander very popular. The entire plant is toxic, including smoke from burning cuttings and water in which the flowers are placed. There have been deaths from use of the branches as skewers for roasting hot dogs. Symptoms begin 1–2 hours after ingestion, and include nausea, vomiting, abdominal cramps, diarrhea, confusion, and blurred vision. In serious ingestions, the heart rhythm may be disturbed.

2. Foxglove is a European import that has toxic leaves and toxic tubular pink or purple flowers (Fig. 115). Poisonings occur from ingestion of the plant parts or from foxglove tea. The symptoms are the same as those from oleander ingestion.

3. Water hemlock ("beaver poison") is found in salt and freshwater marshes and along riverbanks (Fig. 116). A member of the carrot family, the plant grows to 6 feet and has clusters of whitish, heavily scented flowers, and a bundle of tuberous roots. It is easily confused with wild parsnip, celery, or sweet anise. When injured, the stem and trunk exude a yellow oil that smells like celery or raw parsnip. The entire plant is toxic. Symptoms begin 15–60 minutes after ingestion, and include excessive salivation, abdominal pain, diarrhea, and vomiting. In serious ingestions, the patient may suffer seizures and may collapse and have difficulty breathing. Death may occur.

4. Castor bean is a treelike shrub that may grow to 15 feet with clusters of spiny seed pods, which contain seeds with coats that resemble pinto beans (Fig. 117). The seeds contain a potent toxin that causes immediate mouth burning and abdominal pain, followed by vomiting, diarrhea, abnormal heart rhythms, and collapse.

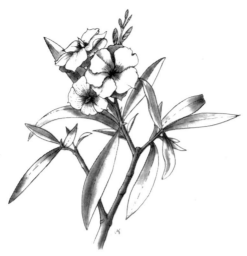

FIGURE 114. *Oleander.*

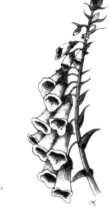

FIGURE 115. *Foxglove.*

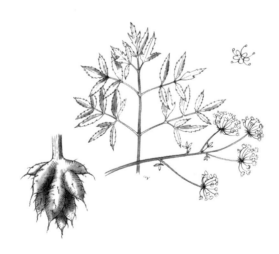

FIGURE 116. *Water hemlock, with tuberous roots.*

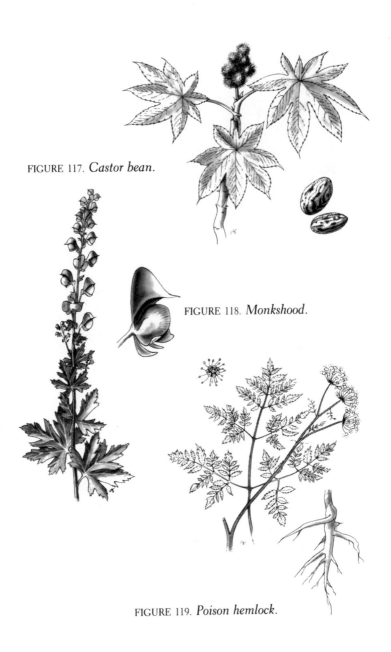

FIGURE 117. *Castor bean.*

FIGURE 118. *Monkshood.*

FIGURE 119. *Poison hemlock.*

5. Monkshood is a flowering plant with tuberous roots and blue helmet-shaped flowers (Fig. 118). The leaves and roots are particularly toxic. Ingestion causes immediate mouth and throat burning, followed by vomiting, diarrhea, headache, muscle cramps, sweating, drooling, blurred vision, and confusion. In serious ingestions, there may be abnormal heart rhythms and collapse.

6. Poison hemlock is a marsh plant that grows to 9 feet with leaves that resemble a carrot top (Fig. 119). The white flowers are clustered and smell like urine if they are crushed. The seeds and white unbranched tuberous roots are also toxic. The symptoms are similar to those from water hemlock ingestion, without significant abdominal pain or diarrhea, and death may follow seizures or paralysis with breathing failure.

7. Pokeweed is a widely distributed plant with clusters of white flowers and plentiful round purple berries (Fig. 120). Ingestion of the root (commonly mistaken for horseradish) or the berries (a favorite for children) causes the intoxication. Symptoms include sore mouth, tongue, and throat (delayed by 2–3 hours), thirst, nausea, vomiting, abdominal cramps, and diarrhea (which may be bloody). The illness may be profound, lasting for up to 2 days, particularly if the roots were ingested.

8. Rhododendrons are common flowering plants that contain a number of toxins (Fig. 121). Poisoning has occurred following ingestion of honey made from the flower nectar. Symptoms include mouth burning, followed by drooling, vomiting, diarrhea, headache, and numbness and tingling. Serious ingestions cause weakness, blurred vision, seizures, and collapse.

9. Jimsonweed (Fig. 122) has white or purple flowers, with prickly seed pods. Adults may ingest a tea made from the leaves or flowers. The entire plant is toxic. Symptoms include dry mouth, rapid heartbeat, hot and dry skin, weakness, difficulty in walking, dilated pupils, and inability to urinate. Severe poisonings cause fever and collapse.

10. Skunk cabbage is a marsh and forest plant that grows to 6

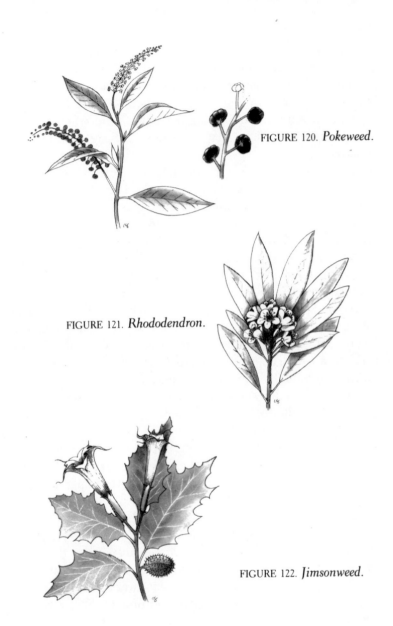

FIGURE 120. *Pokeweed.*

FIGURE 121. *Rhododendron.*

FIGURE 122. *Jimsonweed.*

feet and has broad pleated leaves (Fig. 123). The entire plant is toxic and causes symptoms similar to those that follow ingestion of monkshood, but generally much less severe.

11. Pyracantha is a thorned shrub with white flowers and clusters of small red berries (Fig. 124). Ingestion of the berries in large quantities causes nausea and diarrhea. Birds sometimes eat fermented pyracantha berries and become intoxicated. Scratches from the thorns may cause a burning skin irritation.

12. *Amanita phalloides* (death cap) is a gilled mushroom with a shiny yellow to greenish cap found in the western United States (Fig. 125). The entire mushroom is toxic, and cannot be detoxified by cooking. Symptoms occur 6–12 hours after ingestion, and include abdominal pain, persistent nausea/vomiting/diarrhea, low blood pressure, and rapid heartbeat. The patient

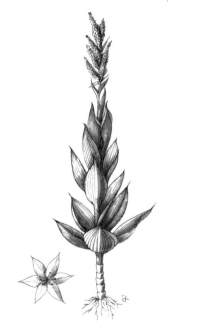

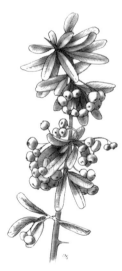

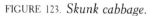

FIGURE 123. *Skunk cabbage.*   FIGURE 124. *Pyracantha.*

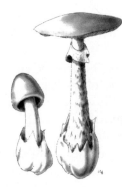

FIGURE 125. *Amanita phalloides (death cap)*.

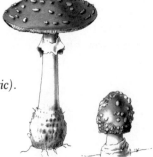

FIGURE 126. *Amanita muscaria (fly agaric)*.

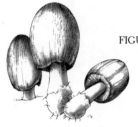

FIGURE 127. *Coprinus atramentarius (inky cap)*.

may appear normal for the next few days, but then rapidly shows signs of massive liver destruction, which include jaundice (yellow skin and eyeballs, darkened urine), easy bleeding, and altered mental status. Fatalities are frequent with this species and with *Galerina autumnalis*.

Most nonfatal mushroom toxins act rapidly to produce symptoms (nausea, vomiting, diarrhea, headache) within 1–4 hours. Severe abdominal pain and headache approximately 6 hours after ingestion is likely due to *Gyromitra esculenta*. Typically, diarrhea and vomiting caused by ingestion of *Amanita phalloides* are delayed by 6–12 hours. However, because most unknowledgeable mushroom foragers eat a mixture of different species, a rapid onset of symptoms does not rule out a potentially disastrous ingestion. Approximately 7 to 10 species of the several thousand varieties of wild mushrooms in the United States can cause death by ingestion.

13. *Amanita muscaria* (fly agaric) is a gilled mushroom with a variably colored cap (yellow, red, warty, etc.) (Fig. 126). Most poisonings are intentional, as persons brew and drink *Amanita* tea for its hallucinogenic effects. Symptoms occur 30 minutes to 2 hours after ingestion, and include euphoria, difficulty in walking, dizziness, hallucinations, and blurred vision. Severe ingestions can result in seizures and coma.

14. *Coprinus atramentarius* (inky cap) is a gilled fungus with a conical cap that liquefies and turns black when picked (Fig. 127). If alcohol is consumed within 24–72 hours after ingestion of the fungus, the victim suffers abdominal pain, vomiting, sweating, facial flushing, and headaches. *Cortinarius rainierensis* may cause the victim to have enormous thirst and increased urination 3–17 days after ingestion, due to a toxic effect on the kidneys.

Many other plants (wild and house plants) can cause illnesses if consumed in sufficient quantities (one appleseed will not poison you). When in doubt as to the identity, quantity of a plant ingested, or the potential toxicity of the plant, it is wisest to immediately consult a certified Poison Control Center or a physician.

TOXICITY OF COMMON PLANTS

The following list divides common plants into four groups:

T: Toxic (see a physician or notify a Poison Control Center)
O: Toxic oxalate (plant juices contain oxalates; ingestion may cause irritation of the mouth and throat, nausea, diarrhea, and difficulty breathing; see a physician or notify a Poison Control Center)
I: Irritant (ingestion may cause abdominal pain, nausea, vomiting and diarrhea, *or* contact with the skin may cause irritation)
N: Nontoxic

Acorn (T)
Akee unripe fruit (T)
Algerian ivy (I)
Alocasia (O)
Aloe vera (I)
Amaryllis, common (I)
American ivy (O)
Amorphophallis (O)
Angel's trumpet (T)
Anthurium (O)
Apple pit (T)
Apricot pit (T)
Aralia (N)
Arnica flowers and roots (T)
Arrowhead vine (O)
Asparagus fern (N)
Asparagus fern berry (I)
Autumn crocus bulb (T)
Avocado leaves (T)

Azalea (T)
Baby's breath (N)
Bamboo palm (N)
Baneberry berries, roots, stock, and sap (T)
Barberry (I)
Beaver poison (T)
Beechnut seeds (I)
Begonia (N)
Belladonna (T)
Betel nut seeds (T)
Bird of paradise seeds and pods (I)
Birdsnest fern (N)
Bittersweet (T)
Black alder berries (I)
Black cherry bark, leaves, and seeds (T)
Black locust (I)

Black nightshade leaves and green fruit (T)
Bleeding heart (T)
Bloodroot (T)
Blue cohosh (T)
Boston ivy (O)
Boxwood leaves and twigs (I)
Buckeye flowers, seeds, and nuts (T)
Buckthorn (T)
Bull nettle green fruit (T)
Bunchberry (I)
Burning bush (T)
Buttercup (T)
Cactus thorn (I)
Calabar bean (T)
Caladium (O)
California poppy (N)
Calla lily (O)
Camellia (N)
Cardinal flower (T)
Carnation (I)
Cassava root (T)
Cast iron plant (N)
Castor bean seeds (T)
Celandine (I)
Century plant (I)
Cherry pit (T)
Chinaberry (T)
Chinese evergreen (N)
Chokecherry (T)
Christmas rose (T)
Chrysanthemum (T)
Clematis (T)
Climbing lily (T)

Coffee senna (I)
Coffee tree (N)
Coleus (N)
Colocasia (O)
Coumnea (N)
Coral berry (I)
Corn cockle seeds (T)
Cornstalk plant (N)
Cotoneaster (T)
Cowbane (T)
Crape myrtle (N)
Creeping Charlie (T)
Crocus: autumn, meadow (T)
Croton (N)
Croton seeds (T)
Crowfoot (T)
Crown of thorns (I)
Cyclamen (I)
Daffodil bulbs (I)
Dahlia (N)
Daisy (I)
Daphne (T)
Deadly nightshade (T)
Death camas bulbs and roots (T)
Delphinium (T)
Desert rose (T)
Devil's ivy (O)
Dieffenbachia (O)
Dogwood (N)
Donkey's tail (N)
Dracunculus (O)
Dragon tree (N)
Dumbcane (O)
Dutchman's breeches (T)
Easter cactus (N)

Easter lily (N)
Elderberry (T)
Elephant's ear (O)
Emerald duke (O)
Emerald ripple (N)
English ivy (I)
European bittersweet (T)
European spindle tree (T)
False hellebore (T)
Fava bean and pollen (T)
Fetter bush (T)
Fiddleleaf fig (N)
Fig tree (N)
Fishberries dried fruit (T)
Fishtail palm (O)
Fool's parsley (T)
Forget-me-not (N)
Forsythia (N)
Four o'clock roots and seeds (I)
Foxglove (T)
Fuchsia (N)
Garden sorrel (O)
Gardenia (N)
Geranium, California (I)
Glacier ivy (I)
Gloriosa (T)
Glory lily (T)
Gloxinia (N)
Goldenchain tree (T)
Golden seal (T)
Golden shower (I)
Grape ivy (N)
Groundsel (T)
Hawaiian ti plant (N)
Hawthorn berry (N)

Heart ivy (I)
Heart leaf (O)
Hemlock tree (N)
Henbane, black (T)
Hibiscus (N)
Holly berry (I)
Honeysuckle berry (N)
Horse bean and pollen (T)
Horse chestnut (T)
Horse nettle green fruit (T)
Hyacinth bulb (I)
Hydrangea (T)
Ice plant (N)
Indian tobacco (T)
Inkberry (T)
Iris root (I)
Jack-in-the-pulpit (O)
Jade plant (N)
Jasmine (N)
Jessamine (T)
Jequirty bean (T)
Jerusalem cherry leaves and
    unripe fruit (T)
Jetberry bush berries (T)
Jimsonweed (T)
Jonquil bulbs (I)
Kentucky coffee tree (I)
Laburnum leaves and seeds (T)
Lady's slipper (N)
Lantana (T)
Larkspur (T)
Laurel, American (T)
Laurel, black (T)
Laurel, English (T)
Laurel, mountain (T)

Laurel, sheep (T)
Lichen (T)
Lily-of-the-valley (T)
Lipstick plant (N)
Lupine (T)
Maidenhair fern (N)
Majesty (O)
Manchineel fruit (I)
Mandrake (I)
Mango skin and sap (I)
Marble queen (O)
Marigold, cowslip (I)
Marijuana (T)
Marsh marigold (T)
May apple (I)
Meadow saffron (T)
Mescal (T)
Mexican jumping bean (T)
Mexican prickle poppy seeds
    and oil (T)
Mimosa (T)
Mistletoe berries (T)
Monkey pod nuts (I)
Monkshood (T)
Moon cactus (N)
Moonseed roots and fruit (I)
Morning glory seed (T)
Mother-in-law's tongue (N)
Mother of pearls (N)
Mountain ash berry (N)
Mountain laurel (T)
Mulberry, red (green berries
    and sap) (T)
Naked ladies (T)
Narcissus bulbs (I)

Natal palm (N)
Nephthytis (O)
Nerve plant (N)
Nightshade (T)
Norfolk Island pine (N)
Nutmeg seeds (T)
Old man cactus (N)
Oleander leaves (T)
Olive tree (N)
Orchid (N)
Oregon grape (N)
Pansy flower (N)
Paradise palm (N)
Parlor ivy (O)
Parlor palm (N)
Passion vine (N)
Peach pit (T)
Peanut cactus (N)
Pear pit (T)
Pellionia (N)
Peony flower (N)
Peperomia (N)
Periwinkle (T)
Petunia (N)
Peyote (T)
Pheasant's eye (T)
Philodendron (O)
Phlox (N)
Physic nut seeds (T)
Plum pit (T)
Poinsettia (I)
Poison hemlock (T)
Poison ivy (I)
Poison oak (I)
Poison sumac (I)

Pokeberry (T)
Pokeweed (T)
Potato (except tuber) (T)
Pothos (O)
Prayer bean (T)
Privet, common/California (T)
Pussy willow (N)
Pyracantha (I)
Rabbit's foot fern (N)
Ragwort (T)
Rainbow plant (N)
Red sage (T)
Rhododendron (T)
Rhubarb leaves (O)
Ripple ivy (I)
Rosary bean/pea (T)
Roses (N)
Rubber plant (N)
Saddleleaf (O)
Sand briar green fruit (T)
Scotch broom seeds and
   leaves (T)
Sentry palm (N)
Shamrock plant (O)
Skunk cabbage (O)
Snakeberry berries, roots,
   stock, and sap (T)
Snakeroot, white (T)
Snapdragon (N)
Snowberry berries (I)
Snowdrop (I)
Soapberry (I)
Spanish broom seeds and
   leaves (T)
Spindle bush (T)

Spider plant (N)
Sprengeri fern (I)
Squill (T)
Staghorn fern (N)
Star anise, Japanese (T)
Star of Bethlehem (I)
Stinkweed (T)
String of beads/pearls (T)
Swedish ivy (N)
Sweet pea (T)
Swiss cheese plant (O)
Sword fern (N)
Thornapple (T)
Tobacco (green) (T)
Tomato leaves (T)
Toyon leaves (T)
Tulip bulb (O)
Tung nut seeds (T)
Umbrella plant (T)
Venus flytrap (N)
Vinca (T)
Virginia creeper (O)
Wahoo (T)
Walnut, green shells (T)
Wandering jew (inchplant) (N)
Water arum (O)
Water hemlock (T)
Wild cherry (T)
Wild garlic (I)
Wild grape roots (T)
Wild onion (I)
Wild sage (T)
Wild tobacco (T)
Wild tomato green fruit (T)
Windsor bean and pollen (T)

Wintersweet (T)
Wisteria pods (I)
Witch hazel (T)
Wood rose (T)
Yellow jessamine (T)

Yellow nightshade fruit (T)
Yew (T)
Yucca (N)
Zinnia (N)

PART FIVE

MISCELLANEOUS

INFORMATION

This section provides information not specifically covered elsewhere in the book. I have tried to answer the questions most frequently asked of the wilderness physician.

Water Disinfection

W ATER *purification* is the removal of chemical pollutants by filtration through activated charcoal or active resin compounds. This usually improves the taste, but does not decrease the incidence of infectious disease, because microorganisms are not removed. Water *disinfection* is the treatment of water with chemicals, boiling, or filtration to remove agents of infectious disease, such as bacteria or cysts.

If at all possible, carry disinfected water with you. If you must drink water from a stream or lake, try to use small tributaries that descend at right angles to the main direction of valley drainage. Clean melted snow is of less risk than ice taken from the surface of a lake or stream. The principal offending agents in contaminated water or on unwashed food that cause illness and diarrhea are the bacteria *Salmonella, Shigella, E. coli,* and *Campylobacter,* and the flagellate protozoan *Giardia lamblia.* Drinking non-disinfected water in parts of Africa, India, and Pakistan can cause dracunculiasis (guinea worm disease). In countries where water is improperly disinfected, the traveler should stick to bottled or canned carbonated beverages, beer, and wine. All containers should be wiped clean to remove external moisture and dirt. All ice should be considered contaminated. Do not urinate or defecate into or near your water supply. Build a latrine 8–10 inches deep into the ground at least 100 feet and downhill from the water supply.

Water may be disinfected by using any of the following methods:

1. Boil the water for 5–10 minutes plus 1 minute for each 1,000 feet of altitude above sea level. *Giardia* cysts are instantly killed in water heated to 140–160°F (60–71°C). Bacteria and

viruses are less sensitive to heat, and require 5–10 minutes' boiling at sea level for killing. Remember, the temperature at which water boils varies with altitude because of the surrounding barometric pressure. Barometric pressure is expressed in terms of the height (in inches or millimeters) of a column of mercury (Hg) that exerts a pressure equal to that of a column of air with the same size base. At sea level (barometric pressure 760 mm Hg), water boils at 212°F (100°C); at 5,000 feet (632 mm Hg), 203°F (95°C); at 10,000 feet (522 mm Hg), 194°F (90°C); at 14,000 feet (446 mm Hg), 187°F (86°C). Boiling water is effective for disinfection at any altitude likely to be attained by a wilderness enthusiast.

2. Add 1 tablet of fresh tetraglycine hydroperiodide (Potable Aqua, Globaline, Coughlan's) to 1 quart of water and allow the water to stand for ½ hour. If the water is cloudy, use 2 tablets. If the water is cold, allow 1 hour after adding the tablets before drinking. A few grains of sodium thiosulfate per quart of water kills the iodine taste. (Any fruit flavorings which contain vitamin C should be mixed in after full time for disinfection has elapsed.) Because a 50-tablet bottle of tetraglycine hydroperiodide contains only 0.4 gram of iodine (1⁄50 the lethal dose), this method is very safe. If military surplus iodine tablets are used, they should be steel gray in color and not crumble when pinched by two fingers. Discard older, crumbled tablets. Also, no matter what chemical disinfection system is used, allow disinfected water to seep around the cap and threads of the canteen or water bottle, in order to disinfect them too.

3. Add 8–10 drops (0.5 ml) of standard 2% iodine tincture per quart of water and allow the water to stand for ½ hour. If the water is not at least 68°F (20°C), this technique may not eliminate *Giardia*. If the water is cold, allow it to stand for 1 hour before drinking. If you have extra time and do not like the iodine taste, use 4–5 drops of iodine and allow the water to stand for 8 hours or overnight.

4. Fill a one- or two-ounce glass bottle with iodine crystals (4–8 grams), then fill the bottle with water. Shake vigorously, then allow the crystals to settle to the bottom. This will create a saturated solution of iodine. Pour at least half of this liquid (*not the remaining crystals*) through a fine filter (such as Teflon) into a quart of water and allow the water to stand for ½ hour. If the water temperature is not at least 68°F (20°C), this technique may not eliminate *Giardia*. The crystals may be reused up to 1,000 times. Remember that 2 grams of iodine represent a potentially lethal dose if ingested, so *it is absolutely essential to keep the iodine crystals out of the hands of children*. A pregnant woman or a person with thyroid disease or iodine allergy should consult a physician before using any iodine compound for water disinfection. A commercial iodine crystal system that can be reused to disinfect up to 2,000 liters of drinking water is sold as Polar Pure Water Disinfectant (Polar Equipment; see page 333).

5. Filter the water through a category three (as set for purification by the Environmental Protection Agency) water treatment device. Two recommended devices are the First-Need (General Ecology Inc.) 0.4 micron filter and the Katadyn 0.2 micron filter. These have pores small enough to filter out *Giardia* cysts and some bacteria, but not viruses. The lightweight Timberline Filter is advertised to effectively filter *Giardia* cysts.

6. Do not rely on Halazone (p-dichlorosulfamyl benzoic acid) or other chlorine (bleach) products to disinfect water. Halazone is relatively inactive in hot, cold, or alkaline water; it has a brief shelf life (5 months at 90°F/32°C); cannot be stored effectively in the heat; loses potency rapidly (75% loss after 2 days) upon exposure to air; and is not always effective against *Giardia* cysts. Superchlorination followed by dechlorination (using concentrated hydrogen peroxide) is an effective technique that is available as the Sierra Water Purifier (4 in 1 Water Systems Co.; see page 332). This is a more complicated method that requires understanding and experience.

Motion Sickness

MOTION sickness (seasickness) can be a disabling problem for sailors, fishermen, divers, and air travelers. It is caused by fluid movement in the labyrinth of the middle ear, which plays a major part in the control of equilibrium. It is made worse by alcohol ingestion, emotional upset, noxious odors (for example, diesel fumes), and inner ear injury or infection. Most people adapt to motion after a few days, but may require medication until they are adjusted to the environment.

Signs and symptoms of motion sickness include pale skin, sweating, nausea, and weakness. Vomiting may provide temporary relief, but prolonged salvation does not occur until the inner ear labyrinth acclimatizes to motion, or someone intervenes with medications. To manage motion sickness:

1. Keep your eyes fixed on a steady point in the distance. If on board a ship, stay on deck. Splash your face with cold water.

2. Take meclizine (Antivert, Bonine) 25 mg orally, or dimenhydrinate (Dramamine) 50 mg orally, every 6–12 hours as necessary to control motion sickness. To be most effective, the first dose of medication should precede the environmental change by 1 hour. Astemizole (Hismanal) is a nonsedating antihistamine that appears to suppress motion sickness as a side effect in some individuals. The dose is 10 mg by mouth every 24 hours.

3. Place a transdermal scopolamine patch (Transderm-Scōp) on the skin behind the ear. This patch releases the drug slowly through the skin and is effective against motion sickness for up to 3 days. Side effects include drowsiness and blurred vision (with a dilated pupil) in the eye on the side of the patch. The patch should be positioned at least 3 hours before rough seas are encountered.

First Aid Kits

FIRST aid kits should be designed according to the environment to be encountered, number of travelers, medical training of the party leaders, and distance from sophisticated medical care. I would like to suggest a few items that should be included to deal effectively with the most common problems. Remember, it is usually easier to bring the patient to the hospital than to carry the hospital with you.

These are not camping lists, so I will not discuss the need for adequate shelter, food, toiletries, etc. If your basic survival supplies (pay heed, winter campers!) are inadequate, you will probably have the opportunity to use your medical kit.

In all cases, what you will carry depends upon your predetermined needs. For instance, day hikers need not carry a portable traction splint, but rock climbers on a lengthy expedition should have one along. Scuba divers should carry a bottle of isopropyl alcohol or vinegar. Select those items that make sense for your group. Carry a realistic quantity of supplies; you should be prepared to treat more than one person. Specific medications to choose from are described in Appendix One and throughout the book in the appropriate sections. Remember to bring along pediatric doses (in liquid form if necessary) when traveling with children.

First aid supplies should be packed to be readily accessible and marked clearly to allow rapid identification. A number of excellent storage sacks, such as the ProMed pack (ProMed; see page 332) or Harper fannypack (Mount Tam Sports; see page 333) are available. On boating, rafting, or diving adventures, carry medical supplies in a plastic or metal container equipped with a rubber O-ring gasket for a tight waterproof seal. Use Ziploc bags within the kit for extra protection. An excellent basic medical kit is available from Adventure Medical Kits (see page 332).

One or two first aid report forms should be carried. Preprinted forms are available from The Mountaineers, 306 Second Avenue, Seattle, Washington 98119. Designed for use on mountain or back-country expeditions, they are a convenient way to record a victim's medical condition and treatment, while serving as a good checklist for proper evaluation. Space is provided for a written rescue request to be carried out by messenger in an emergency.

Before the trip, show all members of the expedition where the medical supplies are stored and explain how they are to be used.

BASIC SUPPLIES

medical guidebook
first aid report form
pencil or pen with notepad
elastic bandages (Band-Aid or Coverlet), assorted sizes, cloth
    adhesive preferable
butterfly bandages or strips for wound closure (Steri-Strip or
    Coverstrip), assorted sizes
2" x 2" sterile gauze pads (packets of 5 minimum) .
4" x 4" sterile gauze pads (packets of 5 minimum)
8" x 10" sterile gauze pads (packets of 5 minimum)
nonstick sterile bandages (Telfa or Metalline), assorted sizes
prepackaged individual sterile oval eye pads
metal or plastic eye shield
1", 2", and 4" rolled gauze (Co-wrap or Elastomull)
2", 3", and 4" elastic wrap (Ace)
cravat cloth (triangular bandage)
1" rolled cloth adhesive tape
rolled duct tape
molefoam
moleskin
Spenco 2nd Skin
steel sewing needle
paper clip

safety pins
needle-nose pliers with wire cutter
sharp folding knife
disposable scalpel, no. 11, and no. 12 or no. 15
paramedic or EMT shears (scissors)
splinter forceps (tweezers)
low-reading hypothermia (rectal) thermometer
oral thermometer
wooden tongue depressors ("tongue blades")
liquid soap
cotton-tipped swabs (Q-Tips)
sterile eyewash, 1 oz.
safety razor
syringe (10 ml) and 18-gauge intravenous catheter (plastic portion) for wound irrigation
tincture of benzoin
oil of cloves
hydrocortisone cream, ointment, or lotion, 0.5–1%
bacitracin ointment
silver sulfadiazine 1% (Silvadene) cream
benzalkonium chloride 1:750 solution (Zephiran)
povidone-iodine 10% solution (Betadine)
buffered aspirin 325 mg tablets
ibuprofen 200 mg tablets
acetaminophen (Tylenol) 325 mg tablets
codeine 30 mg tablets (with or without acetaminophen)
antacid
metered-dose bronchodilator (albuterol or metaproterenol)
decongestant tablets
decongestant nasal spray
prednisone 10 mg tablets
sodium sulamyd or gentamicin eye drops
penicillin VK 250 mg tablets
dicloxacillin 250 mg tablets
ampicillin 250 mg tablets

erythromycin 250 mg tablets
cephalexin 250 mg tablets
ciprofloxacin 500 mg tablets
tetracycline 500 mg tablets
trimethoprim with sulfamethoxazole double-strength tablets
prochlorperazine (Compazine) suppositories 25 mg
promethazine (Phenergan) suppositories 25 mg
insect repellent
sunscreen
sunblock
allergic reaction kit: epinephrine (EpiPen and EpiPen Jr., or
   Ana-Kit)
diphenhydramine 25 mg capsules
waterproof flashlight or headlamp
CYALUME fluorescent light sticks (American Cyanamid Co.,
   Wayne, New Jersey)
Adolph's meat tenderizer (unseasoned)
4¼" x 36" SAM Splints (minimum 2); wire splints
aluminum finger splints

FOREST AND MOUNTAIN ENVIRONMENTS

water disinfection equipment/chemicals
acetazolamide (Diamox) 250 mg tablets
the Extractor
calamine lotion
Space Emergency Blanket
whistle
dexamethasone (Decadron) 4 mg tablets
powdered electrolyte mix (Gatorade)
instant chemical cold pack(s)
hand warmer (mechanical or chemical)
Kendrick Traction Device (splint)

BOATING AND DIVING ENVIRONMENTS

motion sickness medicine
acetic acid (vinegar) 5%
isopropyl alcohol 40–70%
hydrogen peroxide
Vosol otic solution

RECREATIONAL EQUIPMENT SUPPLIERS

Eddie Bauer
Fifth and Union
P.O. Box 3700
Seattle, WA 98124

L. L. Bean, Inc.
Freeport, ME 04033

Cabela's
812 Thirteenth Avenue
Sidney, NE 69160

Recreational Equipment, Inc.
P.O. Box C-88125
Seattle, WA 98188

MEDICAL AND/OR RESCUE EQUIPMENT SUPPLIERS

California Mountain Co., Ltd.
P.O. Box 6602
Santa Barbara, CA 93160

Carolina Biological Products
P.O. Box 187
Gladstone, OR 97207

Dixie USA, Inc.
P.O. Box 55549
Houston, TX 77255

Dyna-Med
6200 Yarrow Drive
Carlsbad, CA 92008-0996

ProMed
P.O. Box 322
Orem, UT 84057

Res-Q-Med
3506 F Street
Philadelphia, PA 19134

Zeal G. H., Ltd.
8 Lombard Street
London SW 19
England

PRODUCT SUPPLIERS

Adventure Medical Kits
P.O. Box 2586
Berkeley, CA 94702
(first aid kits)

Denver Splint Co., Inc.
6065 S. Quebec Street, No. 200
Englewood, CO 80111
(Rhino-Rocket)

Eptek, Inc.
301 Orange Street
Millville, NJ 08332
(Heat Wave thermal packs)

4 in 1 Water Systems
2801 Rodeo Road, Suite B-518
Santa Fe, NM 87505
(Sierra Water Purifier)

Jianas Brothers Packaging
2533 Southwest Boulevard
Kansas City, MO 64108
(Oral Rehydration Salts)

John Wagner Associates
205 Mason Circle
Concord, CA 94520
(Mycoal Grabber hand warmer)

Jordan David Safety Products
P.O. Box 400
Warrington, PA 18976
(skin protection products)

Kenyon Consumer Products
200 Main Street
Kenyon, RI 02836
(thermal wear)

Metallized Products, Inc.
37 East Street
Winchester, MA 01890
(Space Emergency Blanket, emergency strobes)

Mount Tam Sports
Box 111
Kentfield, CA 94914
(Harper fannypack)

Northern Outfitters
1083 North State
Orem, UT 84057
(thermal wear)

Polar Equipment
12881 Foothill Lane
Saratoga, CA 95070-
(Polar Pure Water Disinfectant)

Sawyer Products
Box 188
Safety Harbor, FL 34695
(the Extractor; insect repellents; first aid kits)

Seaberg Co., Inc.
P.O. Box 734
South Beach, OR 97366
(SAM Splint)

Immunizations

B ECAUSE the spectrum of infectious diseases changes with time and location, travelers to or between foreign countries should be aware of the necessity for immunizations. A detailed updated list of required immunizations by country may be obtained in the annual publication entitled "Health Information for International Travel" (Centers for Disease Control, 1600 Clifton Road, NE, Atlanta, Georgia 30333). In this monograph, specific vaccinations (cholera, yellow fever) are listed as "required by the country" in three categories: I) vaccination certificate required of travelers arriving from countries; II) vaccination certificate required of travelers arriving from infected areas; III) vaccination certificate required of travelers arriving from a country any part of which is infected. Also noted by country is malaria risk. General rules and standards for vaccination are discussed, including special topics such as vaccination during pregnancy, vaccination of persons with altered immunocompetence (ability to fight infections), and vaccination of persons with severe febrile (fever) illnesses. Other excellent references for required and recommended immunizations worldwide are the *World Immunization Chart* (IAMAT, 417 Center Street, Lewiston, New York 14092), *Immunization Alert* (P.O. Box 406, Storrs, Connecticut 06268), and the yearly *International Travel Health Guide* (Travel Medicine, Inc., 351 Pleasant Street, Suite 312, Northampton, Massachusetts 01060). The *International Travel Health Guide* also lists vaccination centers in the United States.

Vaccinations may be given under the supervision of any licensed physician. All travelers should carry a completed International Certificate of Vaccination with proper signature and validation for all vaccinations administered. Failure to secure validation at an authorized city, county, or state health department renders the certificate invalid, and may force a traveler to be revaccinated or quarantined. The form (stock number 017-001-004405) is available from the Superintendent of Documents, U.S. Government Printing Office, Washington, D.C. 20402).

TETANUS

All travelers who will be away from medical care for more than 48 hours should have adequate tetanus immunization. The recommendations are as follows:

1. A person previously immunized should receive a booster dose of tetanus toxoid if his last dose was not administered within the past 10 years. If there is a good chance that the traveler will suffer an injury during the trip, he should take a booster if the last dose was not administered within the past 5 years.

2. Nonimmunized individuals should become immunized with a series of 3 injections (requires 3–6 months).

3. Low-risk (for tetanus infection) wounds are those that are recent (less than 6 hours old), simple (linear), superficial (less than ½ inch deep), cut with a sharp edge (knife or glass), without signs of infection, and free of contamination with dirt, soil, or body secretions. High-risk wounds are those that are old (greater

than 6 hours old), crushed or gouged, deep (greater than ½ inch deep), burns or frostbite, with signs of infection, and contaminated. If a person suffers a wound, the following are standard recommendations:

Victim	Low-Risk Wound (not heavily contaminated)	Contaminated Wound (tetanus-prone)
NEVER IMMUNIZED	*Tetanus toxoid* *Tetanus immune globulin*	*Tetanus toxoid* *Tetanus immune globulin*
IMMUNIZED		
Last booster within 5 years	*No shot*	*No shot*
Last booster within 10 years	*No shot*	*Tetanus toxoid* *Tetanus immune globulin*
Last booster over 10 years	*Tetanus toxoid*	*Tetanus toxoid* *Tetanus immune globulin*

POLIOVIRUS, DIPHTHERIA, PERTUSSIS (WHOOPING COUGH), MEASLES, MUMPS, RUBELLA (GERMAN MEASLES)

Immunization against poliomyelitis, diphtheria, pertussis, measles, mumps, and rubella should be obtained prior to travel. These are routinely administered during childhood in the United States. Because of the incidence of these infectious diseases in developing countries, such immunizations are mandatory prior to travel. Polio is still common in developing nations. Unimmunized adults (age greater than 18 years) should receive a series of 3 injections of the inactivated (virus) Salk vaccine, not the oral (Sabin) vaccine, which is recommended for children. Persons under the age of 18 years who have never been immunized should receive 3 doses of oral polio vaccine 1 month apart. Persons who travel to high-risk areas who were immunized as children should receive 1 booster dose of oral polio vaccine.

SMALLPOX

The last reported case of smallpox was in 1977. Therefore, smallpox immunization is no longer required for international travel. However, there is a chance that isolated cases still occur (without reporting) in parts of India, the Himalaya, and in equatorial Africa. Travelers to these areas should inquire about the latest recommendations from the Centers for Disease Control, Atlanta, Georgia.

CHOLERA

Cholera is an intestinal infection caused by the microorganism *Vibrio cholerae*, which induces painful diarrhea and extreme fluid losses through the gastrointestinal tract. A person whose stomach contains normal gastric acid is not at much risk for acquiring cholera. Most countries do not require vaccination. However, some countries require cholera immunization for travelers entering from a territory that still reports the disease. Two injections are administered 1 week apart, and immunity is acquired after a 6-day waiting period. In special cases (high risk, by virtue of living in unsanitary conditions or persons with insufficient gastric acid), an additional booster injection may be required a month after the primary series. The vaccine is good for 6 months, so frequent booster shots are necessary. Infants should not be immunized. The vaccine appears to provide 50% effectiveness in reduction of the disease. To be maximally effective, cholera and yellow fever vaccines should be administered 3 weeks apart.

YELLOW FEVER

Yellow fever is acquired in tropical Africa and South America, where victims may suffer the bite of the *Aedes aegypti* mosquito (urban environment) and/or other mosquitoes (jungle environment). Vaccination is effective against the disease. A single injection is administered and immunity is acquired after a 10-day waiting period. The vaccine is good for 10 years. Infants younger than 6 months and pregnant women should not be routinely immunized, unless they are at high risk for contracting the disease. Yellow fever vaccinations must be given at an officially designated Yellow Fever Vaccination Center, and the certificate must be validated at the same center.

MENINGOCOCCUS

The meningococcus is a bacterium (*Neisseria meningitidis*) that can cause meningitis, particularly in children and young adults. Because of an epidemic of meningococcal meningitis in Nepal in 1983 and subsequent frequent cases in that country, it is a wise idea for travelers, particularly hikers or backpackers, to be immunized. The vaccine is given in 1 or 2 injections, with protection for 1 year achieved 1–2 weeks after administration.

HEPATITIS

A vaccine for immunization against viral hepatitis type B (serum hepatitis) is recommended by some authorities for travel in underdeveloped countries. A series of three injections requires 6 months. Pooled immune serum globulin (ISG, or gamma globulin) is administered to prevent or diminish the effects of viral hepatitis type A (infectious hepatitis). Hepatitis A virus is spread through contamination of water and food and is often encountered in developing nations and areas of poor hygiene. The administration of ISG interferes with the antibody response stimulated by other live virus vaccines, so it should be administered 2–4 weeks after the other vaccines. Because the effects of ISG disappear after 6 months, it should be administered just prior to the trip. Boosters are required for prolonged travel in endemic areas.

BUBONIC PLAGUE AND RABIES

Preexposure vaccines are available for immunization against bubonic plague and rabies. These are administered only to persons whose travels or occupations place them at high risk. In most countries where plague is reported, the risk is greatest in rural mountain or upland regions. Vaccination is generally considered for those who will reside in regions where plague is endemic, where avoidance of rodents and fleas is impossible. The vaccine is injected in 2 doses 1 month apart, followed by a booster dose after 6 months. Pre- and postexposure rabies vaccination are discussed on page 303.

MALARIA

Malaria is discussed in detail beginning on page 121.

TYPHOID FEVER

A vaccine is available for immunization against typhoid fever. Immunization is recommended only for travelers who visit tropical regions known to harbor the disease. A 2-injection series given 4 or more weeks apart is required, followed by booster injections at 1- to 3-year intervals, depending on the local disease risk. A new single-injection vaccine with fewer side effects has recently been tested in Nepal and South Africa; an oral vaccine produced in Switzerland may not be as effective, but is gaining popularity.

TYPHUS FEVER

Typhus vaccine is no longer available in the United States and is not recommended for the foreign traveler.

INFLUENZA AND PNEUMOCOCCAL PNEUMONIA

Vaccines are available against influenza virus and pneumonia caused by *S. pneumoniae* (pneumococcus). In general, these vaccines are recommended for elderly (over 65 years) or infirm travelers (those with cancer or with chronic heart, kidney, liver, or lung disease; persons without a spleen; alcoholics; diabetics; persons with sickle-cell anemia) who would be debilitated by either of these two illnesses. These vaccines are not routinely recommended for children. Influenza vaccine is administered in 1 or 2 injections to children (particularly those receiving long-term aspirin therapy) and adults in October and November prior to the flu season (December through March), with a maximum duration of effect of 6 months.

With regard to influenza, vaccination of high-risk persons prior to flu season is essential. Each year, the vaccine contains the influenza virus strains that are felt to be most prevalent in the United States. Inactivated (killed-virus) influenza vaccine should not be given to persons who are sensitive to egg products. Amantadine hydrochloride (Symmetrel) is a prescription oral drug that is moderately effective in preventing influenza A; however, because it confers no protection against influenza B, it is not considered a substitute for appropriately timed immunization. "Whole" vaccines should not be given to children under 13 years of age. They should be given "split" vaccines, which have been chemically treated to reduce adverse reactions.

PHYSICIANS ABROAD

A traveler to a foreign country may become ill enough to require the services of a physician. The International Association for Medical Assistance to Travelers (IAMAT) is a nonprofit organization that provides a list of approved doctors who adhere to international standards, which include standardization of fees. IAMAT also distributes free of charge updated material on immunization requirements, malaria and other tropical diseases, and sanitary (food and water) and climatic conditions around the world. The directory of affiliated institutions can be obtained by writing to IAMAT, 736 Center Street, Lewiston, New York 14092 (716-754-4883). Other international medical assistance programs include:

Air Ambulance Network, Inc.
P.O. Box 160189
Miami, FL 33116
305-387-1708

Health Care Abroad
923 Investment Building
1511 K Street, NW
Washington, DC 20006
800-336-3310

Intermedic
777 Third Avenue
New York, NY 10017
212-486-8974

International SOS Assistance
P.O. Box 11568
Philadelphia, PA 19116
800-523-8930

International Travelers Assistance Association
P.O. Box 10623
Baltimore, MD 21204
800-723-5309

Nationwide/Worldwide Emergency Ambulance Return (NEAR)
1900 N. MacArthur Boulevard
Oklahoma City, OK 73127
800-654-6700

Physicians Air Transport International
P.O. Box 67
Northampton, MA 01601
413-586-5503

Travel Assistance International
133 F Street, NW, Suite 300
Washington, DC 20004
800-821-2828

World Care Travel Assistance Association, Inc.
2000 Pennsylvania Avenue, NW, Suite 7600
Washington, DC 20006
800-521-4822

Transport of the Injured Victim

THE rescuer may have to decide whether to carry a victim to medical attention or to make camp, send for help and/or signal, and wait for evacuation. With some flexibility for special circumstances, these guidelines should be followed:

1. Never move a victim unless you know where you are going. If you are lost and caring for an injured victim (or yourself), prepare a shelter. Try to position yourself so that visual distress signals can be fashioned in an open field, in the snow, or near a visible riverbank. Keep the victim covered and warm. Remember that the victim is frightened and needs frequent reassurance. If the victim cannot walk, you must attend to his bodily functions. A urinal may be constructed from a wide-mouth water bottle. Defecation is somewhat more complicated, but may be assisted

by cutting a hole in a blanket or sleeping pad placed over a small pit dug in the ground.

2. Unless you are in danger, never leave a victim who is unconscious or confused.

3. If possible, send someone for help and wait with the victim, rather than perform an exhausting and time-consuming solo or duo extrication. If someone is to be sent for help, choose a strong traveler and provide him with a written request that details your situation (for example, number of victims, injuries, need for supplies, specific evacuation method required). While you certainly do not want to underestimate the seriousness of the situation, don't request a helicopter evacuation for someone with a sprained ankle who can easily be carried out on a stretcher. Anyone sent to obtain assistance should contact the closest law enforcement agency, which will seek the appropriate rescue agency.

4. Conserve your strength. Don't create additional victims with heroic attempts at communication or feats of strength and exertion.

5. Attempt to transport a victim only if awaiting a rescue party will be of greater risk than immediate movement, if there are sufficient helpers to carry the victim (as a general rule, it takes 6–8 adults to carry one injured person), and if the distance is reasonable (under 5 miles). A victim who is carried on an improvised stretcher over difficult terrain usually gets a rough ride, which should be avoided if possible. Always test your system on a noninjured person before you use it on the victim.

The method of evacuation used to transport a victim will depend upon the degree of disablement and what is available to the rescuer(s). To conserve the energy of all party members, victims of minor injuries should travel under their own power as much as possible, but should never travel unattended. One healthy and strong person should accompany anyone who must leave the group for medical reasons.

If the victim has suffered an injury that does not allow him to walk out, then mechanical transport must be improvised. A single person who cannot walk, but who does not need to be on a litter (one with, for example, a broken ankle, mild exhaustion, or moderate mountain sickness) may be carried on the back of a strong rescuer using a rope seat. This is fashioned by passing a long one-inch rope or strap across the victim's back and under the arms, and crossing the rope in front of his chest. The victim then is loaded piggyback onto the rescuer's back, and the rope ends are passed forward over the shoulders of the rescuer, under his arms, and around to the rescuer's back, then in between and through the victim's legs from the front, and around the outside of the victim's legs just under the buttocks, to be tied snugly in front of the rescuer's waist (Fig. 128). A rope seat is far preferable to a standard fireman's carry, which is very fatiguing.

Other simple ways to carry a victim include the four-hand seat, backpack carry, ski pole/tree limb backpack carry, and coiled rope seat. In the first method, two rescuers interlock hands. Each

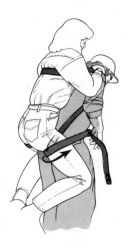

FIGURE 128. *Fashioning a rope (webbing) seat.*

rescuer first grasps his right wrist with his left hand. Holding the palms down, each rescuer then firmly grasps the left wrist of the other rescuer with his right hand, interlocking all four hands. The victim sits on the four-hand seat. In the second method, leg holes can be cut into a large backpack, so that a victim can sit in it like a small child would in a baby carrier. In the third method, two rescuers with sturdy backpacks stand side by side. Pack straps are looped down from each pack, and ski poles or tree limbs are slung across through the loops, or the poles are placed to rest on the padded hip belts. The poles should be padded so that the victim can sit on the rigid seat, steadying himself by draping his arms around the shoulders of his rescuers (Fig. 129). The coiled rope seat is created by coiling a rope, then fixing the coil at one segment. The coil's loops are split and used to position the victim upon the rescuer's back (Fig. 130).

Litters (which resemble ladders) may be fashioned from tree limbs or ski poles fastened with twine, rope, clothing, or pack straps. A rope stretcher is constructed by stretching a 150–200-foot rope on the ground and determining the midpoint. At the midpoint, fold the rope back upon itself. Measure 3 feet from the bend, and fold each half of the rope back again to the outside.

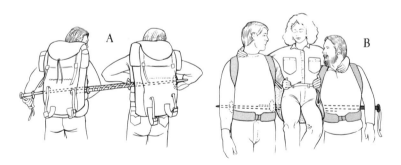

FIGURE 129. *Fashioning a ski pole seat. (A) The poles are slung between rescuers wearing backpacks. (B) A victim can sit comfortably on the padded ski poles.*

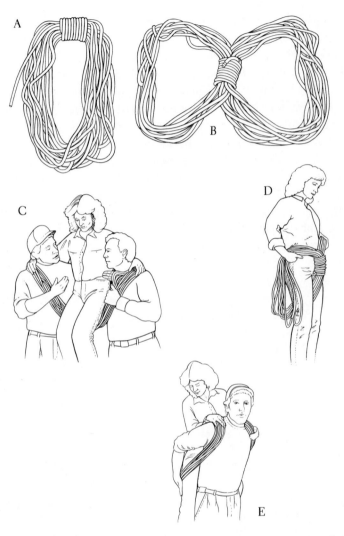

FIGURE 130. *Creating a coiled rope seat. (A) The rope is coiled and the loops secured. (B) The loops of the coil are divided into equal sections at the point of fixation. (C) The loops can be used by two rescuers to carry a victim. (D) Alternatively, the victim can step through the split loops, so that (E) a single rescuer can carry the victim.*

This creates the central "rungs" of a "ladder" that will be 3 feet wide. Repeat the process of folding the rope back upon itself in 3-foot segments, moving away from the central rungs in each direction and laying out a series of evenly spaced parallel loops. About 16 or 18 loops (rungs) should create a ladder approximately the same length as the patient. Take the two remaining long ends of the rope, and lay them perpendicular to the rungs, alongside the bends in the rope (Fig. 131A). Use the long ends to secure the loops together (completing the long sides of the ladder) by tying a clove hitch or other secure knot onto each consecutive bend in the rope 2–3 inches inside the bend, so that a small loop remains to the outside of the knot (Fig. 131B). Each pair of knots should be separated by 3–4 inches. After all the knots are tied, the rope ends are threaded through the small outside loops as the remaining lengths are circled around the outside of the stretcher and finally tied off (Fig. 131C).

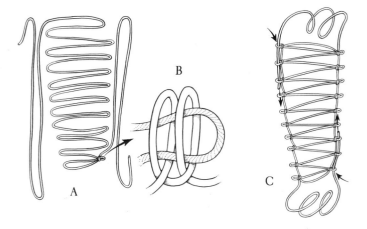

FIGURE 131. *Making a rope stretcher. (A) Having laid a series of parallel loops, lay the lengthwise segments perpendicularly alongside. (B) Use a clove hitch to secure the loop ends. (C) The remaining long ends of the rope are passed through the outside loops to form the perimeter of the stretcher, and are tied off to complete the process.*

Test the stretcher with an uninjured person before trusting it to bear the weight of the victim. Be certain to fasten the victim securely into the stretcher, so that he doesn't fall out. Pad all injuries to make the victim as comfortable as possible. Positioning on a stretcher is very important. In general, keep the injury uphill, to keep extra weight and jostling from causing extra pain. If the chest is injured, keep the victim lying on his side with the wounded side (lung) down. If the victim has altered consciousness, is nauseated, or is vomiting, he should be kept on his side, to protect the airway (see page 18). If the victim has suffered a face, head, or neck injury, he should be transported with the head slightly elevated (see page 54). Victims with shock (see page 53), bleeding, or hypothermia (see page 221) should be carried with the head down and feet elevated. Victims with chest pain and/or difficulty breathing, which might indicate a heart attack or heart failure (see page 46), should be carried with the upper body elevated.

All victims should be covered above and below with blankets, clothing, sleeping bags, or whatever else is available for warmth. Handle all suspected hypothermics *gently*. A victim secured to a stretcher should never be left unattended. Constantly reassure the victim. If the terrain is steep, be sure to keep the feet of the victim downhill. Remember that litter transport is exhausting for the rescuers and should not be entertained if the distance to be covered is more than a few miles.

HELICOPTERS

Because people get into trouble on glaciers, rock faces, and far out to sea, an increasing number of rescues involve aircraft, particularly helicopters. Most helicopters used for medical evacuation can land at altitudes of up to 10,000 feet and are limited by visibility, landing space, and weather conditions. Persons on the ground should be aware of the limitations of maneuverability, and should obey certain rules when involved with a helicopter rescue:

1. Prepare and brightly mark a proper landing site if possible. The ideal location is on level ground (bare rock is best; snow is worst) and has access from all sides. Clear an area 100 yards long by 100 feet wide of all debris which could interfere with landing or be scattered by gusts from the propellers. The absolute minimum ground diameter for landing is 100 feet. A smoky fire or smoke signal should be placed near the landing site so that the pilot can judge the wind (pilots prefer takeoffs and landings to be directed into the wind). If this is not possible, stand away from the landing site where the pilot can see you, and hold up an improvised wind flag, or position yourself with the wind behind your back, and point with both arms at the landing site. At night, if you have lights, shine them on objects that will alert the pilot to unseen danger (such as the poles of power lines).

2. Unless otherwise instructed, stay at least 150 feet from a helicopter with rotors spinning. Look away as the ship lands, so as not to be struck in the face or eyes by flying debris. Protect the victim. Secure all loose objects or clear them from the landing area.

3. Always approach or leave a helicopter at a 30–45 degree angle from the front, in sight of the pilot and crew. Never approach the helicopter from ground higher than the landing spot, to avoid walking into a rotor. Stay away from the tail rotor, as it is nearly invisible when rotating.

4. Keep your head down! You may not perceive that the rotor blade is dipping (up to 4 feet from the center attachment) until it chops your head off. Don't hold any objects (particularly your arms) above your head. Protect your eyes from dust kicked up by the rotor wash.

5. Do not smoke a cigarette near a helicopter.

6. Follow the pilot's instructions. Do not enter, leave, or load a helicopter until he gives the command.

7. Do not stand under or anywhere near a helicopter during takeoff or landing. All persons near the landing site should stay at a safe distance in a single group, clearly visible to the pilot.

8. If a cable or rope is lowered, allow it to touch the ground before you handle it, to avoid a shock from static electricity. Never tie the rope or cable to an immovable object on the ground (this could cause a crash).

9. All persons should wear hard hats and eye protection, if available.

Ground-to-Air Distress Signals

I F a party is trapped or lost, and helicopter or airplane search parties are likely to be in the region, it may help to attempt to signal the aircraft. One way that this may be done is by creating ground-to-air distress signals, either by marking an open field or a riverbank that is visible from the air by stamping out large (8–10 feet) designs in the snow (in an open area), or by attracting attention with display patterns of clothing, rocks, fire rings, etc. Figure 132 illustrates the standard ground markings for communication. The 3 signals that are recognized (and remembered) by most pilots are: three of anything — distress; large X — unable to proceed; and an arrow — proceeding in this direction. *Three fires (set 100 feet apart) placed in a triangular configuration is a sign of distress to a passing pilot.* Remember, ground-to-air patterns should be large, composed of straight lines, and made up of colors that contrast sharply with the natural colors of the environment (royal blue is best). Small battery-powered emergency strobes are available from Metallized Products, Inc. (see page

333). Heliograph mirrors are small signal reflectors that can be accurately aimed to reflect sunlight at a distant object (such as an aircraft).

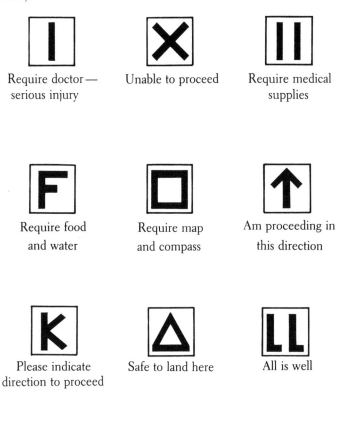

Require doctor — serious injury	Unable to proceed	Require medical supplies
Require food and water	Require map and compass	Am proceeding in this direction
Please indicate direction to proceed	Safe to land here	All is well
No	Yes	I do not understand

FIGURE 132. *Ground-to-air distress signals.*

Lost Persons

Persons lost in the wilderness often act in a predictable manner. Rapid location of a lost person can make the difference between life and death. These general guidelines may assist you in a search. Remember:

1. Lost persons tend to follow the path of least resistance (open fields, trails, roads, dry streambeds).

2. A person who is lost tends to travel downhill and to seek apparent short-cuts toward civilization or a familiar location.

3. Persons tend to avoid barriers and obstacles (lakes, large rivers, boulder fields, dense brush).

4. At night, a lost person tends to travel toward lights.

5. In bad weather, persons tend to seek shelter with overhead protection.

6. Small children tend to seek shelter when tired.

Procedures

SUBCUTANEOUS INJECTION

Subcutaneous (just below the skin) injection of epinephrine is used to manage a severe allergic reaction. The injection may be performed with a preloaded syringe (already containing the medicine in the barrel), or may require that the medicine be drawn up for administration. After you wash your hands, follow these instructions:

1. Select the proper syringe and needle. For the treatment of an allergic reaction, a syringe that holds 1 milliliter (ml) is necessary, commonly equipped with a 25 or 27 gauge needle (the

larger the gauge number, the smaller the diameter of the needle).

2. Never touch the metal of the needle with your hands.

3. If the medication is in a preloaded syringe, be sure to see that the amount of medicine does not exceed the dose you want to administer. Be certain not to inject too much medicine.

4. If the medicine is in a glass vial, flick the vial a few times with your finger to drive the air bubble to the top, and then snap the vial open at the line marked on the glass at the neck (Figs. 133A, 133B). Draw the proper amount of medicine to be administered up into the syringe (Fig. 133C). In the case of epinephrine, this will be 0.3–0.5 ml for an adult and 0.01 ml per kg (2.2 lb) for a child (not to exceed 0.3 ml).

5. If the medication is in a glass bottle with a rubber top, wipe the top of the bottle with alcohol, stick the needle through the rubber, and draw up the desired amount of medication. If you cannot draw the medicine out of the bottle, you may need to inject some air into the bottle first (use the same entry into the bottle to inject air in and to draw medicine out).

6. Before injection, point the needle upward, tap the syringe a few times to drive the air bubbles to the top, and squirt out any air that is in the syringe (Figs. 133D, 133E). You should be left with only medicine. Try not to inject any air.

7. Wipe off the skin with alcohol or with soap and water (if no alcohol is available) where you intend to administer the medicine. The easiest place to inject epinephrine is on the lateral arm at the shoulder.

8. Pinch the skin up between your fingers, and quickly plunge the needle in just under the skin at a 15–30 degree angle to the skin (Fig. 133F). With the needle in the skin, gently pull back on the plunger, to see if blood enters the syringe (if it does, you have inadvertently entered a blood vessel, and you should draw back the needle until no blood is returned). If no blood is returned, then firmly push the plunger and inject the medicine. Quickly remove the needle from the skin, and gently massage the injection site.

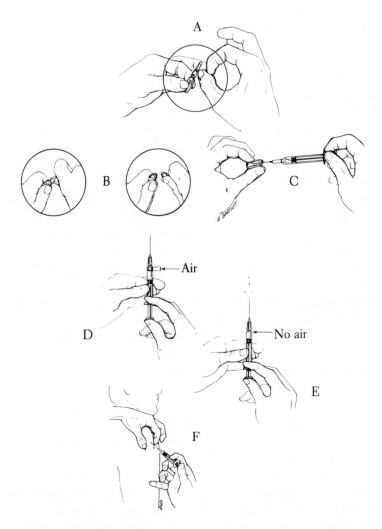

FIGURE 133. *Administering an injection. (A) Flick the air bubble to the top of the vial. (B) Break off the top of the vial at the narrowing or line. (C) Draw the medicine into the syringe. (D) Holding the needle straight up, gently push the plunger until (E) no air is left. (F) Pinch up a fold of skin and briskly stick the needle through the skin.*

FISHHOOK REMOVAL

If a fishhook enters the skin, gently scrub the skin which surrounds the entry point with soap and water. After the skin is clean, apply gentle pressure along the curve toward the point while pulling on the hook. If the hook is not easily removed, this means that the barb is caught in the tissue (Fig. 134A). In this case, the hook must usually be removed by pushing it through the skin. This should be done (because of the increased risk of infection) if it will take more than 8 hours to get to a doctor. With a steady firm motion, push the hook through the skin so that the barb appears (Fig. 134B). Cut off the shaft or the barb (take care to cover the area to prevent the detached barb from flying into someone's eye), and pull the remainder of the hook back out of the skin (Figs. 134C, 134D). Another technique is to pass a shoelace or length of rolled gauze through and around the bend of the hook. The hook can then be yanked from the skin while

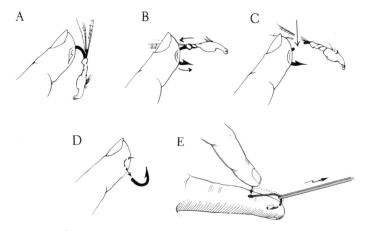

FIGURE 134. *Fishhook removal. (A) The barb is embedded in the finger. (B) The hook and barb are pushed through the skin. (C) The shaft of the hook is cut. (D) Both pieces are easily extracted. (E) "Press and yank" method of fishhook removal.*

the eyelet of the hook is pressed into the victim's skin to disengage the barb (Fig. 134E).

Vigorously wash the wound and leave it open with a simple dry dressing. Do not seal in the dirt and bacteria with any grease or home remedies (see page 197). If the hook was dirty (or was holding a dirty worm), begin the victim on dicloxacillin, penicillin, erythromycin, or cephalexin. If a hook enters the skin anywhere near the eye, do not attempt removal; tape the hook in place so that it cannot be snagged and take the victim immediately to see a doctor.

SPLINTER REMOVAL

Splinters can be removed by gently cutting away the skin near the entrance, until a firm grasp can be made with a small tweezers or with the fingers. If a splinter enters the finger under the fingernail, cut a small V-shaped wedge out of the nail, so that the splinter can be grasped. If a splinter cannot be removed for a period of longer than 24 hours, begin the victim on penicillin, erythromycin, or cephalexin.

APPENDIXES

Appendix One

Commonly Used Drugs and Doses

BEFORE administering any medication, *always ask the recip-ient if he suffers from allergy to medications*. If so, do not administer the drug or anything that you feel is similar to it. Use medications only if you have a solid understanding of what you are treating. Many of these drugs are used to suppress symptoms (such as abdominal pain, nausea and vomiting, headache) of potentially serious disorders. In these cases, do not overmedicate the victim if you need to watch for a worsening condition. Particularly in children, always investigate the problem to be sure you are not masking a serious problem with a drug effect.

The drugs are listed by purpose. I have tried to enumerate a number of products that are available over the counter; however, many of the drugs mentioned here require a prescription. *Always have a doctor or pharmacist explain the actions and side effects of any drug you obtain.* I have listed some drugs that persons may carry for preexisting conditions, so that the rescuer may have a better understanding of his patient's medical history.

Doses are listed in absolute amount (generally, for adults) or in amount to be given per body weight or per age (generally, for children). For determination of weight, 1 kilogram (kg) equals 2.2 pounds (lb). The drug should be administered orally unless otherwise specified. Because children generally require a fraction of the dose used for adults, they may need to have the drug in special tablet or liquid form. Exercise extreme caution and do not administer drugs to pregnant women, infants, or small children unless absolutely necessary.

Drugs have many side effects. The most common of these are noted.

Drugs are listed in the following order:

For relief from a severe allergic reaction (page 362)
For relief from a mild allergic reaction or hay fever (page 363)
For relief from severe asthma (page 364)
For relief from mild (or chronic) asthma (page 365)
For treatment of chest pain (angina) (page 366)
For treatment of chronic (congestive) heart failure (page 366)
For treatment of seizures (epilepsy) (page 367)
For relief from pain (page 367)
For relief from fever (page 368)
For relief from muscle aches or minor arthritis (page 368)
For relief from itching (page 368)
For relief from toothache (page 368)
For relief from motion sickness (page 369)
For relief from nausea and vomiting (page 369)
For relief from diarrhea (page 370)
For relief from constipation (page 371)
For relief from ulcer pain (page 371)
For relief from indigestion or gas pains (page 372)
For relief from heartburn (reflux esophagitis) (page 372)
For relief from nasal congestion (page 373)
For relief from cough (page 373)
For relief from sore throat (page 374)
Cold formulas (page 374)
Skin medications (page 374)
For sleep (page 376)
Insect repellents (page 376)
Sunscreens (page 377)
Antibiotics (page 377)

DRUGS AND PREGNANCY

In general, it is best to avoid taking any medications when pregnant. However, women can certainly become ill during pregnancy, so it is important to know what can be administered safely, and what should be absolutely avoided. Fortunately, many of the drugs that are labeled "potentially hazardous" have only been proven hazardous in laboratory animals, frequently in relative doses that far exceed their common use in humans.

The following list reflects recommendations compiled from the current medical literature. Whenever possible, a pregnant woman contemplating use of medications should seek the advice of her physician.

No Recognized Hazard	Avoid If Possible	Hazardous
ANTIBIOTIC / ANTIFUNGAL		
penicillin	trimethoprim-sulfa	tetracycline*
cephalosporins	metronidazole	ciprofloxacin
erythromycin	nitrofurantoin	norfloxacin
clotrimazole	quinine	doxycycline*
miconazole	chloroquine	
nystatin	primaquine	
proguanil	quinacrine	
ampicillin/amoxicillin		
paromomycin		
PAIN MEDICATION		
acetaminophen	codeine	ibuprofen
		naproxen
		aspirin
		indomethacin
VACCINE		
influenza (killed)	polio (oral)	smallpox
hepatitis B (killed)	polio (injection)	measles
tetanus toxoid	typhus	mumps
diphtheria toxoid	tuberculosis	varicella
tetanus immunoglobulin	typhoid	rubella
hepatitis A immunoglobulin	cholera	
hepatitis B immunoglobulin	yellow fever	
ANTIALLERGY		
chlorpheniramine	hydroxyzine	diphenhydramine†

No Recognized Hazard	Avoid If Possible	Hazardous
epinephrine (in critical situation)		brompheniramine dimenhydrinate cyclizine

ANTINAUSEA / ANTI–MOTION SICKNESS

trimethobenzamide prochlorperazine promethazine Dramamine	meclizine Transderm-Scōp	

OTHER

prednisone dexamethasone betamethasone prednisolone theophylline metaproterenol albuterol	epinephrine isoproterenol diazepam† acetazolamide triazolam loperamide diphenoxylate	phenacetin dapsone tolbutamide Pepto-Bismol

* Can cause staining of teeth and altered bone development in fetus.
† During first trimester.

ALLERGIC DRUG REACTION

If a person develops an allergic reaction to a drug (shortness of breath, swollen tongue, difficulty talking, skin rash, etc.), immediately discontinue the drug, and follow the instructions on page 58.

FOR RELIEF FROM A SEVERE ALLERGIC REACTION

Epinephrine (Adrenalin) 1:1,000 aqueous solution: adult dose 0.3–0.5 ml injected subcutaneously (see page 352).

This may be repeated 2 times at 20-minute intervals. The pediatric dose is 0.01 ml per kg (2.2 lb) body weight injected subcutaneously, not to exceed 0.3 ml. DO NOT USE EPI-NEPHRINE IF THE PATIENT IS OLDER THAN 45 OR HAS A KNOWN HISTORY OF HEART DISEASE. DO NOT AD-MINISTER EPINEPHRINE TO A PREGNANT FEMALE UNLESS THE SITUATION IS ABSOLUTELY LIFE THREATENING (because it might decrease circulation to the baby).

Side effects: rapid heartbeat, nervousness.

Diphenhydramine (Benadryl): adult dose 25–50 mg every 4–6 hours; pediatric dose 1 mg per kg (2.2 lb) body weight every 4–6 hours.

Side effect: drowsiness.

Metaproterenol (Alupent inhaler): adult dose 2 puffs every 3–6 hours as needed.

Side effects: rapid heartbeat, nervousness.

Albuterol (Ventolin inhaler): adult dose 2 puffs every 3–6 hours as needed.

Side effects: rapid heartbeat, nervousness.

Prednisone: adult dose 50–80 mg the first day. Each day, the dose should be decreased by 10 mg (that is, 50 mg day 1, 40 mg day 2, 30 mg day 3, etc.). The pediatric dose is 1 mg per kg (2.2 lb) body weight the first day, ½ mg per kg day 2, ¼ mg per kg day 3. Administer with food or with an antacid if possible.

For a bad skin reaction to poison ivy, poison oak, or poison sumac, see the instructions on page 183. For a severe sunburn, see the instructions on page 178.

Precaution: Do not administer prednisone to a person with a history of bleeding ulcers.

FOR RELIEF FROM A MILD ALLERGIC REACTION (NO SHORTNESS OF BREATH OR FACIAL SWELLING) OR HAY FEVER

Diphenhydramine (Benadryl): Same as for relief from a severe allergic reaction (above).

Diphenhydramine (25 mg) with pseudoephedrine (60 mg) (Benadryl Decongestant): adult dose 1 tablet every 8 hours.

Terfenadine (Seldane): adult dose 60 mg every 12 hours. This antihistamine rarely causes drowsiness. Do not use in children less than 12 years of age.

Astemizole (Hismanal): adult dose 10 mg every 24 hours. This antihistamine rarely causes drowsiness. Do not use in children less than 12 years of age. A beneficial side effect may be that this drug prevents motion sickness.

Prednisone: adult dose 50 mg the first day. Each day, the dose should be decreased by 5 mg (that is, 50 mg day 1, 45 mg day 2, 40 mg day 3, etc.). The pediatric dose is 1 mg per kg (2.2 lb) body weight the first 3 days; ½ mg per kg days 4, 5, and 6; ¼ mg per kg days 7 and 8. Prednisone should only be given if a person is incapacitated by allergies and does not improve with other medications.

Triprolidine with pseudoephedrine (Actifed): adult dose 1 tablet every 8 hours; pediatric dose (6–12 years of age) ½ tablet every 8 hours.

Side effect: drowsiness.

FOR RELIEF FROM SEVERE ASTHMA

Epinephrine (Adrenalin) 1:1,000 aqueous solution: adult dose 0.3–0.5 ml injected subcutaneously (see page 352). The pediatric dose is 0.01 ml per kg (2.2 lb) body weight injected subcutaneously, not to exceed 0.3 ml. This may be repeated 2 times at 20-minute intervals. DO NOT USE EPINEPHRINE IF THE PATIENT IS OLDER THAN 45 OR HAS A KNOWN HISTORY OF HEART DISEASE. DO NOT ADMINISTER EPINEPHRINE TO A PREGNANT FEMALE UNLESS THE SITUATION IS ABSOLUTELY LIFE THREATENING (because it might decrease circulation to the baby). *Primatine Mist (inhaler)* is an inhaled mixture of epinephrine and alcohol available over the counter. *This preparation should not be used in*

substitution for injected epinephrine in cases of severe asthma.
Terbutaline (Brethine tablets): adult dose 2.5–5 mg every 6–8 hours.

Metaproterenol (Alupent inhaler): adult dose 2 puffs every 3–6 hours as needed.

Metaproterenol (Alupent tablets): adult dose 20 mg every 4–6 hours; pediatric dose (6–9 years of age or less than 60 lb) 10 mg every 4–6 hours.

Albuterol (Ventolin inhaler): adult dose 2 puffs every 3–6 hours as needed.

Albuterol (Ventolin tablets): adult dose 2–4 mg 3–4 times a day.

Cromolyn sodium (Intal inhaler): adult and pediatric dose 2 puffs every 4–6 hours; not for use in children less than 5 years of age.

Theophylline: adult dose 100–200 mg every 6–8 hours; pediatric dose 4 mg per kg (2.2 lb) body weight every 6–8 hours.

Prednisone: adult dose 50 mg the first day. Each day, the dose should be decreased by 5 mg (that is, 50 mg day 1, 45 mg day 2, 40 mg day 3, etc.). The pediatric dose is 1 mg per kg (2.2 lb) body weight the first 3 days; ½ mg per kg days 4, 5, and 6; ¼ mg per kg days 7 and 8. Prednisone should be given only if the child is severely ill and has no real improvement with epinephrine.

FOR RELIEF FROM MILD (OR CHRONIC) ASTHMA

Metaproterenol (Alupent inhaler): same as for relief from severe asthma (above).

Metaproterenol (Alupent tablets): same as for relief from severe asthma (above).

Albuterol (Ventolin inhaler): same as for relief from severe asthma (above).

Albuterol (Ventolin tablets): same as for relief from severe asthma (above).

Theophylline: same as for relief from severe asthma (above).

Cromolyn sodium (Intal inhaler): same as for relief from severe asthma (above).

Ipatropium bromide (Atrovent inhaler): adult dose 2 puffs every 4–6 hours as needed; do not exceed 12 puffs in 24 hours; do not use in children less than 12 years of age.

Beclomethasone dipropionate (Vanceril inhaler): adult dose 2 puffs every 4–6 hours, not to exceed 20 puffs in 24 hours; pediatric dose (6–12 years of age) 1 or 2 puffs every 6 hours, not to exceed 10 puffs in 24 hours. Rinse the mouth after each use.

FOR TREATMENT OF CHEST PAIN (ANGINA)

Nitroglycerin ¹/₁₅₀ *grain (0.4 mg):* adult dose 1 tablet dissolved under the tongue (alternative: nitroglycerin lingual aerosol, 0.4 mg metered dose per spray) for the treatment of anginal pain. This may be repeated every 10 minutes for 2 additional doses. Side effects include dizziness (low blood pressure) and headache. If a person uses nitroglycerin and becomes faint, he should lie down and have his legs elevated, until his skin color returns to normal and he feels better (usually, in a minute or two). If chest pain and weakness persist, this may indicate a heart attack (see page 46).

FOR TREATMENT OF CHRONIC (CONGESTIVE) HEART FAILURE

Furosemide (Lasix) diuretic (promotes urination): adult dose 1–4 tablets (20–80 mg) each day for the fluid retention associated with heart failure. DIURETICS SHOULD NOT BE USED FOR FLUID RETENTION NOT ASSOCIATED WITH HEART FAILURE, SUCH AS THAT FROM HIGH ALTITUDE, OR FOR WEIGHT REDUCTION.

Digoxin (Lanoxin): adult dose 0.125–0.25 mg each day. This drug increases the force and efficiency with which the heart contracts.

FOR TREATMENT OF SEIZURES (EPILEPSY)

Diphenylhydantoin (Dilantin): adult dose 300–400 mg per day; pediatric dose 2.5 mg per kg (2.2 lb) body weight twice a day.

Phenobarbital: adult dose 60–120 mg 3 times a day; pediatric dose 1–1.5 mg per kg (2.2 lb) body weight 3 times a day.

Carbamazepine (Tegretol): adult dose 400–1200 mg a day in 2–3 divided doses; pediatric dose 10–20 mg per kg (2.2 lb) body weight each day in 2–3 divided doses.

FOR RELIEF FROM PAIN

Acetylsalicylic acid (aspirin): adult dose 650 mg (10 grains, 2 tablets) every 4–6 hours; pediatric dose 60 mg (1 grain) per year of age (not to exceed 600 mg) every 4–6 hours.

Side effects: stomach irritation. Do not administer to a person with an ulcer or upset stomach. Take with food if possible.

Ecotrin (enteric coated aspirin): These are coated to prevent stomach irritation and should be used whenever aspirin is given to someone with known ulcer disease. If coated aspirin is not available, aspirin can be administered with a dose of antacids.

Acetaminophen (Tylenol): adult dose 650 mg (2 tablets) every 4–6 hours; pediatric dose: up to 1 year, 60 mg; 1–3 years, 60–120 mg; 3–6 years, 120 mg; 6–12 years, 240 mg — each dose, every 4–6 hours.

Codeine: adult dose 30–60 mg every 6–8 hours; pediatric dose 0.5–1.0 mg per kg (2.2 lb) body weight every 4–6 hours. *Codeine is a narcotic and has side effects of drowsiness and inability to perform dangerous tasks that require coordination. Narcotics such as codeine should be given to a child only under the guidance of a physician, nurse, or emergency medical technician–paramedic (EMT-P).*

Acetaminophen (325 mg) with codeine (30 mg): adult dose 1–2 tablets every 4–6 hours.

FOR RELIEF FROM FEVER

Acetylsalicylic acid (aspirin): same as for relief from pain (above).

Acetaminophen (Tylenol): same as for relief from pain (above).

Ibuprofen (Motrin, Advil, Nuprin): adult dose 400–600 mg every 4–6 hours; pediatric dose 5–10 mg per kg (2.2 lb) body weight every 4–6 hours, not to exceed 400 mg.

DO NOT USE ASPIRIN TO CONTROL FEVER IN A CHILD UNDER THE AGE OF 17, to avoid the rare complications of Reye's syndrome (postviral encephalopathy and liver failure).

FOR RELIEF FROM MUSCLE ACHES OR MINOR ARTHRITIS

Acetylsalicylic acid (aspirin): same as for relief from pain (above).

Nonsteroidal anti-inflammatory drugs:

Ibuprofen (Motrin, Advil, Nuprin): adult dose 400–600 mg every 4–6 hours.

Naproxen (Naprosyn): adult dose 250–500 mg every 6–8 hours.

Side effects: upset stomach. Do not take on an empty stomach.

FOR RELIEF FROM ITCHING

Diphenhydramine (Benadryl): same as for relief from a mild allergic reaction (above).

Hydroxyzine hydrochloride (Atarax): adult dose 25–50 mg every 8 hours; pediatric dose: up to 6 years, 10 mg every 8 hours; 6–12 years, 10–25 mg every 8 hours.

FOR RELIEF FROM TOOTHACHE

Benzocaine-phenol-alcohol (Anbesol, Numzit): for topical application to the gums.

Oil of cloves: for topical application to the gums.

FOR RELIEF FROM MOTION SICKNESS

Dimenhydrinate (Dramamine): adult dose 50 mg every 4–6 hours; pediatric dose (8–12 years of age) 25 mg every 4–6 hours.
Side effect: drowsiness.

Meclizine HCl (Antivert, Bonine): adult dose 25–50 mg 1–2 times per day. DO NOT GIVE THIS DRUG TO CHILDREN UNDER THE AGE OF 12.
Side effect: drowsiness.

Cyclizine (Marezine): adult dose 50 mg every 6 hours as necessary:
Side effect: drowsiness.

Scopolamine (Transderm-Scōp transdermal therapeutic system): adult dose — apply one patch on the hairless area behind the ear. A single patch is good for 3 days. Take care to wash the hands carefully after application of the patch, to avoid getting any medication in the eyes. THIS PRODUCT IS NOT YET APPROVED FOR CHILDREN UNDER THE AGE OF 12.
Side effects: blurred vision, dry mouth, decreased sweating. Divers who use this preparation should be alert to the danger of heat illness while topside in constrictive wet suits.

Astemizole (Hismanal): adult dose 10 mg every 24 hours. Although not advertised for this purpose, astemizole appears to prevent motion sickness as a side effect.

FOR RELIEF FROM NAUSEA AND VOMITING

Prochlorperazine (Compazine): adult dose 5–10 mg every 8–12 hours (by suppository 25 mg twice daily). DO NOT GIVE THIS DRUG TO CHILDREN. Side effects include neck spasm, difficulty in swallowing and talking (inability to control the tongue), difficulty with eye movement, and muscle stiffness. If these occur, discontinue use of the drug, and administer diphenhydramine (Benadryl) 50 mg every 6 hours for 4 doses (pediatric dose 1 mg per kg [2.2 lb] body weight every 6 hours for 4 doses).

Promethazine (Phenergan): adult dose 25 mg every 6–8 hours (by suppository 12.5–25 mg every 12 hours); pediatric dose 0.25–0.5 mg per kg (2.2 lb) body weight every 6–8 hours by mouth or per rectum (suppository).

Side effects: similar to those with prochlorperazine (Compazine), and may be treated as above with diphenhydramine (Benadryl).

Cyclizine hydrochloride (Marezine): adult dose 25–50 mg every 6–8 hours.

FOR RELIEF FROM DIARRHEA

Diphenoxylate (Lomotil): adult dose 2 tablets 2–4 times per day. DO NOT GIVE THIS DRUG TO CHILDREN.

Loperamide (Imodium): adult dose 2 capsules initially, followed by 1 capsule after each loose bowel movement, not to exceed 8 capsules. DO NOT GIVE THIS DRUG TO CHILDREN.

Bismuth subsalicylate (Pepto-Bismol): adult dose 2 tablespoons or 2 tablets every ½–1 hour, not to exceed 8–10 doses; pediatric dose: 3–6 years, 1 teaspoon or ½ tablet; 6–10 years, 2 teaspoons or 1 tablet; 10–14 years, 4 teaspoons or 1½ tablets; may repeat dose in children every 1 hour, not to exceed 4 doses. THIS DRUG SHOULD NOT BE GIVEN TO PERSONS WHO ARE SENSITIVE TO ASPIRIN-CONTAINING PRODUCTS. Note that it may cause a black discoloration of the tongue and of bowel movements.

Kaolin-pectin (Kaopectate): adult dose 4–8 tablespoons after each loose bowel movement; pediatric dose: 3–6 years 1–2 tablespoons; 6–12 years 2–4 tablespoons; older than 12 years 4 tablespoons after each loose bowel movement.

Antibiotics: See page 377.

FOR RELIEF FROM CONSTIPATION

Mineral oil: adult dose 1–2 tablespoons; pediatric dose (older than 5 years) 1–2 teaspoons.

Dioctyl sodium (Colace): adult dose 50–100 mg twice a day; pediatric dose 0.3 mg per kg (2.2 lb) body weight once or twice a day. The dose should be adjusted to the response. This drug is a stool softener.

Milk of magnesia: adult dose 1–2 tablespoons at bedtime. This drug is a mild laxative.

Lactulose syrup, USP (Duphalac): adult dose 1–2 tablespoons daily.

Bisacodyl (Dulcolax): adult dose 5 mg tablet or 10 mg suppository. This drug is a moderate laxative.

Psyllium mucilloid (Metamucil): 1–2 packets per day dissolved in water. This drug increases the bulk of the stool, and should be ingested with at least 1–2 pints of liquid.

FOR RELIEF FROM ULCER PAIN

Antacid (Mylanta II): adult dose 2 tablespoons or 2 tablets (chewed) 1 and 3 hours after meals, at bedtime, and as needed. This is a mixture of aluminum hydroxide, magnesium hydroxide, and simethicone.

Rolaids: adult dose 1–2 tablets (chewed) after meals as necessary. These contain dihydroxy-aluminum sodium carbonate. Because of the relatively high sodium content, THESE SHOULD NOT BE USED ROUTINELY BY PATIENTS WITH CHRONIC HEART FAILURE (see page 42).

Cimetidine (Tagamet): adult dose 300 mg 3 times a day with meals and at bedtime. This drug decreases the secretion of gastric acid.

Ranitidine (Zantac): adult dose 150 mg twice a day. This drug decreases the secretion of gastric acid.

Propantheline (Pro-Banthine): adult dose 7.5–15 mg 3 times a day before meals and at bedtime. This drug is used to control gastric acid secretion and to reduce bowel activity (decrease cramping).

Sucralfate (Carafate): adult dose 1 tablet (gram) one hour before meals and at bedtime. This drug binds to the ulcer crater in the stomach, and requires the presence of acid to work properly. Therefore, antacids should not be ingested within ½ hour before or after sucralfate.

Omeprazole (Prilosec): adult dose 1 capsule (20 mg) a day to diminish gastric acid secretion.

FOR RELIEF FROM INDIGESTION OR GAS PAINS

Antacid (Mylanta II): same as for relief from ulcer pain (above).

Simethicone (Mylicon-80): adult dose 1–2 tablets (chewed) after meals and at bedtime.

FOR RELIEF FROM HEARTBURN (REFLUX ESOPHAGITIS)

Antacid (Mylanta II): same as for relief from ulcer pain (above).

Gaviscon or Gaviscon II: adult dose 1–2 tablets (chewed) or 1–2 tablespoons after each meal and at bedtime. This is a mixture of aluminum hydroxide, magnesium trisilicate, sodium bicarbonate, and alginic acid.

Metaclopramide hydrochloride (Reglan): adult dose 10 mg up to 4 times a day, 30 minutes before meals and at bedtime. This drug is used by persons who do not respond to antacids. An uncommon side effect is a "dystonic reaction," in which a person has stiffened neck muscles and difficulty swallowing and speaking. If this occurs, the victim should be given diphenhydramine (Benadryl) in a dose similar to that for an allergic reaction (see page 363).

FOR RELIEF FROM NASAL CONGESTION

Pseudoephedrine (Sudafed): adult dose 30–60 mg every 6–8 hours; pediatric dose 1 mg per kg (2.2 lb) body weight every 6–8 hours.

Phenylephrine hydrochloride 0.25% nasal spray (Neo-Synephrine ¼%): adult dose 2–3 drops or sprays twice a day; pediatric dose (older than 6 years) use 0.125% (half-strength) 2 drops twice a day. DO NOT USE THIS DRUG FOR MORE THAN 3 CONSECUTIVE DAYS, to avoid "rebound" swelling of the nasal passages from chemical irritation and sensitization to the medicine.

Oxymetazoline hydrochloride 0.05% (Afrin): adult dose 2–3 drops or sprays twice a day; pediatric dose (older than 6 years) use 0.025% (half-strength) 2 drops twice a day. DO NOT USE THIS DRUG FOR MORE THAN 3 CONSECUTIVE DAYS, to avoid "rebound" swelling of the nasal passages.

FOR RELIEF FROM COUGH

Glyceryl guaiacolate (Robitussin) expectorant: adult dose 1 teaspoon every 3–4 hours; pediatric dose ½ teaspoon every 3–4 hours.

plus codeine (cough suppressant): Robitussin-AC

plus codeine, pseudoephedrine (decongestant): Robitussin-DAC

plus pseudoephedrine: Robitussin-PE

plus dextromethorphan (cough suppressant): Robitussin-DM

Codeine: adult dose 15–30 mg every 4–6 hours. This is the most potent cough suppressant.

CoTylenol Liquid Cold Formula: adult dose 2 tablespoons every 6 hours; pediatric dose (6–12 years) ½–1 tablespoon every 6 hours. Two tablespoons contains dextromethorphan hydrobromide 30 mg (for cough), acetaminophen 650 mg (for fever, aches), chlorpheniramine maleate (antihistamine) 4 mg, pseudoephedrine hydrochloride (decongestant) 60 mg.

Dextromethorphan hydrobromide-guaifenesin (Vicks Cough Syrup): adult dose 2–3 teaspoons every 4–6 hours; pediatric dose: 2–6 years, 1 teaspoon every 6 hours; 6–12 years, 1–2 teaspoons every 6 hours.

FOR RELIEF FROM SORE THROAT

Benzocaine-hexylresorcinol (Sucrets Antiseptic Throat Lozenges)

Benzocaine-cetylpyridinium (Cēpacol lozenges, Vicks lozenges)
Dose: follow the package directions.

COLD FORMULAS

Contac: phenylpropanolamine (decongestant), chlorpheniramine (antihistamine).

Contac Severe Cold Formula: pseudoephedrine (decongestant), chlorpheniramine, acetaminophen (for fever, aches), dextromethorphan (for cough).

Chlor-Trimeton: chlorpheniramine.

Chlor-Trimeton Decongestant: chlorpheniramine, pseudoephedrine.

Coricidin: chlorpheniramine, aspirin.

Coricidin "D": phenylpropanolamine, chlorpheniramine, aspirin.

CoAdvil: ibuprofen, pseudoephedrine.

Co-Tylenol: see for relief from cough (above).

Dristan: phenylephrine (decongestant), chlorpheniramine, aspirin, caffeine.

Dristan Time Capsule: phenylephrine, chlorpheniramine.
Dose: follow the package directions.

SKIN MEDICATIONS

Bacitracin antiseptic ointment: apply thinly to the skin twice a day.

Bacitracin-polymixin B sulfate-neomycin (Neosporin or Mycitracin) antiseptic ointment: apply thinly to the skin twice a day.

Silver sulfadiazene (Silvadene cream): soothing antiseptic cream for burns; apply to the skin once or twice a day. Do not use in children younger than 2 years; avoid use on the face.

Lidocaine HCl 2.5% anesthetic ointment: used for relief from pain due to scrapes; apply to the skin and leave in place for 10 minutes prior to scrubbing. DO NOT APPLY IF THE AREA TO BE COVERED IS GREATER THAN 5% OF THE TOTAL BODY SURFACE AREA (an area approximately 4–5 times the size of the victim's fingers and palm).

Benzalkonium chloride (Zephiran) antiseptic solution (1:750 dilution in water): may be used full strength to clean unbroken skin, but should be diluted 1:2 or 1:3 with water to swab an open wound or animal bite (to kill rabies virus).

Benzalkonium 0.1%-lidocaine HCl 2.5% (Bactine solution): very mild antiseptic-anesthetic combination available over the counter. May be used to swab animal bites.

Hexachlorophene scrub (pHisoHex): use gently as a scrubbing soap on cuts, scrapes, and infected skin. Do not use on children under 1 year of age.

Povidone-iodine (Betadine) antiseptic solution: use in a 1:10 dilution with water to gently scrub cuts and scrapes. Povidone-iodine (Betadine) surgical scrub (soap) should not be used as a substitute.

Tolnaftate (Tinactin) antifungal cream, lotion, or powder: apply to the skin 2–3 times a day for athlete's foot or jock itch.

Clotrimazole (Lotrimin) antifungal cream, lotion, or powder: apply to the skin 2–3 times a day for athlete's foot or jock itch.

Zinc undecylenate (Desenex) antifungal cream, lotion, or powder: apply to the skin 2–3 times a day for athlete's foot or jock itch.

Calamine lotion: apply thinly as a drying agent 2–3 times a day to skin affected with poison ivy, poison oak, or poison sumac.

Pramoxine (Prax, PrameGel): topical anti-itch medication for skin rashes due to plant allergy, insect bites, or sunburn; apply 2–3 times a day.

Calamine-diphenhydramine (Benadryl)-camphor-alcohol lotion (Caladryl): apply thinly as a drying agent 2–3 times a day to skin affected with poison ivy, poison oak, or poison sumac. This also helps to kill the itch. Avoid this product if you are skin-sensitive to diphenhydramine.

FOR SLEEP

Diphenhydramine (Benadryl): adult dose 50 mg at bedtime.
Flurazepam (Dalmane): adult dose 15–30 mg at bedtime.
Triazolam (Halcion): adult dose 0.125–0.25 mg at bedtime. This is shorter-acting, and may be a better choice at high altitude.

INSECT REPELLENTS

Choose a product with one or more of these four active ingredients: N,N-diethyl-meta-toluamide (DEET); butyl 3,4-dihydro-2,2-dimethyl-4-oxo-2H-pyran-6-carboxylate (Indalone); 2-ethyl-1,3-hexanediol (EHD; Rutgers 612); dimethyl phthalate (DMP).

Good choices include: *Ben's 100* (100% DEET), *Cutter spray* (18% DEET, 12% DMP), *Cutter stick* (33% DEET), *Cutter cream* (52% DEET, 13% DMP), *Muskol spray* (25% DEET), *Muskol lotion* (100% DEET), *OFF spray* (25% DEET), *Deep Woods OFF cream* (30% DEET), *Deep Woods OFF liquid max. strength* (100% DEET), *6–12 Plus spray* (25% EHD, 5% DEET), and *Repel spray* (40% DEET). Do not use repeated applications or concentrations of DEET greater than 15% on children under the age of 6 years. In adults, 75–100% DEET may cause skin rash or rare serious reactions.

Permanone is 0.5% permethrin; this is for spray application to clothing and is an excellent tick repellent. Sawyer Products Deet

Plus (16.6% DEET plus MGK 264 synergist) is an effective lotion that may be applied to skin to repel ticks, mosquitoes, gnats, flies, and fleas.

SUNSCREENS

SPF: sun protective factor (higher number indicates greater protection).

Butyl methoxybenzoylmethane 3% plus padimate O 7%: Photoplex.

Para-aminobenzoic acid (PABA)-alcohol: Presun (SPF 4, 8, or 12).

Padimate O-oxybenzone: Chap Stick Sunblock (SPF 15), Coppertone Supershade (SPF 15), Block Out (SPF 10 or 15), Bain de Soleil (SPF 15), Eclipse (SPF 10 or 15), Sundown (SPF 15).

Padimate O: Bain de Soleil (SPF 2, 4, 6, or 8), Eclipse (SPF 5), Sea and Ski (SPF 2, 4, or 6), Sundown (SPF 4 or 8).

Padimate O-aloe: Hawaiian Tropic (SPF 4, 6, or 8).

Water-resistant preparations: BullFrog 15 or 36, PreSun 29, Sundown 30, Vaseline 15, Solbar 50, Aloegator 40.

Side effects: skin irritation, yellow discoloration of skin and clothing, allergic reactions. Persons sensitive to PABA should use a non-PABA product, such as Piz-Buin or Uval.

ANTIBIOTICS

Phenoxymethyl penicillin (Penicillin VK): adult dose 250–500 mg every 4–6 hours; pediatric dose: 2–6 years, 125 mg every 6–8 hours; 6–10 years, 250 mg every 6–8 hours.

Dicloxacillin: same dose as phenoxymethyl penicillin.

Ampicillin: same dose as phenoxymethyl penicillin.

Amoxicillin: adult dose 250–500 mg every 8 hours; pediatric dose 7–10 mg per kg (2.2 lb) body weight every 8 hours.

Cefadroxil (Duricef): adult dose 500 mg to 1 gm twice a day.

Cephalexin (Keflex, Keflet): adult dose 250 mg every 4–6 hours or 500 mg every 12 hours; pediatric dose as for phenoxymethyl penicillin. *AVOID USE with penicillin allergy; 5–10% of persons allergic to penicillin are allergic to cephalexin.*

Erythromycin: same dose as phenoxymethyl penicillin. A frequent side effect is diarrhea (particularly with the higher dose). This drug is the first alternative for penicillin in penicillin-allergic persons.

Doxycycline (Vibramycin): adult dose 100 mg twice a day for treatment or once a day for prevention of infectious diarrhea. (Doxycycline should not be given to pregnant women or small children up to the age of 7, because this drug may cause permanent dark discoloration of the teeth.)

Trimethoprim-sulfamethoxazole (Septra or Bactrim DS [double strength]): adult dose 1 pill twice a day for infectious diarrhea or bladder infection; 1 pill once a day for prevention of traveler's diarrhea. The pediatric dose for an ear infection or severe infectious diarrhea (*Shigella*) is 1 teaspoon of the pediatric suspension per 10 kg (22 lb) body weight every 12 hours (twice a day), not to exceed 4 teaspoons (the adult dose) per dose.

Ciprofloxacin (Cipro): adult dose 500 mg twice a day for 3 days to treat infectious diarrhea. This drug should not be given to children under the age of 18 or to pregnant women.

Metronidazole (Flagyl): adult dose 250 mg 3 times a day. DO NOT DRINK ALCOHOL WHEN TAKING THIS MEDICATION AND FOR THREE DAYS AFTERWARD. THE INTERACTION CAUSES SEVERE ABDOMINAL PAIN, NAUSEA, AND VOMITING.

Tetracycline: adult dose 500 mg 4 times a day. This drug should not be given to pregnant women or small children up to the age of 7, because this drug may cause permanent dark discoloration of the teeth.

Appendix Two

Sources of Information About Wilderness Medicine

The following is a list of organizations and literature to direct the reader who is interested in further information.

ORGANIZATIONS

Divers Alert Network. Duke University Medical Center, Durham, NC 27710.

International Association for Medical Assistance to Travelers (IAMAT). 736 Center Street, Lewiston, NY 14092.

The Mountaineers. 715 Pike Street, Seattle, WA 98101.

National Association for Search and Rescue. P.O. Box 50178, Washington, DC 20004.

National Outward Bound Training Institute. 384 Field Point Road, Greenwich, CT 06830.

North American Mycological Association. 157 W. Ninety-fifth Street, New York, NY 10025.

Survival Education Association. 9035 Golden Given Road, Tacoma, WA 98445.

U.S. Department of Natural Resources. Olympia, WA 98504.

U.S. Forest Service Fire and Aviation Management. P.O. Box 96096, Washington, DC 20013.

The Undersea Medical Society. 9650 Rockville Pike, Bethesda, MD 20014.

The Wilderness Medical Society. P.O. Box 397, Point Reyes Station, CA 94956.

LITERATURE

AMA *Handbook of Poisonous and Injurious Plants*. American Medical Association, 1985, Chicago.

The Audubon Society Field Guide to North American Mushrooms, by G. Lincoff. Alfred A. Knopf, 1981, New York.

The Avalanche Book, by Betsy Armstrong and Knox Williams. Fulcrum, Inc., 1986, Golden, CO.

Bear Attacks. Their Causes and Avoidance, by Stephen Herrero. Winchester Press, 1985, Piscataway, NJ.

Dangerous Marine Animals of the Indo-Pacific Region, by Carl Edmonds. Wedneil Publications, 1975, Newport, Australia.

Giardia and Giardiasis, ed. by S. L. Erlandsen and E. A. Meyer. Plenum Press, 1984, New York.

Going Higher — The Story of Man and Altitude, by Charles Houston. Little, Brown, 1987, Boston.

Health Information for International Travel, Centers for Disease Control. Superintendent of Documents, U.S. Government Printing Office, Washington, DC. Yearly.

Human Poisoning from Native and Cultivated Plants, by J. M. Arena and J. W. Hardin. Duke University Press, 1974, Durham, N.C.

Hyperbaric and Undersea Medicine, ed. by Jefferson C. Davis, M.D. Medical Seminars, Inc., 1981, San Antonio.

Journal of Wilderness Medicine, Wilderness Medical Society, Chapman and Hall, London.

Management of Wilderness and Environmental Emergencies, ed. by Paul S. Auerbach, M.D., and Edward C. Geehr, M.D. C.V. Mosby, 1989, St. Louis.

Medical Care for Mountain Climbers, by P. Steele. Heinemann Medical Books, 1976, London.

Medicine for Mountaineering, ed. by James A. Wilkerson, M.D. The Mountaineers, 1985, Seattle.

Mountaineering First Aid, by Jan Carline, Steven Macdonald, and Marty Lentz. The Mountaineers, 1985, Seattle.

Mountain Sickness: Prevention, Recognition, and Treatment, by Peter Hackett, M.D. American Alpine Club, 1980, New York.

Outdoor Emergency Care, by Warren D. Bowman, Jr. National Ski Patrol System, Inc., 1988, Lakewood, CO.

Photosensitivity Diseases. Principles of Diagnosis and Treatment (2nd edition), by L. Harber and D. Bickers. B. C. Decker, Inc., 1989, Toronto.

Poisonous and Venomous Marine Animals of the World (2nd revised edition), by Bruce W. Halstead, Darwin Press, 1988, Princeton.

Restraint and Handling of Wild and Domestic Animals, by Murray E. Fowler. Iowa State University Press, 1978, Ames.

Snake Venom Poisoning, by Findlay Russell. Scholium, 1983, New York.

Tom Brown's Field Guide to Wilderness Survival, by Tom Brown, Jr. Berkley Books, 1983, New York.

Trauma Management for Civilian and Military Physicians, by S. Wiener and J. Barrett. W. B. Saunders, 1986, Philadelphia.

Wilderness Search and Rescue, by Tim J. Setnicka. Appalachian Mountain Club, 1980, Boston.

Winter First Aid Manual, by Warren D. Bowman, Jr. National Ski Patrol System, 1984, Denver.

World Immunization Chart. IAMAT, Lewiston, NY (annual).

Your Guide for Plant Safety, by Olga Woo. San Francisco Bay Area Regional Poison Center, 1985, San Francisco.

GLOSSARY

abdomen: the part of the body between the chest and the pelvis

abrasion: a scraped area of skin

abscess: a localized collection of pus surrounded by inflamed tissue

acclimatize: to adapt to a new altitude, climate, environment, or situation

acidotic: in a state of abnormal reduced alkalinity; overwhelmed by acid; related to decreased pH

acute: sudden in onset

airway: passage for air into the lungs including the mouth, nose, pharynx, larynx, trachea, and bronchi

alkaline: having the properties of a base; related to high pH

allergy: exaggerated reaction (sneezing, runny nose, itching, skin rash, difficulty in breathing) to substances that do not affect other individuals

ambulatory: able to walk

amnesia: loss of memory

amputate: to cut from the body

analgesia: relief from pain

anaphylaxis: hypersensitivity to substances following prior exposure, resulting in a severe allergic reaction

anemia: deficiency in red blood cells

anesthesia: loss of sensation

aneurysm: abnormally dilated blood vessel

angina pectoris: episodic chest pain caused by insufficient oxygen supply to the heart

antibiotic: drug used to kill bacteria

antibody: body substance, produced by specialized cells, that combines with and neutralizes foreign substances or toxins

antiemetic: drug used to control nausea and vomiting

antihistamine: drug used to inactivate histamine

anti-inflammatory: drug used to prevent or correct inflammation

antiseptic: substance that limits or stops the growth of microscopic germs

antivenin: drug used to inactivate the effects of animal or insect venom

anus: posterior opening from the intestine to the outside world

aorta: ‘the large artery that carries oxygenated blood from the heart to be distributed to the body

appendectomy: surgical removal of the appendix

appendicitis: inflammation of the appendix

appendix: wormlike appendage of the bowel, located in the right lower quadrant of the abdomen

aqueous: mixed with or related to water

arrest: sudden stop

arterial: pertaining to an artery

artery: muscular- and elastic-walled blood vessel that carries oxygenated blood from the heart to the body

arthritis: inflammation of the joints

arthropod: invertebrate animals with jointed limbs of the phylum Arthropoda; insects, spiders, and crustaceans

aspirate: to draw by suction; to inhale into the lungs

asthma: labored breathing caused by narrowing of the smaller air passages (past the bronchi) in the lungs, associated with shortness of breath, wheezing, cyanosis, and coughing

atherosclerosis: hardening of the arteries

aura: a sensation of lights or sounds that occurs prior to a migraine headache or seizure

barotitis: disorders of the ear due to increased or decreased atmospheric pressure

bile: green fluid produced by the liver and stored in the gallbladder, where it is released into the duodenum to aid in the digestion and absorption of fats

bilirubin: a pigment formed from the destruction of red blood cells

blister: fluid-filled elevation of the epidermis

bowel: intestine

bronchitis: inflammation of the bronchial tree

bronchodilator: drug used to relax and widen the bronchi

bronchus: main passageway from the trachea to the smaller air passages in the lungs

bruise: injury that does not break the skin, with rupture of small blood vessels that causes blue or purplish discoloration

bursa: fluid-filled sac that allows smooth motion of muscles or tendons over a bone or joint

bursitis: inflammation of a bursa

buttocks: the seat of the body; the rump

calorie: the amount of energy necessary to raise the temperature of one gram of water by 1°C; one food calorie (or kilocalorie) is equal to 1,000 energy calories

cancer: malignant tumor; uncontrolled growth of cells that invade normal body tissues for no reason and serve no purpose

canker sore: small painful ulcer of the mouth

cannula: small tube for insertion of fluid or air

carbonaceous: rich in carbon; black like soot

carbon dioxide: gas that combines with water to form carbonic acid; formed by the combustion and decomposition of organic substances

carbon monoxide: odorless, colorless gas product of incomplete combustion

cardiac: pertaining to the heart

cardiopulmonary: pertaining to the heart and lungs

carotid artery: chief artery that travels up the neck and carries blood to the head and brain

cartilage: elastic tissue that is transformed into bone

cartilaginous: composed of cartilage

caustic: corrosive; capable of destroying by chemical action *central nervous system:* the brain and spinal cord

cerebral: pertaining to the brain

cervical: pertaining to the neck

chilblain: inflammation, swelling, and blistering of the skin caused by exposure to the cold

cholecystitis: inflammation of the gallbladder

chronic: of long duration

colic: acute pain caused by spasm, obstruction, or twisting of a hollow organ

colitis: inflammation of the colon

colon: the large intestine

coma: a state of profound unconsciousness

comatose: in a coma

comminuted: in multiple pieces; shattered

compound fracture: broken bone accompanied by torn skin

conjunctiva: membrane that covers the insides of the eyelids and extends over the whites of the eyes

convulsion: seizure; abnormal involuntary contraction or series of contractions of the muscles

COPD: chronic obstructive pulmonary disease, caused by scarred lung tissue.

core: center; involving the abdomen and chest organs

cornea: the transparent covering of the eyeball over the iris and pupil that allows light to enter the eye

corticosteroid: one of a number of hormones produced by the adrenal glands

costochondritis: inflammation of the cartilage that attaches the ribs to the sternum

CPR: cardiopulmonary resuscitation, with artificial breathing and chest compressions

cravat: triangular cloth bandage

crepitus: a crackling sound or feeling

culture: to grow in a prepared laboratory medium

cyanosis: blue or purple discoloration of the skin due to inadequate oxygen in the blood *cyst:* an abnormal sac containing gas, fluid, or solid material.

decompression: loss of pressure; contributes to diving-related "bends"

debridement: surgical removal of torn, contaminated, or devitalized tissue

dehydration: depletion of body fluids

dermatitis: inflammation of the skin

dermis: layer of skin just underneath the epidermis which contains sensitive nerve endings, blood vessels, and hair follicles

diagnose: to identify a disease

diaphragm: muscular wall that separates the chest from the abdomen

dilatation: stretching to normal or beyond normal dimensions

dinoflagellate: marine plankton

discharge: liquid released from an organ or tissue surface

dislocation: displacement of bones at a joint

diuretic: medicine that promotes urination

diverticulitis: inflammation of a diverticulum

diverticulum: small outpouching from a hollow organ (such as the large intestine)

dressing: bandage; covering for a wound

duodenum: first part of the small intestine

edema: swelling caused by the accumulation of fluid

electrolyte: soluble inorganic chemical (such as sodium or potassium) found in body fluids

embolism: sudden obstruction of a blood vessel by an embolus

embolus: abnormal particle (solid or gas) circulating in the bloodstream

encephalopathy: disease of the brain that often results in abnormal mentation

endemic: native to

endotracheal: through the trachea

envenom: to poison with venom

epidermis: outermost layer of the skin

epigastrium: area lying over the stomach; central upper area of the abdomen

epilepsy: disorder associated with disturbed electrical discharges in the central nervous system that cause convulsions

esophageal reflux: return of food and acid from the stomach into the esophagus; major cause of heartburn

esophagitis: inflammation of the esophagus

esophagus: muscular tube from the pharynx to the stomach

eustachian tube: a tube of bone and cartilage that connects the middle ear with the upper throat and allows equalization of pressure on both sides of the eardrum

exhale: to breathe out

expectoration: sputum, phlegm, or mucus; the act of spitting out saliva or mucus from the air passages via the mouth.

extremity: arm and hand (upper extremity) or leg and foot (lower extremity)

facial: pertaining to the face

fallopian tube: small tube that conducts the egg from the ovary to the uterus

feces: solid human bodily waste discharged through the anus

feculent: pertaining to or resembling feces

femoral artery: large artery that carries blood to the leg

femur: large bone of the thigh

fibrillation: unsynchronized quivering

flagellate: possessing a flagellum

flagellum: whiplike organelle ("tail") for locomotion

flail chest: series of detached ribs that cannot move properly to assist with breathing

flatulence: the presence of excessive gas in the bowel

flatus: gas generated in the digestive system and discharged via the anus

follicle: skin cavity in which the root of a hair lies

fracture: to break; a broken object

frostbite: freezing of the tissues

gallbladder: muscular hollow organ that stores bile produced by the liver

gangrene: tissue death due to loss of blood supply; may be caused by injury or infection

gastroenteritis: inflammation or irritation of the stomach and/or intestine

gastrointestinal: pertaining to the stomach and intestine; digestive system

gauge: the diameter of a hypodermic needle expressed as a standard number

genitals: external organs of reproduction

gland: a specialized group of cells that either selectively removes substances from the blood, concentrates or alters substances in the blood, and/or creates and releases special substances into the blood

glaucoma: disease of the eye associated with increased pressure within the eyeball

glucose: type of sugar used by the body for energy

gonorrhea: sexually transmitted disease caused by the bacterium *Neisseria gonorrhea*

graft (skin): piece of skin taken from one area of the body to cover a defect or burn in another area

grain: a measure of weight equal to 0.0648 gram

gram: a measure of weight equal to 15.432 grains

grand mal seizure: convulsion manifested by violent generalized muscle contractions, clouded consciousness, and a period of confusion after the event

hallucinate: to see visions or imaginary perceptions

heartburn: burning discomfort behind the sternum related to irritation or spasm of the lower portion of the esophagus

Heimlich maneuver: technique for removal of an object caught in the upper airway

helminth: intestinal worm-shaped parasite

hemoglobin: iron-containing oxygen-carrying pigment in red blood cells

hemorrhage: bleeding

hemorrhoid: dilated vein found at the anal margin

hepatitis: inflammation of the liver

hernia: protrusion of part or all of an organ through a wall of the space in which it is normally contained

hiatal hernia: protrusion of part of the stomach through the diaphragm

histamine: chemical compound that plays a major role in allergic reactions

hives: raised red skin wheals associated with allergic reactions

hormone: chemical substance formed in the body that is carried in the bloodstream to affect another part of the body; an example is thyroid hormone, produced by the thyroid gland in the neck, which affects growth, temperature regulation, metabolic rate, and other body functions

hydrate: to cause to take up water

hyper- (prefix): excessive

hyperbaric: pertaining to increased atmospheric pressure

hypertension: elevated blood pressure

hyperthermia: elevated core body temperature

hyphema: collection of blood in the chamber of the eye between the lens and the cornea

hypo- (prefix): insufficient; underneath

hypodermic: under the skin

hypoglycemia: low blood sugar

hypothermia: low core body temperature

ileum: the last (and longest) segment of the small intestine

iliac: pertaining to the ilium

ilium: the upper bone that forms the side of the pelvis

immobilize: to prevent freedom of movement

immune: not susceptible to

immunity: condition of being able to resist a certain disease

immunization: the process of developing immunity

impetiginize: to involve with impetigo

impetigo: contagious skin disease caused by *Staphylococcus* or *Streptococcus* bacteria, characterized by weeping, crusting, and areas of pus

incarcerate: to confine; to entrap

infarction: area of tissue death caused by obstruction of blood circulation

inflammation: response to cell injury that involves dilation of small blood vessels, redness, warmth, pain, and migration of white blood (pus) cells to the region; part of the healing process that removes noxious substances and damaged tissue

infrared: light that lies outside of the visible spectrum, with wavelengths longer than that of red light

inhale: to breathe in

inspiration: the act of breathing in

intestine: the digestive tube that passes from the stomach to the anus; the small intestine (bowel) consists of the duodenum, jejunum, and ileum; the large intestine (bowel) consists of the cecum (with attached appendix), colon (ascending, transverse, descending, and sigmoid), and rectum

intoxication: state of poisoning

intravenous: into a vein

irrigate: to rinse

-itis (suffix): inflammation of

jaundice: yellow pigmentation of the tissues and body fluids

jejunum: the segment of the small intestine that follows the duodenum and precedes the ileum

kg (abbreviation): kilogram

kilocalorie: one food calorie, or 1,000 calories; the energy necessary to raise the temperature of 1 kilogram of water by 1°C

kilogram: 1,000 grams; 2.2 pounds

lacerate: to tear or cut roughly

lateral: away from the midline; outer

larynx: the portion of the trachea that contains the vocal cords; the voice box *lb (abbreviation):* pound

lethargy: drowsiness or aversion to activity, caused by disease

ligament: fibrous connective tissue that attaches bone to bone

liter: volume of water that weighs 1 kilogram; 1.0567 quarts

localized: confined to a specific area

lumbar: pertaining to the lower back

lymph: amber nutrient fluid that contains white blood cells; circulates in lymphatic system and is involved with injuries, infections, and cancers

lymphatic: related to lymph glands, cells, or fluid; small vessel that transports lymph fluid

lymph node: collection of lymph cells that function as a gland

mandible: lower bone of the jaw

manipulate: to move mechanically with the hands

melena: dark-colored, tarry stools, due to the presence of blood altered by intestinal juices

meningitis: inflammation of the covering of the brain and upper spinal cord

mental status: condition of alertness and comprehension

metabolism: the energy-producing and energy-utilizing processes that occur in the human body

mg (abbreviation): milligram

micron: measure of length equal to one millionth of a meter

microorganism: small life form that requires a microscope to be visualized

migraine: recurrent severe headaches generally accompanied by nausea, vomiting, and dizziness

milligram: 1/1000 of a gram

milliliter: 1/1000 of a liter

ml (abbreviation): milliliter

mononucleosis: infectious disease characterized by an abnormal increase in monocytes (one type of white blood cells) in the blood, weakness, fever, sore throat, and enlargement of the spleen and lymph nodes in the neck *mottled:* covered with colored spots or blotches

mucus: slippery secretion created by mucous membranes (such as those that line the nose, throat, and mouth) for lubrication and some protection against bacteria

myocardial: pertaining to the heart muscle

myoglobin: iron-containing oxygen-carrying pigment present in muscle tissue

nanometer: one billionth of a meter

narcosis: altered mental status ranging from confusion to coma

nebulize: to reduce to a fine spray

neurological: pertaining to the nervous system

nm (abbreviation): nanometer

nonsteroidal: not containing steroids

organ: part of the body with a specific function

otitis: inflammation or infection of the ear

ounce: measure of weight equal to 28.35 grams; ⅟₁₆ pound

ovulation: release of an egg from the ovary

oxygen: colorless, odorless gas necessary for combustion and life

oxygenate: to supply with oxygen

oz (abbreviation): ounce

ozone: triatomic form of oxygen (O_3) that is formed by electric discharge through air

pallor: pale skin color

palpate: feel with the hands

palpitation: abnormal beating of the heart felt by the victim

pancreas: gland that produces and secretes digestive juices and insulin hormone

pancreatitis: inflammation of the pancreas

pediatric: pertaining to children

pelvic: related to the pelvis

pelvis: strong basin-shaped bone structure that provides support for the spine, hips, and legs

peptic: related to digestive juices

peritoneum: lining of the abdominal organs and cavity

peritonitis: inflammation of the peritoneum

petit mal seizure: form of epilepsy characterized by brief periods of confusion without major abnormal muscle activity

pharyngitis: inflammation of the pharynx; sore throat

pharynx: throat

phlegm: mucus secreted in the respiratory passages

photophobia: aversion to light

photosensitivity: sensitivity to light, particularly to ultraviolet radiation

plankton: microscopic plant life found in natural bodies of water

pleura: lining that covers the lungs and the inside of the chest cavity

pleural space: small space between the pleura that covers the lung and that which lines the inside of the chest wall; normally, this space is filled with negative pressure, which allows the lung to expand with the chest wall

pleuritis: inflammation of the pleura

pneumonia: infection of the lung characterized by fever, cough, shortness of breath, and the production of purulent or bloody sputum

pneumothorax: collapsed lung with air in the pleural space

potable: drinkable (preferably disinfected)

prognosis: projected outcome

prone: lying flat with face down

prophylactic: for the purpose of prophylaxis

prophylaxis: measures designed to maintain health and to prevent disease

protozoan: microscopic unicellular or acellular animal

pubic: pertaining to the region of the pubis

pubis: the lowermost and anterior bone of the pelvis

pulmonary: pertaining to the lungs

pupil: contractile round opening in the center of the iris of the eye through which light is transmitted to the lens

purulent: foul

pus: white, yellow-green, or cream-colored creamy fluid that is formed by decomposing tissue, white blood cells, and tissue juices

quadrant: one of the four quarters into which a region can be divided

radial artery: the main artery that travels through the wrist to supply the hand

radiation: emission of energy in the form of waves or particles

radiation of pain: pain that travels from one region to another, such as from the hand to the shoulder

rebound tenderness: pain in the abdomen that is worse upon release of pressure than it is upon compression

recompression: the method whereby increased atmospheric pressure is used to treat victims of air embolism or decompression sickness

reflux: backward flow

reflux esophagitis (heartburn): inflammation of the esophagus caused by backward flow of acid from the stomach

respiratory: pertaining to the organs of breathing or the act of breathing

resuscitate: to revive from death or unconsciousness

retina: the posterior inside surface of the eye, which receives a light image and transmits it to the brain via the optic nerve

saline: salty (solution); "normal saline" (liquid compatible with most human tissues) is 0.9% sodium chloride in water

saturate: to soak; to dissolve to the highest possible concentration

seizure: epileptic convulsion

serum: the fluid component of the blood after the cells are removed

shock: a clinical state manifested by profound depression of all body functions caused by insufficient blood and nutrient supply to the tissues; low blood pressure, cool clammy skin, altered mental status, and collapse

silica: silicon dioxide

soft tissue: body tissue that is not composed of bone or cartilage; generally refers to skin, muscle, and fat; generally excludes internal organs

spasm: involuntary muscular contraction

sphincter: muscular ring that serves as a junction between two tubes, such as the anal sphincter.

spirochete: curled or spiraled microorganism capable of causing infectious disease.

sprain: incomplete stretching or tearing of ligaments

sputum: phlegm composed of saliva and discharges from the respiratory passages

status: unchanging situation, such as status asthmaticus (severe, unchanging asthma) or status epilepticus (nonceasing convulsions)

sterile: uncontaminated by infectious agents

sternocleidomastoid: prominent neck muscle that connects the mandible to the collarbone and sternum

sternum: breastbone

steroids: hormones, vitamins, body constituents, and drugs with a specific chemical structure

strain: incomplete stretching or tearing of tendons or muscles

stridor: harsh vibrating noise heard in the upper airway during breathing

sub- (prefix): underneath

subconjunctival: under the conjunctivae

subcutaneous: under the skin

sublingual: under the tongue

supine: lying flat with face up

suture: to sew with surgical thread or nylon; thread or nylon used to sew a wound closed

symphysis: a barely movable junction of two bone surfaces connected by a fibrous cartilage pad

syndrome: a collection of signs and symptoms that, taken together, constitute a particular disease or abnormality

synthesize: to create or compose

syringe: device used to inject fluids into or remove them from the body

systemic: affecting the entire body

tendon: fibrous tissue that attaches muscle to bone

tension pneumothorax: collapsed lung under pressure from air in the pleural space

tetanus: an infectious disease caused by the bacterium *Clostridium tetani,* characterized by severe muscle contractions and inability to open the mouth (lockjaw); the bacterium that causes tetanus

thermoregulatory: in control of temperature

thrombophlebitis: inflammation of the veins that causes the formation of blood clots

tissue: group of cells that combine in the body to serve a specific function

tourniquet: a device used to control blood flow by impeding or preventing circulation

toxin: poisonous substance

trachea: main passageway for air from the pharynx to the bronchi

tracheostomy: surgical opening created in the neck into the trachea to allow breathing when the upper airway is obstructed

trauma: mechanical injury

traumatic: related to mechanical injury

triage: sorting of patients by priority

tumor: abnormal growth of tissue that arises in the body without purpose; may be benign (noncancerous) or malignant (cancerous)

tympanic membrane: eardrum

ulcer: erosion, open sore

ultrasonic: beyond the normal range of sound waves

ultraviolet: light beyond the violet end of the visible spectrum with a wavelength shorter than that of visible light

unconscious: unaware; unarousable

ureter: muscular tube that carries urine from the kidney to the bladder *urethra:* passage that carries urine from the bladder to the external opening in the genital region

vaccinate: to inject a special preparation for the purpose of achieving immunity from disease

vaginitis: irritation of the vagina

varicose: abnormally swollen or dilated

vascular: pertaining to the blood vessels

vein: blood vessel that carries blood from the body back to the heart

venom: poison secreted from venom glands in animals and insects; usually introduced into the victim with a bite or sting

venous: pertaining to the veins

ventricle: one of two large chambers of the heart

vertebra: one of the bony segments that form the spinal column (backbone)

vertigo: dizziness; sensation of whirling motion

vessel: container; a blood vessel may be an artery, vein, or capillary

Index

Abdomen, examination of, 11
Abdominal pain, 98–117
  aortic aneurysm and, 112–113, 117
  appendicitis and, 107–108, 114
  bowel obstruction and, 109
  colitis and, 170
  diverticulitis and, 110–111
  in epigastrium, 99, 101–104
  in flank, 101
  gallstones and, 104–106
  gastroenteritis and, 103, 165–166
  general evaluation of, 98–99
  heart attack and, 101
  heartburn and, 47, 172–173, 372
  hepatitis and, 175–176, 338
  hernia and, 109–110
  kidney infection and, 213, 214
  kidney stones and, 116–117, 214
  in left lower quadrant, 100, 110–111
  in left upper quadrant, 100, 106–107
  liver injury and, 35, 104
  in lower abdomen (central), 101, 112–118
  ovarian infection and, 113–114
  ovulation, ovarian cyst, or torsed ovary and, 114
  pancreatitis and, 103–104
  physical examination for, 99–101
  in right lower quadrant, 100, 107–110
  in right upper quadrant, 100, 104–106
  spleen injury and, 106–107

  ulcer and, 101–103, 174–175, 371–372
  with vaginal bleeding, 114–115
  vaginitis and, 115
Abrasions, 198
Abscesses, 156, 158, 188–190
  sty, 151–152
Acclimatization, 240, 245, 248–249
Acute mountain sickness (AMS), 247–248
Air embolism, 293–294
Airway:
  inhalation injury and, 91, 92, 95–97
  obstruction of, 18–23
Allergic reactions, 23, 58–59, 191
  to drugs, 359, 362
  hay fever, 161–162, 363–364
  hives, 186–187
  to insect bites, 278–279
  medications for, 362–364
  scombroid poisoning and, 274–275
Altitude-related problems, 244–250
  acute mountain sickness, 247–248
  cerebral edema, 247
  flatus expulsion, 250
  fluid retention, 249–250
  general information on, 245
  prevention of, 248–249
  pulmonary edema, 245–246
  snow blindness, 149–150
  sore throat, 250
Amanita muscaria, 312, 313
Amanita phalloides, 311–313
Amputation, 88–89

Breathing, 23–25
  evaluation of, 9, 38–39
  mouth-to-mouth, 24–25
Breathing problems:
  airway obstruction, 18–23
  broken nose and, 153
  chest injury and, 35, 36, 37
  hyperventilation, 216–217
  inhalation injury, 91, 92, 95–97
  See also Lung disorders, serious
Bronchitis, 43, 44, 46–47, 160–
  161
Bruises, 194–195
Bubonic plague, 303, 339
Buddy-taping, 74, 75, 87
Burns, 23, 90–95, 214
  antibiotics and, 94–95
  blisters in, 91, 93, 191–192
  first-degree, 90, 92, 93
  inhalation injury, 91, 92, 95–97
  lightning, 291
  second-degree, 90–91, 93–94
  sunburn, 92, 177–178
  tar, 95
  third-degree, 91, 93, 94
  treatment for, 91–94
  wet vs. dry dressings for, 94
Bursitis, 209, 210
Butterfly bandage, 199, 200

Canker sores, 157
Carbon monoxide poisoning, 244
Cardiac arrest, 26, 46, 227
Cardiopulmonary resuscitation
  (CPR), 26–30
  of children, 29, 30, 31
  hypothermia and, 227
Castor beans, 306, 308
Cat bites, 201, 204, 301, 302
Caterpillars, 287–288
Catfish, 271
Cerebral edema, high-altitude
  (HACE), 247
Cervical spine. *See* Neck
Chemical inhalation, 95, 97

Chest:
  bandaging of, 37–38, 202
  examination of, 11
Chest injuries, 23, 35–39
  broken rib, 23, 35, 39, 82
  bruised lung, 23, 37
  flail chest, 35, 38, 39
  pneumothorax, 23, 35, 36, 37–
    38, 294
  treatment for, 37–39
Chest pain, 45–48, 366
  angina and, 45–46, 47, 366
  heart attack and, 42, 46, 47,
    101
  noncardiac causes of, 46–48
Chilblains, 232
Children, 6, 12
  administering medication to, 359
  asthma in, 40, 41
  cardiopulmonary resuscitation of,
    29, 30, 31
  choking in, 22
  ear infection in, 140
  fever in, 135–136, 140
  head injury in, 57
  near-drowning and, 298, 300
  pulse in, 9, 25
Chills, 136
Chlamydia, 213
Choking, 21–23
Cholecystitis, 104–106
Cholera, 337
Chronic obstructive pulmonary disease (COPD), 43–44
Ciguatera fish poisoning, 276
Coiled rope seat, 344, 345, 346
Cold, common, 159–160, 374
Cold, injuries and illnesses due to,
  221–232
  frostbite, 229–231
  frostnip, 231
  immersion foot (chilblains), 232
  See also Hypothermia
Cold sores, 157
Cold-water drowning, 31, 228

Eyelids:
  foreign body under, 144–145
  injury to, 151
  sty in, 151–152
Eyes, 144–152
  black, 196
  bleeding in, 146, 147–148
  glaucoma and, 151
  protective sunglasses for, 149–150
  red or pink, 148
  removal of contact lenses from, 147
  retinal injury and, 150–151
  snow blindness and, 149–150

Facial injury, 19, 31, 70–71, 153–154
Fainting, 134
  due to heat, 237–238
  See also Unconsciousness
Fatigue headache, 138
Feet:
  athlete's foot and, 192
  bandaging of, 202
  heat-related swelling of, 237
  immersion foot and, 232
Female reproductive system, disorders of, 113–115
Femoral fracture or dislocation, 83–85
Fever, 134–136, 368
Fever blister, 157
Figure-of-eight bandage, 76–77, 207, 208
Fingernails, blood under, 196, 197
Fingers:
  bandaging of, 202
  fracture or dislocation of, 71–73, 74, 75
Fires, wildland, 240–244
  carbon monoxide poisoning in, 244
  encounters with, 242–243
  most common medical problems in, 243–244

risk for, 241
  standard procedures for, 241–242
First aid kits, 327–334
  basic supplies for, 328–330
  for boating and diving environments, 331
  for forest and mountain environments, 330
First aid principles, 8–12
Fish handler's disease, 186, 187
Fishhook removal, 355–356
Flail chest, 35, 38, 39
Flatus, 172, 250, 372
Flu, 160, 340
  stomach, 103
Fluids:
  altitude-related retention of, 249–250
  diarrhea and, 163–164
  muscle cramps and, 236–237
  requirements for, 7–8, 228–229, 238–239
Fly agaric, 312, 313
Food poisoning, 166
Forearm fracture, 73
Foreign objects:
  in ear, 143–144
  embedded in body, 52
  under eyelid, 144–145
Foreign travel:
  infectious diseases and, 121–126
  locating physicians in, 340–342
  traveler's diarrhea and, 166–168
Four-hand seat, 344–345
Foxglove, 306, 307
Fractures and dislocations, 26, 62–87
  of ankle, 87, 88
  bleeding due to, 48–49
  of collarbone, 76–77
  of elbow, 73–75
  of forearm, 73
  of hip or thigh, 83–85, 86
  of jaw, 70–71